QUARANTINE!

QUARANTINE!

East European Jewish Immigrants
and the New York City
Epidemics of 1892

HOWARD MARKEL

The Johns Hopkins University Press
Baltimore and London

© 1997 Howard Markel
All rights reserved. Published 1997
Printed in the United States of America on acid-free paper
06 05 04 03 02 01 00 99 98 97   5 4 3 2 1

The Johns Hopkins University Press
2715 North Charles Street
Baltimore, Maryland 21218-4319
The Johns Hopkins Press Ltd., London

Library of Congress Cataloging-in-Publication Data will be found
at the end of this book.
A catalog record for this book is available from the British Library.

ISBN 0-8018-5512-8

In memory of my grandparents,

Louis and Miriam Lumberg,
Issie and Sarah Markel,

who first taught me about the
American Immigration Experience

Contents

Figures and Tables

Figures

Tables

Preface and Acknowledgments

As a medical student I rarely, if ever, considered the stigma of disease and its effects on a particular patient or family. For the most part, like my eager peer group, I focused on memorizing the immense volume of material our professors decreed necessary to "become a physician." After I began my internship and residency in pediatrics at the Johns Hopkins Hospital, I learned an inestimable amount of information on the art and science of medicine during many long days and nights. Yet I must confess that my most significant "clinical" lesson originated from a far more personal source. It was during the years of 1987 to 1988 that I first began to appreciate, through the eyes of my late wife, Dr. M. Deborah Gordin, the singularly isolating experience serious illness imposes. Debby was diagnosed with cholangiocarcinoma, a rare cancer of the bile ducts of the liver, one month before our wedding in August 1987. She died, tragically, only thirteen months later at the age of thirty.

What struck me most clearly during that impossible year was the palpable loneliness and helplessness disease frequently engenders. Even a disease as "socially acceptable" and noncommunicable as cancer has the potential to frighten healthy people away. Caregivers of the ill, I learned firsthand, also complain of isolation from the so-called healthy or normal world. Friends, relatives, and colleagues frequently avoided both of us, especially as Debby's illness progressed. This is not at all to say that we were bereft of love and support; we both relied heavily on the strength of our families and friends during the ordeal. Nevertheless, I do recall my dismay at those who showed their discomfort with Debby's terminal cancer by their absence. Entries from the daily diary I kept during those months are filled with envy for those who were healthy, feelings of intense yet misdirected anger, and the sense of being "quarantined," cut off entirely from normal human society simply because I was the husband of a dying woman. This sense of social isolation, obviously, was all the more real to Debby.

After Debby's death, I completed my residency and stayed on at Johns Hopkins for fellowship training in adolescent medicine and doctoral studies at the Institute of the History of Medicine. In graduate school, I became interested in American urban history, the history of public health, and immigration history during the nineteenth and twentieth centuries. A principal focus of these studies was how issues of class, gender, race, and cultural

beliefs shape the experience of disease. Illness, I began to appreciate, is typically protean in its social as well as its pathological manifestations.

For a variety of reasons that will become clear later in this book, I decided
to center my historical research on New York City. In the Rare Book Room
of the William H. Welch Library on a steamy Baltimore mid-July day in 1991,
I turned to the volume of the *Annual Reports of the Health Department of
the City of New York* detailing the events for the year 1892. In terse prose that
belied the excitement and chaos it detailed, Dr. Charles F. Roberts, a junior
sanitary inspector for the New York City Health Department, described two
serious epidemics that occurred that year. Both of these epidemics—the
first, typhus fever, and the second, cholera—were believed to have been imported by impoverished, newly arrived East European Jewish immigrants.
The conquest of these diseases, according to Dr. Roberts, was largely due to
the Health Department's massive quarantine efforts.

As my investigation of the details of these epidemics unfolded, a clear
intellectual dichotomy arose from my dual training as a historian of medicine and as a physician. As a social historian, I base my analysis on the theory
that diseases are socially constructed or framed; in other words, social historians study how nonbiological factors, such as class or cultural beliefs, influence a population's response to issues of disease, public health, and health
care across time.[1] In this role I attempt to gather as much data as possible
about a particular era's social institutions, cultural perceptions, daily activities, and other demographic markers in order to create a clear and complete
snapshot of the past. Unfortunately, such snapshots or historical images are,
by definition, taken from a distance, separated by both time and experience.

Physicians, on the other hand, frequently begin their diagnostic inquiries
on the socially microscopic level, with the individual patient, in order to
reach more general conclusions about health and disease. For example, in
my own clinic I am aware that culture and society have major effects on
my patients' health and I recognize the need to factor those influences
into my diagnostic thinking. More typically, however, I spend the majority of
my time with patients, asking them specific questions about their individual
aches, pains, and symptoms, proceeding to their individual medical, social,
and sexual histories, and then, performing a physical examination. For the
practicing physician—and for his or her patients—it is often vital to concentrate on the more biological factors of disease during such encounters.

Because of the personal contact and commitment required in a successful
patient-doctor relationship, it is rather difficult for me to consider life events
such as an individual's birth, illness, or death solely as demographic indica-
tors of a society's health or history. Instead, I view these as *unique* events

with very specific ramifications for the patient (and his or her family). There is a difference, too—even if very slight—from the life events of others who may live during the same time period and under similar conditions. To be sure, the physician, like the historian, must make generalizations from these events in order to approach an understanding of them; nevertheless, they remain to the people experiencing them quite unique. The central question that arose in my mind, then, was how best to incorporate the social and cultural historian's task of recording the daily lives and perceptions of large groups of ordinary people with the physician's focus on the individual patient's interpretation of the experience of illness.[2]

It was another clinical experience that framed my study of quarantine and the stigma of disease. A large portion of my clinical practice at the time I was in graduate school consisted of patients with human immunodeficiency virus (HIV) and acquired immune deficiency syndrome (AIDS). During my three years as a physician treating patients with AIDS, the most frequent concern of patients I encountered—aside from queries about medications, laboratory tests, and acute medical complaints—was over the development of public health policies that might further isolate HIV-infected people from the healthy society. The fear of potential infringements on their personal liberties was consistently articulated by my patients using the term *quarantine*. I often attempted to explain the futility of establishing a quarantine for a sexually transmitted disease like AIDS. Yet I know that my carefully measured, doctorly responses did little to allay their fears of being "quarantined" in some fashion. My patients, many of whom had been exposed to social ostracism long before the diagnosis of HIV, quite reasonably worried that the biological stigma of HIV/AIDS would only reinforce and multiply the many levels of social isolation they experienced in their everyday lives.

Working with these courageous people, it became apparent that issues of sexuality, assignment of blame, poverty, substance abuse, and cultural or social biases had definite effects on the delivery of these patients' health care, treatment outcomes, and means of disease prevention. More apparent to me, however, was the fact that each of my patients had unique experiences of illness despite having the "same" disease. One obvious difference was that each patient was affected differently by the disease's physical manifestations; more moving were the most human expressions of illness, the individual's life story, and how he or she adapted to a life-threatening disease, the stigma of disease, and the resulting isolation.

So, too, was it with the stories of the East European Jewish immigrants in New York City's Lower East Side in 1892. As I read through the detailed account of the epidemics, I was fascinated by the bold, stark tables listing, name by name, the fate of each victim: "Abram Dikar, Age 20, recovered from typhus fever after quarantine on North Brother Island . . . Fayer Mermer, Age 40, dead of typhus fever . . . Max Fengermann, Age 20, dead of typhus fever. . . ."[3] These East European Jewish surnames reminded me of reading my grandparents' *landsmanshaftn*[4] annual report. The public health document was more than a list of those who had the misfortune to contract a horrible disease. The familiarity of the names and my grandparents' recollections of immigrating to the United States in the early 1920s urged me to look beyond the tables of mortality and morbidity. A personal dividend of these studies has been the opportunity to learn more about my cultural heritage as a second-generation East European Jewish American. The world of my grandparents seems much clearer and far less distant as a result. Because of my own experiences of witnessing the isolation of disease, I was especially intrigued with documenting these epidemics and quarantines from the viewpoint of the stigmatized immigrants.

To come full circle, as a medical educator I am often asked by medical students and more than a few colleagues about my work as a "clinician-historian." In many ways this book is one answer to these questions. It is an attempt to show the linkages between medical practice and social and cultural history. In order to document the quarantine year of 1892–93, I attempted to engage in a dialogue, albeit a one-sided one, with the historical sources. The Yiddish press, immigrant diaries, immigrant society minutes, Jewish social agency reports, American newspapers, government documents, and the other materials I consulted provide a very real sense of how late-nineteenth-century New Yorkers experienced and understood epidemic disease and quarantine. On reflection, my historical research and clinical work are really not that dissimilar; both endeavors involve a great deal of time and energy spent collecting "historical" data from the perspective of the ill individual and any other source that facilitates an understanding or diagnosis.

There were, of course, many people who were instrumental in the completion of this book and I am delighted to take this opportunity to thank them. At the Johns Hopkins Hospital and School of Medicine, Drs. Barton Childs, Catherine DeAngelis, and the late Frank A. Oski encouraged me to continue my historical research in concert with my medical training as a pediatrician. Dr. Catherine DeAngelis provided the wherewithal to organize a combined fellowship in general pediatrics, adolescent medicine, and graduate work in the history of medicine at Johns Hopkins. At the Johns Hopkins Institute of the History of Medicine, I benefited from my studies under my dissertation advisor, Dr. Gert H. Brieger, and many scholars, including Professors Jerome Bylebyl, Elizabeth Fee, Harry Marks, Daniel Todes, Ronald Walters, Matthew Crenson, John Higham, and Edward T. Morman. I am also indebted to my friends Walton Schalick III, Kate Levin, Susan Abrams, John Given, Marion E. Rodgers, and Denise Rubin, who patiently listened to my ideas and read, and reread, drafts of this book.

Others who took time out of their busy schedules to read critically various drafts of this book include Alan M. Kraut, Kenneth M. Ludmerer, Bert Hansen, the late Irving Howe, Allan Brandt, Daniel M. Fox, the late David C. Rogers, Victor Navasky, Sherwin Nuland, Guenter Risse, Steven C. Martin, Neil A. Holtzman, Eric T. Juegnst, and John J. Hanley, and my editor at the Johns Hopkins University Press, Jacqueline Wehmueller. Daniel Epner helped with the Yiddish translations cited in this work. I could not have utilized the wonderful historical resources of the Yiddish press without his patience, instruction, and guidance. All English transliteration of Yiddish or Hebrew words that appear in this book are the recognized spellings as suggested by the YIVO Institute for Jewish Studies.

I received the help and advice of the staffs of the Welch and Eisenhower Libraries at Johns Hopkins, the National Archives, the Library of Congress, National Library of Medicine, Columbia University, Yale University, New York Public Library, New-York Historical Society, YIVO Institute for Jewish Studies, New York City Municipal Archives, the American Jewish Historical Archives, the Steamship Historical Association Archives, the University of Michigan, and the New York Academy of Medicine.

Most of the research for this book was supported by generous funding from the Johns Hopkins University Department of Pediatrics and Department of the History of Science, Medicine, and Technology and a National Research Service Award from the Ethical, Legal, and Social Implications of the Human Genome Project Program, National Center for Human Genome Research, National Institutes of Health (grant no. 5F32 HG00037-02). These grants and fellowships allowed me the time and freedom to pursue a Ph.D. and conduct historical research. Earlier versions of Chapters 4 and 5 appeared in the *Bulletin of the History of Medicine* 67 (1993): 691–95 and (1995): 420–57. I thank the Johns Hopkins University Press for permission to incorporate these materials into this book.

In July 1993, I joined the faculty of the University of Michigan Medical School, where I teach clinical pediatrics, medical history, literature and medicine, and medical ethics. The Department of Pediatrics and Communicable Diseases is a supportive home for my work as a clinician-historian. In Ann Arbor I have benefited greatly from my colleagues Horace Davenport, Joel Howell, Ronald Holmes, Arthur J. Vander, Robert P. Kelch, Jean Robillard, Nicholas Steneck, Richard Judge, Gina Morantz-Sanchez, Martin Pernick, Timothy Johnson, and Andrew Achenbaum. Finally, I must acknowledge the important role my parents, Samuel and Bernice Markel, and my grandparents, Louis and Miriam Lumberg and Issie and Sarah Markel, played in my life and education.

The Concept of Quarantine

My doctor told me that I was [isolated] in an infectious disease ward—that in adjacent rooms were people with tuberculosis and cholera. They put a person with a compromised immune system in a ward with the world's most contagious diseases. The doctor said it was not a medical decision but an administrative one. My room had five beds; it was the male HIV room. Physically, it was not clean—the bed frame next to mine was covered with dried vomit. For meals, a glass cabinet was built into the wall, and from the hallway a nurse would open a door and put the food in. Then I had to retrieve the food from the other side. Once or twice a day, a nurse came in to check my vital signs, and she wore a mask, gloves, a surgical cap, and a disposable covering over her uniform. I never saw her face. For the first and only time in my life, I considered suicide.

—Lawrence Berner, a fifty-year-old American with HIV/AIDS living in Japan, recalling his stay at the Tokyo-Komagome Hospital in 1989

Calls for quarantine appear in our daily newspapers and popular magazines as a panacea for epidemic diseases such as AIDS, pneumonic and bubonic plague, Ebola virus, and drug-resistant tuberculosis.[1] Unlike other once-heartily endorsed tools or doctrines of medicine such as the use of purgatives for humoral imbalances, the concept of quarantine is no mere footnote in an antiquated medical text or an artifact in a museum. It remains, for many, a viable method for the prevention and containment of epidemic diseases.

Historians have long been fascinated by epidemics and have pursued that fascination through a distinguished body of scholarship. An epidemic, as suggested by Charles Rosenberg, is a particularly useful means of studying social responses to disease because it is an event, not a trend: "It elicits immediate and widespread response. It is highly visible and, unlike some aspects of humankind's biological history, does not proceed with imperceptible effect until retrospectively 'discovered' by historians and demographers."[2] Indeed, the "unique historical moment" of an epidemic allows one to study the effects of "a randomly occurring stimulus against which the varying reactions of [a population can] be judged."[3] As historian Asa Briggs suggested in 1961, epidemics are a useful means of testing "the efficiency and resilience of local administrative structures" and in exposing "relentlessly political, social, and moral shortcomings . . . rumors, suspicions and at times violent social conflicts."[4]

It is not surprising that epidemics have long been of interest not only to historians, physicians, and public health workers but also to novelists, playwrights, screenwriters, and journalists. Epidemics are, after all, a dramatic unfolding of events; they are stories of discovery, reaction, conflict, illness, and resolution. One of the most common social responses to epidemics, across time and national boundaries, has been the quarantine.[5]

If we look at quarantine as part of the typical progression of an epidemic, we begin to appreciate a number of impulses that often help shape it. These include: (1) the social response of avoiding the ill, or those perceived to be ill, particularly if the disease is thought to be easily transmitted from person to person (i.e., contagious); (2) negotiations over how the epidemic disease in question is understood by both experts and the community at large, especially in terms of cause, prevention, and amelioration; (3) the complex political, economic, and social battles that guide or obstruct a community's quarantine efforts; and (4) the extent to which ethnicity and perceptions about a social group associated with a contagious disease frame the social responses of quarantine.

Formalized practices of avoiding and isolating the ill have long been a major response to periodic visitations of contagious diseases. Some of the earliest recorded examples of such isolation and corresponding sanitary procedures can be found in the Old Testament. Medical historian Fielding H. Garrison identified the ancient Hebrews as the "founders of prophylaxis." To cite but a few examples, clear instructions on isolating lepers, disinfecting the home, and other procedures are discussed in the Books of Leviticus and Numbers. In Deuteronomy we find decrees on how one should properly dispose of his or her excreta. A now-forgotten function of the ram's horn or shofar, traditionally sounded during the Jewish High Holidays, was its ancient use as a signal that a case of diphtheria or another highly contagious disease had been noted in the community.[6]

Although the ancient Greeks had markedly different views of contagion and disease from those of modern medicine, there is ample evidence in the historical writings of Thucydides (c. 460–c. 400 B.C.) and the medical treatises of Hippocrates (c. 460–c. 370 B.C.) that they avoided the contagious.[7]

The Roman authority on medicine, Galen of Pergamon, occupied much of his professional life during the second century A.D. with the study of anatomy and internal causes of disease; yet he, too, warned that there were specific diseases (plague, tuberculosis, skin and eye infections) that made it "dangerous to associate with those afflicted."[8] Some three and a half centuries later, in A.D. 549, the Byzantine emperor Justinian enacted one of the first laws calling for the delay and isolation of travelers from regions of the world where the plague was known to be raging. Similar forms of detention for plague directed against sailors and foreign travelers were also widely practiced in seventh-century China and other parts of Asia and Europe during the Middle Ages. Not surprisingly, there was early recognition of the critical relationship between the transmission of epidemic diseases and the pattern and extent of human migrations.[9]

The word *quarantine* originates from the Italian words *quarantina* and *quaranta giorni*. The term refers to the forty-day period ships entering the Port of Venice were required to remain in isolation before their goods, crew, and passengers were allowed to disembark during the plague-ridden days of the fourteenth and fifteenth centuries. In about 1374, Venice enacted its forty-day quarantine regulation; twenty-nine years later, in 1403, the municipality established the first maritime quarantine station or lazaretto on the island of Santa Maria di Nazareth.

The origins of an enforced forty-day period of detention are vague. It may be based on the Hippocratic doctrine of distinguishing acute and typically contagious diseases (lasting fewer than forty-five days) from more chronic diseases. Other scholars have argued that the frequent use of the number 40 throughout the Old Testament may be the source of its origin. More likely, the time period was used because Renaissance observers noted that, after forty days, people stricken with the plague either died or recovered without further spread to others.[10] From medieval times on, shutting the gates of a city or port to all those suspected of being ill and isolating those sick people discovered to have entered represented the best, and often the only, means available for stemming the tide of an epidemic.

One of the most striking results of the rise of international commerce and travel during the Renaissance and the subsequent three centuries was the progressive spread of contagious and sexually transmitted diseases around the globe. To prevent the entry of contagion, sanitary cordons (quite literally a ring of armed soldiers ordered to guard against diseased fugitives) and quarantines were used in France, Britain, Austria, Germany, Russia, and several other European and Asian nations from the fourteenth through the nineteenth centuries.[11] By the mid-1800s, in response to devastating epidemics of cholera and plague imported from Turkey and Egypt, there was

great pressure by nations with the broadest commercial or colonial interests to create an international board of sanitary or quarantine control. These
International Sanitary Conferences commenced in 1851 and continued well
into the twentieth century.[12]

Yet the exact definition and length of quarantine vary widely, depending
on the era, the location, and the threat of a particular disease. Like the topic
it remains intimately connected with, infectious diseases, quarantine has
many different meanings to different people. At first glance, the interdepen-
dence of quarantine policies and the concurrent medical understanding of
contagious diseases seems intuitive. A closer examination of past epidemics
suggests a far more complex interaction of medical knowledge and actual
practices of disease control. During the first half of the nineteenth century in
the United States, for example, the notion that a tiny microbe might be the
cause of a devastating epidemic was almost laughable to medical experts and
the lay public. Diseases we now commonly attribute to specific germs, such
as plague, cholera, and yellow fever, were held by anti-contagionists to be
caused by constitutional changes in the atmosphere, rotting organic matter,
human and animal waste, and other environmental sources of filth. It was
thought that the "cure" for such evils was cleaning up the environment. This
does not mean, however, that the anti-contagionists were necessarily anti-
quarantine. Their scientific doctrine was far more flexible in practice than in
theory. Quarantines were often mounted even by those who did not believe
in the existence of germs. Serious epidemics of yellow fever in the United
States during the late eighteenth and early nineteenth centuries—a period
of devout anti-contagionism among medical professionals—often inspired
some type of quarantine regulation.

When studying the history of epidemics and quarantines in the United
States over the past two centuries, one of the strongest leitmotifs is the use
of quarantine as a medical rationale to isolate and stigmatize social groups
reviled for other reasons. As psychiatrist and medical historian David F.
Musto asserts, quarantine is far more than the mere "marking off or creation
of a boundary to ward off a feared biological contaminant lest it penetrate
a healthy population"; one cannot limit the consideration of quarantine to
the control of a contagious disease without minimizing and underestimat-
ing the "deeper emotional and broadly aggressive character" of any policy
that dictates separation. The element of blame and stigma associated with
quarantine is especially real for those diseases linked to the poor, the alien,
or the disenfranchised: "When an epidemic illness hits hardest at the lowest
social classes or other fringe groups, it provides that grain of sand on which
the pearl of moralism can form."[13]

A convenient target for the dangerous conflation of epidemic disease and social scapegoating in this country has been the immigrant.[14] The nationality of "undesirable" immigrants has changed over time in the United States but their association with disease, either real or perceived, has not. This has been especially true during periods of economic or political dysfunction, such as the late nineteenth century, when many members of American society espoused sentiments of nativism — the frankly American distrust of all people, institutions, and ideas originating outside the United States.

Ironically, there was little gaiety in the United States during the 1890s despite that decade's familiar sobriquet. It was a period marked by bouts of economic depression and the closing of the western frontier. It was also a period of social upheaval in the form of urbanization, industrialization, rapid transportation, and labor unrest. For many Americans, the personification of all these social evils was the foreign, impoverished, and unkempt immigrant from Russia, Italy, Austria-Hungary, and other European nations.[15] As Irving Howe noted, these "new immigrants" became both "the symptom and the cause of a spreading social malaise" in the United States.[16]

Widespread nativistic and hostile sentiments that cut across lines of class and geographic location were expressed by both native-born and well-assimilated, foreign-born Americans.[17] A number of Americans organized nativist groups and repeatedly urged the U.S. Congress during the late nineteenth and early twentieth centuries to put a halt to unrestricted immigration. This anti-immigrant activism culminated with the Immigration Restriction Act of 1924 and its progeny of laws enacted throughout the 1930s. These restrictive policies essentially closed the gates to immigration for more than forty years. In many respects, the movement to restrict immigration to the United States during this period was a call for quarantine in its broadest sense against undesirable immigrants. The reasons for such a call were not always specifically stated using the language of disease and medicine, but its results were remarkably similar to the medieval quarantines against plague: Foreigners perceived to be dangerous to the community were prevented from entry.

The native-born American of the Gilded Age had many reasons to be concerned about the huge number of immigrants arriving daily at Ellis Island and similar, but smaller, immigration stations around the country. The demographics of this wave of immigration are striking: Between 1881 and 1884, approximately 3 million new refugees arrived — a number nearly equal to the number of immigrants who came to the United States during the entire decade of the 1870s. Between 1885 and 1898, 6 million immigrants arrived; between 1898 and 1920, another 15 million foreigners landed on America's shores.[18]

There was also concern among late-nineteenth-century Americans over the type of immigrant seeking entry to the United States. Clear classifications of "old" and "new" immigrants began to be elaborated. The term *new immigrants* referred specifically to those originating from Eastern and Southern Europe (Russia, Poland, Austria-Hungary, Bulgaria, Greece, Italy, Montenegro, Portugal, Romania, Serbia, Spain, and Turkey) while *old immigrants* originated from Northern Europe (England, Ireland, Scotland, Wales, Belgium, Denmark, France, Germany, the Netherlands, Norway, Sweden, and Switzerland). New immigrants, such as East European Jews and southern Italians, were considered by many Americans to be less assimilable and far more troublesome than their old counterparts. Many were extremely poor and uneducated. The late-nineteenth-century characterization of new immigrants as "wretched refuse" was not only uttered by the nativist in his or her parlor; it also appeared in Emma Lazarus's 1883 poem, "The New Colossus," inscribed on the Statue of Liberty's pedestal in New York Harbor.[19] Between 1819 and 1880, more than 95 percent of immigrants to the United States originated from the old immigrant regions; by 1892, the peak year for immigration during the nineteenth century, the more desirable old immigrants made up less than 50 percent of total immigration. This trend only continued as the twentieth century began.

Perhaps no one articulated the cultural differences between genteel, native-born Americans and the alien hordes better than Harvard Professor William James. In an essay entitled "What Makes a Life Significant?" inspired by an 1896 visit to the Chautauqua grounds in upstate New York, James called the bucolic retreat a "sacred enclosure" where "sobriety and industry, intelligence and goodness, orderliness and ideality, prosperity and cheerfulness, pervade the air." James even qualified why he thought Chautauqua was a "middle-class paradise": "You have no zymotic disease, no poverty, no drunkenness, no crime, no police. You have culture, you have kindness, you have cheapness, you have equality, you have the best that mankind has fought and bled for and striven for under the name of civilization for centuries. You have, in short, a foretaste of what human society might be, were it all light, with no suffering and no dark corners."[20] For many Gilded Age Americans, these "dark corners" represented city slums overcrowded with newly arrived immigrants and the urban poor.

The 1890s was also an era when remarkable advances in scientific knowledge were occurring. Smack in the middle of an exciting era of the "germ theory," new discoveries about the specific causes and possible prevention of tuberculosis, cholera, diphtheria, and other infectious scourges were being made with such rapidity that it reminded the renowned neurosurgeon Harvey Cushing of "corn popping out of a pan."[21] Less enthusiastic was pediatrician Abraham Jacobi, who worried publicly that too many physicians and lay persons were consumed with "bacteriomania." [22] Not unlike the advances being made today in genetics, progress in bacteriology and its applications during the 1890s were far from esoteric; the intricacies and import of bacteriology in daily life were avidly discussed by the general public and widely reported in the daily newspapers, popular magazines, and books written for a lay audience.

By 1892, the maritime definition of quarantine had changed markedly from its medieval origins. As the decade progressed and bacteriology's powerful tenets began to dominate public health and medicine, the process of quarantine was fine-tuned to the natural histories of specific, living, etiologic agents called germs. In America's largest port, New York Harbor, there existed a well-developed system of medical inspection and detention that had few similarities to the medieval doctrines of *quaranta giorni*. Instead, public health authorities defined *quarantine* as the process of inspecting all ships, cargos, and passengers for evidence of contagion. These inspections were conducted at a quarantine station placed in a remote portion of the port, off Staten Island, where all entering ships were required to berth for a cursory period. Passengers and sailors were examined for evidence of contagious diseases. The diseases deemed "quarantinable" by an American quarantine officer of the 1890s were cholera, typhus fever, yellow fever, plague (both bubonic and pneumonic), smallpox, and leprosy.[23] Those discovered to have one of these contagious diseases were admitted to the isolation hospital at the quarantine station, where they were attended by a small staff of physicians, nurses, and orderlies. Treatment was largely supportive and included bedrest, fluids (teas and broths), meals, and the occasional prescription of an opiate-based, pain-relieving medication. Those stricken with the less serious contagious diseases associated with childhood, such as measles, scarlet fever, and mumps, or other medical problems were sent to the U.S. Marine Hospital on nearby Ellis Island.

The health officer of the Port of New York during the late nineteenth century essentially held supreme control over any potentially threatening health issue. If the health officer decided it was necessary, he ordered disinfection of passengers, ship, and cargo with a variety of chemical agents at the shipper's expense. He could also order the detention and isolation of passengers or crew members suspected of being ill with a contagious disease. Sometimes the ship itself was detained at the quarantine station, incurring huge costs for the steamship company. By the 1890s, the period of detention was largely, but not always, dictated by the contagious disease in question — specifically, its period of incubation and infectivity to others as understood by physicians of that era. In reality, the health officer could legally set the detention for any period of isolation he decreed, regardless of the opinions or theories of others. The health officer also had the final authority over the closure of the entire Port of New York for reasons of a public health emergency. Because it would elicit business community enmity in New York and beyond, this option was rarely taken.

The men who held this vast power over the economic and physical health of the Port of New York and similar American seaports during the nineteenth century did not necessarily earn it by years of studying maritime public health. A political appointee of the governor of the state of New York, the nineteenth-century health officer of the port was typically a medical doctor but his training and qualifications varied greatly from appointment to appointment. More often than not political connections proved far more instrumental in his obtaining this powerful position than his medical knowledge or abilities.[24]

In the city of New York, a parallel system of public health and disease control existed in the form of the city's Health Department. When contagious diseases such as cholera, yellow fever, smallpox, or typhus fever appeared in the city itself, the responsibility for inspecting those reported to be ill and overseeing their subsequent removal to the city's quarantine island fell to the department's Division of Contagious Diseases. Sanitary inspectors, physicians, and the Health Department's special police force were invested with the power to remove anyone or to close down anything that they remotely suspected of harboring a contagious disease.

The Health Department of the city of New York was long a leader of municipal health departments across the nation.[25] Like many local health agencies, the department continued to be governed by a politically appointed board of health throughout the nineteenth century. The board typically consisted of prominent businessmen who shared political ideologies with those holding power over the city. In 1892, this control rested largely in the lap of Tammany Hall. Political connections and patronage often had a great deal to do with the selection of physicians and workers for the important jobs in the Health Department during this era. Negotiating a career in the city's Health Department required both a mastery of new technologies and a healthy dose of political savvy.

Municipal public health officials of the late nineteenth and early twentieth centuries had to be as adroit in selling the value of their services as in the actual delivery of them. A common dénouement to a turn-of-the-century American epidemic was the barrage of newspaper articles documenting the heroic and daring work of the Health Department. The professionals at the New York City Health Department were quite familiar with the working New York press; for example, Jacob Riis records in his memoirs daily interactions with prominent members of the Health Department as a police reporter during the 1880s and 1890s.[26] These public health physicians were aware of the power of positive media accounts of their work and made themselves readily available for interviews with reporters covering the hard-boiled police, health, and fire beats for their respective papers. Such attention to public perceptions and political maneuvering was essential for the development of the public health agency's role as a powerful social institution.[27]

During the year 1892, no American locale was more threatened by imported epidemic disease than New York City. New York boasted the busiest port in the country and, after Hamburg, the second busiest in the world. The port was so commercially active that tariffs charged on the goods delivered to it made up over half of the budget of the U.S. federal government.[28] It was also the port of first landing for more than 75 percent of all immigrants coming to the United States.[29] Pandemics of typhus and cholera raging in Asia, Russia, and continental Europe during the summer, combined with the global village created by rapid steamship transportation, made New Yorkers unlikely to rest complacently on the notion that the wide Atlantic Ocean would protect them from diseased newcomers or, worse still, devastating epidemics.

To be sure, the most frequently sounded objection to the wave of immigration to the United States during this period was an economic one—the age-old fear that immigrants would inevitably drive down wages and overuse public assistance, despite excellent evidence to the contrary.[30] A close second objection was tied to racist sentiments against particular immigrant groups. The group in question was predicted to have difficulties assimilating into the American way of life. Too often, anti-immigrant prejudice was cloaked in the concern about an immigrant's untoward political (e.g., anarchist, socialist, or communist) beliefs and the fear of the immigrants' collective potential somehow to taint the American political process or American society itself. As Herman J. Schulteis warned the U.S. Treasury Department in early 1892 on the dangers of admitting Russian Jewish socialists such as labor leader Joseph Barondess into the United States: "We should guard against an invasion of such hordes as we would against an armed host or a pestilence."[31]

One of the most insidious rationales for the nativist's fear of unrestricted immigration, however, surrounds safeguarding the nation's public health against infections potentially transported by immigrants. Regardless of social or medical explanations of a particular infectious disease's etiology, historical analysis of past epidemics in the United States suggests that one of the greatest risk factors for the creation of class- or race-biased public health policies is the association of contagious diseases with a particular undesirable segment of the population, such as newly arrived immigrants.[32] The reaction to such an association has frequently been medical isolation, or

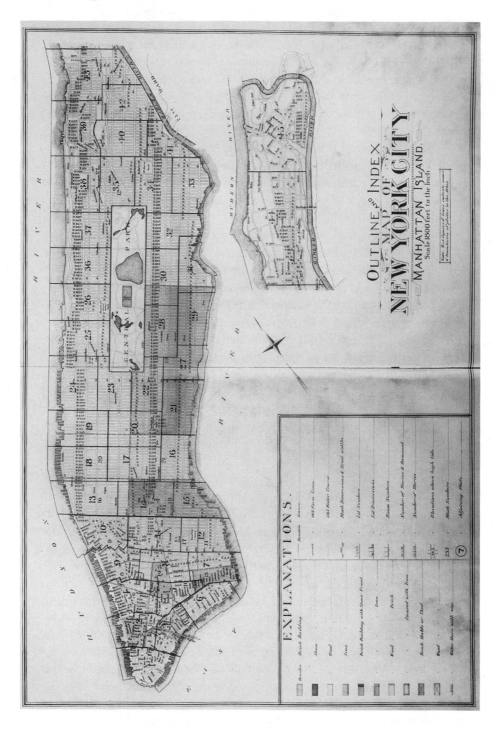

quarantine, and a call for broad immigration restrictions. A neglected risk of linking anti-immigrant sentiment to quarantine policies is the potential for inhumane or inadequate health care justified on the basis of race, socio-economic status, or nationality.

But it is essential to view the institution of quarantine as both a dramatic example of how society responds to the threat of contagious disease *and* an extremely real event for those unfortunate enough to be in one. The isolation of the ill from the healthy, the essential aspect of quarantine, is a double-edged sword; the measure of protection afforded depends exclusively on which edge of the sword you find yourself. Most of us find ourselves pro-tected by the sword of quarantine and we spend little time considering its negative characteristics — such as how cultural perceptions about a scape-goated group guide medical practice or public health policies or how such policies are interpreted by those most affected by them — the isolated scape-goats. It is only by examining such issues and paying attention to the voices of quarantined people that one begins to get a sense of the quarantine's ag-gressive potential for harm.

In New York City in 1892, epidemics of typhus fever and, six months later, cholera were closely associated with newly arriving East European Jewish immigrants. Judging largely by the accounts of white, native-born Americans, the conclusions one might draw include this one: The quaran-tine efforts were virtuous examples of modern medical science and public health. Brave medical men were heralded as scientific warriors in the battle against epidemic disease. The East European Jewish immigrants were com-monly portrayed in these accounts as less than human and a decided health threat to New York City and beyond. A far different picture emerges, of course, when exploring the Yiddish American press, the fount of informa-tion on the New World for East European Jewish immigrants, and similar firsthand Yiddish accounts. Instead of a story describing the honorable work of doctors and the value of quarantine, we find accounts filled with fear de-scribing insensitive and rapid removal from one's home, terrible unsanitary living conditions on isolated islands, and, for some, death.

There are many other social scapegoats in the annals of American his-tory that illustrate how quarantine policies were often based on social as-sumptions and cultural perceptions. The impoverished alien has been an especially common but hardly exclusive target of blame during epidemics. I have chosen to focus on several hundred unfortunate East European Jews in 1892 largely out of personal interest and, more pragmatically, because the

Figure 1.1. Map of New York City, circa 1890. From G. W. Bromley's *Atlas of New York City.* Collection of the New-York Historical Society.

enticing circumstances of East European Jewish immigrants accused of importing epidemic disease into the United States did occur that year and the events were well documented.

My reliance on such a case history approach where the events discussed occurred over a fifteen-month period should not be interpreted as my having constructed a universal explanation of how all policies of quarantine are generated; nor should these events be transformed into an equation such as social scapegoat plus epidemic disease always equals disaster. Rather, I hope to study a brief episode in American history where the conflation of one socially undesirable group with epidemic diseases did lead to a combination of disastrous and positive results. My purpose is to document fully and to interpret one historical moment of quarantine not only from the perspective of the medical officers or social authorities instituting it but also from the essential—and often overlooked—perspective of these victims of quarantine.

The result, I hope, is a textured historical analysis of how the many levels of social, political, economic, legal, and cultural barriers isolate the ill—or those perceived to be ill—long before the dreaded "quarantine" placard is actually hung on their window. These layers of separation reflect the social conflicts and differential medical policies that may emerge from the devastating combination of an undesirable social group with a dreaded contagious disease. The events that constitute this book may, at times, appear horrifyingly cruel; at other times, they may appear to be sound preventive public health measures. The tension between the two ends of the spectrum of quarantine—conquest of disease versus isolation or death of the individual—is purposeful. This tension continues to challenge American society when confronted with epidemic disease and the potential for social scapegoating.

PART I

AVERTING A PESTILENCE

The Typhus Fever Epidemic on New York's Lower East Side

Our things were taken away, our friends separated from us; a man came to inspect us, as if to ascertain our full value; strange looking people driving us about like dumb animals helpless and unresisting; children we could not see crying in a way that suggested terrible things; ourselves driven into a little room where a great kettle was boiling on a little stove; our clothes taken off, our bodies rubbed with a slippery substance that might be any bad thing; a shower of warm water let down on us; without warning we are forced to pick out our clothes from among all the others, with the steam blinding us; we choke, cough, entreat the women to give us time. . . . Those gendarmes and nurses always shouted their commands at us from a distance, as fearful of our touch as if we had been lepers. . . . [Our] last place of detention [before embarking to America] turned out to be a prison, "Quarantine" they called it. . . . Several hundred of us were herded in half a dozen compartments . . . with never a sign of the free world beyond our barred windows; with anxiety and longing and home sickness in our hearts. . . . The fortnight in quarantine was not an episode; it was an epoch, divisible into eras, periods, events.

—*Mary Antin, reflecting on the two weeks she spent in quarantine at the Port of Hamburg, just prior to departing for Boston in 1894*

CHAPTER 1

The Russian Jews of the SS *Massilia*

In February 1892, an epidemic of typhus fever erupted on New York City's Lower East Side. Although only two hundred people contracted the extremely contagious and highly feared disease, its limitation to one area (the impoverished and dirty Jewish Quarter) and to one particular group (newly arrived Russian Jewish immigrants) engendered vigorous calls for quarantine from the New York City Health Department, the U.S. Congress, the U.S. Marine Hospital Service, and numerous newspapers and private citizens.

Typhus fever was no stranger to New York and many other urban centers in America, as there were frequent outbreaks of the lethal contagious disease throughout the nineteenth century. Nevertheless, in February 1892, no deaths from typhus had been reported in New York City since 1888.[1] Despite this decline in mortality, the exact cause and transmission of typhus fever remained a mystery during most of the germ-theory era.[2] Its clinical manifestations, however, were frequently observed and highly feared. Like many acute infectious diseases, typhus fever begins in a vague manner. The victim may complain of muscle pain, headache, nausea, thirst, and the sudden onset of an intensely high fever (104°F to 105°F). As the disease progresses over the first week, the patient experiences dizziness, sleep disturbances, weakness or exhaustion, and a curious body rash — irregular, raised pink-to-purple splotches that disappear with the slightest pressure of one's finger. Sometimes accompanying these symptoms is the "classic typhus odor," which has been described by physicians since the days of the Renaissance as the repulsive smell of rotting straw.

The second and third weeks of a bout of typhus are most alarming to those who observe it and, of course, to those who experience it. At this point, the patient becomes quite delirious, if not crazed, most likely a result of the central nervous system's reaction to the causative organism of typhus fever, *Rickettsia prowazekii*. Charles Murchison, the world's leading medical authority on typhus fever during the late nineteenth century, described the disease's "delirium phase" as dangerous to the patient and, frequently, shocking to the family: "[On occasion] the patient shouts, talks incoherently, and is more or less violent; if not restrained, he will get up and walk around the room, or even throw himself from an open window. This violent state is usually followed by great collapse, or the noisy condition passes into low, muttering delirium."[3] The intense struggle against the infection typically ends within three weeks. A sudden onset, excruciating fevers and pain, a period of crazed delirium, and for two or three out of every ten patients, death—such was the terrifying experience of typhus fever in 1892.

Most late-nineteenth-century American physicians and public health workers associated typhus fever with impoverished living conditions, overcrowding, and unsanitary habits. What was also clear to Gilded Age physicians was typhus fever's rapid and malignant spread from person to person in the event of an epidemic.[4] Not surprisingly, in an era of mass immigration, slum housing, poverty, and intense social revulsion toward immigrants, typhus fever came to be regarded if not as a foreign disease, then certainly as a disease of the urban poor and foreigners.[5]

The 1892 epidemic in New York City was especially remarkable because almost every case of typhus fever, with the exception of some medical attendants, police guards, and close neighbors, occurred among newly arrived Russian Jewish immigrants who had traveled on the same steamship, the *Massilia,* and were temporarily housed under the bond of the United Hebrew Charities of New York City in eight boarding houses on the Lower East Side.[6] The primary mechanism of disease containment was quarantine, whether it was the forced removal of the immigrant Russian Jews and their neighbors afflicted with typhus to the city's contagious disease hospital on North Brother Island; the quarantine of developing typhus cases and their healthy contacts on the Lower East Side; or the temporary detainment of all Russian Jews but not other immigrants at the Port of New York's quarantine station.

The Pale of Settlement

The life of the Jews in Russia was, at best, a difficult and precarious one. Novelist and noted *New York Times* European correspondent Harold Frederic spent the year 1891–92 covering the Russian famine. He often referred to the Russian Jews in his dispatches as "the Pariah Community."[7] Theirs was a life lived separately from other Russians—religiously, socially, economically, geographically, and legally. Indeed, if one were searching for a living metaphor of quarantine or isolation, one could hardly do better than to look at the Russian Jews confined to the Pale of Settlement during the late nineteenth and early twentieth centuries.

A significant amount of this social separation was imposed by the Russian Jewish communities themselves. On a religious level, the Jews were mandated by the teachings of the Torah to think of themselves as distinctly different from other people. The rigid orthodoxy of Judaism advocated the avoidance of all things secular, including literature, music, and art. The Jew-

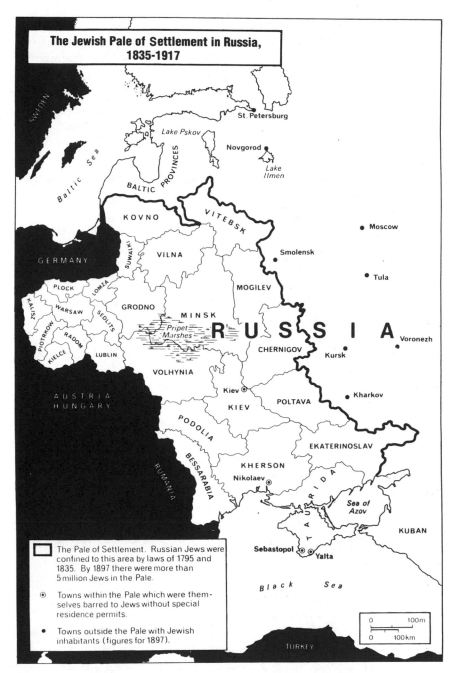

The Jewish Pale of Settlement in Russia, 1835-1917

The Pale of Settlement. Russian Jews were confined to this area by laws of 1795 and 1835. By 1897 there were more than 5 million Jews in the Pale.

⊙ Towns within the Pale which were themselves barred to Jews without special residence permits.

• Towns outside the Pale with Jewish inhabitants (figures for 1897).

Figure 1.1. From Martin Gilbert, *The Atlas of Jewish History* (New York: William Morrow, 1992).

ish religion instilled in its practitioners the fervent belief that a loyal faith in God would bring about a Messianic miracle, the restoration of the Holy Land, and individual salvation in the afterlife, provided the Jews maintained this social separation from the Gentile world and followed the strict precepts of the Torah. On a cultural level, the Russian Jews often spoke Yiddish rather than Russian, making communication between Russians and Jews difficult. Many prominent Russians derided Yiddish as jargon or gibberish, belying the language's rich and expressive power. For example, the Yiddish word *goyim* originates from the Hebrew word for "nations." It subsequently came to mean "other nations" and, later still, "the other" in the sense of those who are not of the Jewish faith. With the slightest change in intonation, however, *goyim* becomes a harsh slur directed at Gentiles.

Another barrier had to do with one of the few interactions Jews might have with their Russian neighbors: mercantile trade.[8] Jewish mastery or so-called exploitation of the Russian peasant class in petty business relations was often a sore spot in the Russian psyche. Its true extent is difficult to estimate. For example, in his report on the inciting causes of immigration from Russia to the United States in 1891, Herman J. Schulteis interviewed several Russian government officials who made exaggerated claims of Jewish dominance over the Russian economy: "They practically monopolize the fur, grain, clothing, and live-stock trades. . . . One-third of them own nearly one-half of the entire wealth of the country."[9] Certainly, some Jewish businessmen were successful even in Czarist Russia, yet contemporary studies of the level of poverty among Russian Jews suggest that the "financial dominance" issue was still another means of justifying the many anti-Semitic edicts of the government.

On a more imposing level, Czar Alexander III and his minister of the interior, Nicholas P. Ignatiev, enforced the Russian Jews' pariah status with harsh economic sanctions and repressive edicts, such as the May edicts of 1882. These laws required the majority of the Jews of Russia to live in the Pale of Settlement, twenty-five provinces of the Russian Empire that included fifteen western districts of Russia and the ten districts of the former Kingdom of Poland. Jews were forbidden from venturing outside their restricted province for a visit or for purposes of settlement unless they had special permission from various Russian authorities. Such permission was difficult to obtain, to say the least. The severity of this imposition takes on graver meaning when one considers the social impact of the Russian famine of 1891–92, the 1892 cholera pandemic, and the resulting desire among Russian Jews to migrate to safer regions.

Other anti-Semitic sanctions ranged from petty annoyances to policies of death and destruction. For example, in 1891, the mayor of Moscow, M. Aleixieff, ordered a ban on the admission of "sick Jews" to Muscovite hospitals. This same mayor expelled ten thousand Jews from Moscow in October 1892 for fear that they might disrupt the daily life of the city. Similar orders were made by a number of provincial governors across the Pale between 1891 and 1892, in imitation of Moscow's official refusal to provide medical services to Jews. Other anti-Semitic sanctions included restrictions on how Jews could

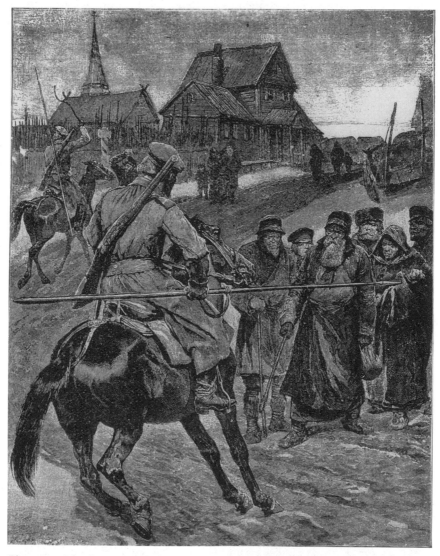

Figure 1.2. The famine in Russia. A Cossack patrol prevents peasants from leaving their village. *Frank Leslie's Illustrated Weekly* 74 (1892).

earn a living, regulations barring Russian Jews from attending colleges and universities or obtaining government jobs, heavy taxes on kosher foods and items needed for ritual devotions such as Sabbath candles and skull caps (*yarmulkes*), and forced conscription in the Russian army for all firstborn Jewish males between the ages of twelve and eighteen for periods as long as twenty-five years.[10]

There was a negative synergy to Czarist Russia's social and legal quarantine of the Jews combined with the Russian Jews' self-imposed isolation from Russian culture and life. In early 1893, Pierre Botkine, the secretary of the Russian legation to the United States, publicly denied all allegations of Russian anti-Semitism in an article he wrote for the popular American magazine *The Century*. Botkine characterized the Russian Jews as a "backward" and "superstitious" lot who wanted to live apart from the Russians. To prove his point, Botkine cited the Jews' refusal to adopt the native tongue, their inability to read or write Russian, and their devotion to a separate God as evidence of their desire to live apart in the Pale.[11] Such outcries against the Russian Jews, simultaneously barred from Russian society and chastised for their subsequent ignorance of it, reminded the Yiddish journalist Abraham Cahan of "the hypocritical miser who kept his gate guarded by ferocious dogs and then reproached his destitute neighbor with holding himself aloof."[12]

Perhaps most trying of all for the Russian Jews was the rising tide of mass orders for expulsion and the violent pogroms that threatened their lives. At the arbitrary whim of a provincial governor, an entire shtetl or village population could be abruptly ordered to resettle to a different area or leave the country entirely. Such decisions were commonly based on a substantial dislike for Jewish residents and a desire to rid the province of their influence. During the enforcement of these orders of exile, Jews were beaten by Russian citizens and army personnel, women were raped, children were spat upon, and many Jews were summarily executed; others were forced to view their cemeteries and synagogues being vandalized, and were exposed to numerous other atrocities without any means of recourse or protection under existing Russian law.[13]

In 1891, U.S. Commissioner of Immigration John B. Weber and neurologist Walter Kempster made a visit to the Russian Pale of Settlement at the request of the U.S. House of Representatives Immigration Committee. The report that Weber and Kempster subsequently sent to President Benjamin Harrison in December of that year noted not only the inhumane persecutions of the Russian Jews but also the international repercussions of such atrocities:

Willing and able to work, they are unable to trade in the country, unable to leave the precincts where they now are, excluded from governmental work, it is no wonder they wish to fly somewhere where they can breathe and have an equal chance in the struggle for existence. The only thing that prevents them from going *en masse* to other countries is their poverty.[14]

In 1911, a subsequent U.S. government inquiry into the emigration situation in Russia was conducted by the Senate Committee on Immigration. The resulting report characterized the year 1892 as one of widespread famine, disease, and overcrowding, and, with the various anti-Semitic laws enacted that year, as "one of the most oppressive for the Jews." This report went on to describe graphically the effect pogroms had on the Russian Jews:

> One cannot estimate the damage done by the pogroms in mere figures. Completely destroying the safety of property, the pogrom ruins credit, brings about economic crisis, and throws tens of thousands of unemployed workmen into the streets. Still more terrible is the effect of the pogroms upon the moral atmosphere prevailing among the Jews. The knowledge that in the full light of day in the sight of everybody, a crowd of the lowest rabble may burst into your house, plundering and murdering, destroying all that you have toiled for, may violate the honor of those who are dearer than life itself, may maim or kill you while those who are set to preserve your security will at best remain passive spectators of these events and at worst may take active part in them, the knowledge that it is useless to struggle, because behind the pogromists armed force is against you — such knowledge paralyses the energy of people, causes them to fly without retrospection, without calculation, only to escape from the threatening horrors of the pogrom.[15]

In this environment of ostracism and oppression, as Irving Howe observed, "neither stability nor peace, well-being nor equality was possible for the Jews of Russia."[16]

The Voyage of the SS Massilia

Odessa had long been a cultural center and desirable place to live for Russian Jews exiled to the Pale of Settlement. Originally a Turkish possession, the city and its surrounding province on the northwestern shore of the Black Sea was annexed by the Russian Empire in 1789. Unlike the harsh and often anti-Semitic provincial governments of other regions in Russia, the local authorities in Odessa had a reputation for being benevolent toward Jewish citizens. For example, Jews in Odessa during the eighteenth and early nineteenth centuries were allowed to establish their own schools, to participate in commercial activities of the province, and to follow their religious beliefs.[17] By the mid-nineteenth century, Odessa was attracting large numbers of Jews who were escaping harsh living conditions or who had been expelled from the provinces of Volhynia, Podolia, Lithuania, and Galicia.

At the end of September 1891, a large group of Jews escaping from the province of Volhynia arrived in Odessa. Although these Jews and their ancestors had lived in their tiny shtetl for generations, they began a long nomadic trek that would take them far away from the Russian Pale. Forcibly evacuated from famine-stricken Volhynia in the late summer by the provincial governor, they traveled on foot to Podolia. They were as unwelcome there as they were in their home province and continued their arduous travels to Odessa, hoping to escape the famine, disease, and tyranny they had left behind.

On October 4, 1891, approximately five days after their arrival in Odessa, the provincial governor issued an order expelling the 1,168 Russian Jews. The edict gave them forty-eight hours to leave what was considered to be one of the friendliest places for Jews to live in Russia. The exiled Jews had few options but to go back where they came from, hardly a desirable choice given the circumstances of their exile, or to leave the country entirely.[18] Quickly arranging their passage out of Odessa and packing what little belongings and clothing they owned, the group of laborers, petty artisans, butchers, draymen, and their families left Russia forever with the hope of emigrating to Palestine. Within earshot of the footsteps of armed Russian soldiers sent to evict them from their cheap boarding houses, the exiled Jews boarded a dilapidated steamer that would take them across the Black Sea to Constantinople. As the Yiddish American newspaper, the *Arbeiter Zeitung*, described it, the 1,168 Jews escaped Odessa "with the greatest of difficulties and the bitterest of pain."[19]

The difficulty and pain were only magnified once the exiled pilgrims landed at Constantinople. Although they carried papers approved by the Odessa authorities giving them dual status as Russian and Turkish subjects, the Jews were denied travel papers by representatives of the sultan of Turkey. A recent law enacted by the Turkish government expressly forbade the passage of Russian Jews through the Ottoman Empire to any other country, based on "sanitary grounds."[20] Instead of making the planned escape to Palestine, the émigrés were forced to hide in the Jewish ghetto of Constantinople, a district described in the Yiddish press as a den of "pestilence, sin and death."[21] There they remained, fugitives without a national identity, for three months while Turkish authorities deliberated their fate.

On Christmas Eve 1891, the Russian Jews were again given expulsion orders, this time endorsed by Turkish officials. Without many choices, they hurriedly escaped to Smyrna. From there the 1,168 Jews were embraced by agents of the Baron de Hirsch Fund, a philanthropic agency founded by the German Jewish financier and multimillionaire Baron Maurice de Hirsch. The fund, with its $2.4 million endowment, was dedicated to helping Jews get out of Russia and settle in the United States, Palestine, and South America.[22]

Not surprisingly, a charity concerned solely with aiding the emigration of Jews out of the Russian Empire to America was subject to intense scrutiny and concern by immigration restrictionists in the United States. Both Terence V. Powderly and Herman J. Schulteis warned the U.S. Treasury Department in 1891 of the Baron de Hirsch Fund's "hypnotic influences" and its aim of obscuring the immigration laws of the United States in order to bring over as many Russian Jewish paupers as possible.[23] An angry *New York Sun* editorial on the subject of "undesirable new immigrants" asked: "Can we afford to honor Baron Hirsch's drafts?"[24] Similarly, Senator William Eaton Chandler, chairman of the Senate Immigration Committee and an avowed opponent of the entry of undesirable Russian Jews and Italians, openly questioned the legitimacy of the Baron de Hirsch Fund from the well of the U.S. Senate.[25]

In Smyrna, the Hirsch Fund agents sent 900 of the exiled Jews to Argentina; the other 268 continued their disastrous exodus, traveling by rail to Marseilles and then boarding the Febre Line steamship *Massilia,* bound for New York City, on January 2, 1892. The ship did not point its bow toward America, however, until after a January 7 stop in Naples, where it picked up 470 Italian passengers also emigrating to the New World. Given the cursory state of immigrant medical inspections at both Marseilles and Naples during the winter of 1892, it seems doubtful that any of the *Massilia* passengers underwent a careful medical examination before embarking for America.[26]

The *Massilia*'s twenty-eight-day voyage across the Atlantic Ocean was especially difficult and long, marked by stormy weather and rough seas. The average length of voyage for most steerage steamers making the crossing from Europe to America during that period was about seven to twelve days. The ship had been launched in 1891, after being built in Dundee by the Scottish shipyard Gourlay Brothers. The *Massilia* was small in size for a transatlantic steamer (340 feet by 25.5 feet), slow in speed, and easily tossed about in the rough waters. Even with two sailmasts to augment its velocity, the ship's single-screw engine only carried the vessel at 11 to 13 knots, about half the speed of the state-of-the-art transatlantic steamships of the day.[27]

Cramped and unsanitary living conditions aboard the ship only made the rough voyage rougher for the immigrants. The steerage compartments consisted of long tiers of berths on either side of the ship with a central area for benches and tables where the passengers took their meals. The fare served on board steerage steamships of that era typically consisted of decaying herring, rotten potatoes, stale black bread with a paltry ration of rancid butter, and tea. In addition to frequent complaints of unappealing food and seasickness, the Jewish immigrants feared ingesting food that was forbidden by Jewish dietary (kosher) laws. Many of the Jewish passengers ate little or

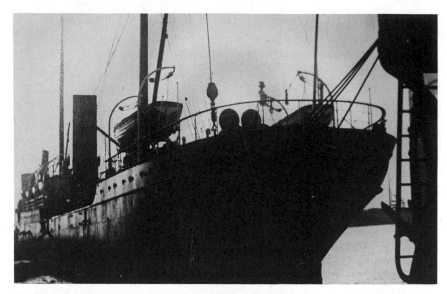

Figure 1.3. SS *Massilia.* Collection of the Peabody Essex Museum, Salem, Mass.

nothing during the *Massilia*'s voyage. Such malnourishment, overcrowded conditions, and the chronic debilitation enforced by bitter travails only increased the passengers' risks of contracting such so-called filth diseases as typhus and cholera.

The berths in the steerage were divided among those traveling as families, single men, and single women. The Febre steamship line later reported that the Russian Jewish immigrants were berthed in separate compartments from the Italians picked up at Naples. Yet all those aboard the *Massilia* were exposed to filthy living conditions in the poorly cleaned steerage. Open troughs served as toilets; they were sporadically flushed with water or cleaned during the voyage. Salt water basins were used for personal washing as well as for cleaning laundry, plates, and utensils.

Perhaps the only respite the "chosen people" aboard the *Massilia* enjoyed were the occasional rare days when the weather was clear enough for them to go up to the open deck. There, huddled together trying to protect themselves from the cold, the immigrants were allowed the luxury of "fresh air."[28] As one marine hospital surgeon stationed at Ellis Island the day the *Massilia* sailed into New York Harbor observed: "The *Massilia* is one of the best ships afloat for the propagation of typhus fever."[29]

Although in retrospect it is evident that the *Massilia* passengers were likely not in the best of health, there is evidence to suggest that the medical inspection process at New York Harbor in January 1892 suffered from a number of flaws that made the importation of an epidemic disease possible. For example, when the ship reached New York Harbor on January 30, 1892, it made a brief but mandatory inspection stop at the quarantine station located off Staten Island at the point of the Narrows. More than eight hundred passengers and crew members aboard the *Massilia* were inspected for evidence of typhus, cholera, plague, yellow fever, smallpox, and leprosy by two physicians in little under an hour.

The rapid and routine medical inspection processes at the New York quarantine station and similar public health outposts were often critically questioned by experienced clinicians. Seldom, however, were improvements (such as hiring more medical inspectors) made during periods when no epidemic disease was threatening. As the Johns Hopkins Hospital superintendent, Dr. Henry Hurd, pointedly asked during the fall of 1892: "How can a physician inspect two thousand persons as they should be in a couple of hours, when it sometimes takes a doctor twice that long to diagnose one patient?"[30]

Adding to the rush and confusion of medical inspection was the striking shift of medical personnel going on at the quarantine station the week the *Massilia* landed in New York. The long-time health officer of the port, Dr. William Smith, had recently been ousted from his position in a bitter political battle. Smith was to be replaced on February 1, 1892, by the Tammany Hall-supported William Jenkins. When the *Massilia* sailed into New York Harbor on January 30, however, there was no official chief of the station and she was inspected by the acting health officer, Dr. E. C. Skinner. After a thirty-five-minute inspection of the vessel, Skinner found nothing "medically remarkable" about the bedraggled, half-starved immigrants and

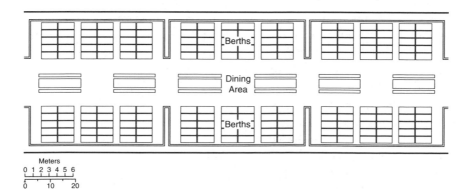

Figure 1.4. Steerage compartment of the SS *Massilia*. Artist's reconstruction based on ship plans from the University of Dundee Archives, Scotland.

admitted the *Massilia* into the Port of New York.[31] A similarly quick process of medical inspection followed at the immigration station on Ellis Island.

Both medical teams at the quarantine station and Ellis Island later justified their rapid inspection of the passengers on the basis of the ship's "clean bill of health" and because no outbreaks of disease were noted during the voyage. This bill of health, however was essentially useless since the papers attesting to the Jewish passengers' health were endorsed by the U.S. consul at Odessa, John Volkmann, some four months earlier and *before* the *Massilia* Jews began their exile in Turkey. Although the ship's log contained information that documented the *Massilia*'s passengers' three-month stay in the typhus-infested districts of Constantinople, this definite risk factor was not given serious consideration by the health officials in New York Harbor.

Falsified or inaccurate consular reports attesting to the health of a particular immigrant ship posed a common and vexing problem to American immigration officials during the early 1890s. Frequently, the consular agent signing the bill of health had no experience in public health or medicine and rarely had an opportunity to inspect the ships or immigrants leaving a particular port. Moreover, as Colonel John Weber observed during his inspection of Russia for the U.S. Immigration Commission during 1891, there were simply too many immigrants per consular agent to make any such bill of health an effective tool for quarantine officers on the American side of the Atlantic.[32] Careful medical inspections and observation of those suspected to be ill at the port of arrival were considered by leading maritime quarantine authorities of the late nineteenth century to be a less-than-perfect means of preventing immigrants from importing infection.[33]

What remains difficult to explain, therefore, is not the failure of the various health officers to diagnose an incubating case of typhus fever as it quickly passed the eyes of a few physicians inspecting hundreds of passengers; this was a virtual impossibility even in the hands of the most experienced physician in 1892. Instead, what is troubling about the state and federal inspection process is that the health officers ignored the acknowledged debilitated condition of the Russian Jewish passengers and their documented history of forced exile in Constantinople. Neither of these factors induced them to perform further medical investigation or to call for temporary observation of the passengers at either the quarantine station or the Ellis Island hospital on the day the *Massilia* sailed into port.

One curious example of the inconsistent public health procedures practiced in the Port of New York was articulated by the commissioner of immigration at Ellis Island, Colonel John Weber. Weber was a strong advocate of open immigration and a prominent "friend" of the East European Jewish immigrant community. Two days after the *Massilia*'s landing, Weber openly protested to the *New York Times* about the "inhuman if not criminal han-dling" of the *Massilia* passengers by its ship's surgeon and the Febre steam-ship line.[34] Weber went one step further to notify the assistant secretary of the treasury A. B. Nettleton on February 19, 1892, about his recollections on the state of health of the Russian Jews aboard the *Massilia*:

> I happened to be standing at the entrance through which they passed on reach-ing here and saw what seemed to me to be a clear case of inhumanity on the part of the ship's surgeon in permitting these cases to be brought down, as it was evi-dent that they should not have been directly transported or transferred but sent directly to a suitable hospital for treatment and care. . . . The passengers of the *Massilia* embraced a number of Russian Jews who came here in an emaciated, worn condition the explanation of which is that they had been expelled from their country and traveled about, many of them since last spring.[35]

According to the Immigration Bureau's annually published regulations, Weber's observations should have prompted further investigation by the health officers at either the quarantine station or Ellis Island, but the ship was not held over for isolation or observation. One month after the *Massilia*'s landing, Weber confidently testified before the Congressional Immigration Committee that he and his staff were in no way responsible for the incursion of typhus fever into New York City.[36]

In fact, only sixty-eight of the *Massilia* passengers were temporarily de-tained by the immigration officials at Ellis Island. Those detained, however, were not considered threats to the public health or in any way ill. Instead, these unfortunate immigrants were held back because of the "Likely to Be-come a Public Charge" exclusionary laws. All but twenty-three of the de-tained immigrants were eventually released under the bond of the United Hebrew Charities Organization and allowed to settle in the United States. The twenty-three immigrants who were barred entry to the United States were excluded solely for economic reasons. Their deportations were jus-tified on the immigration officials' belief that they would require public charity within twelve months of living in the United States. One represen-tative example of these exclusions was an immigrant named Rachel Wein-stein, a thirty-five-year-old seamstress with four young children who had been driven out of Russia. Mrs. Weinstein was described as being in excel-lent health and never having received public support. She was deemed likely to become a public charge, however, because she had no money or family in America and her husband had died during their exile.[37]

A frequently described scene in the American immigration experience is that of a steamship entering New York Harbor under the outstretched arm of the Statue of Liberty. As ships steamed past this magnificent symbol of

America, immigrants on the open decks were known to stand in awe, simply staring at the statue. Men took off their hats in deference; the attention of chattering children became focused and riveted; many women cried. All of their hopes, dreams, and fears seemed intimately tied to her.[38] Unfortunately no written record of the *Massilia*'s voyage, inspection process, or landing at the Hudson piers on Manhattan's Lower West Side survives. Nor can the historian presume to speculate what hopes the immigrants may have borne or what fears must have been in the minds of these storm-tossed, potentially ill immigrants as they faced inspections, temporary lodging on the Lower East Side, the crushing need to find their own places to live and jobs to keep food on the table, and the challenges of adjusting to a new land and mode of life. We probably can assume, however, that they could not have known the threat of typhus fever they may have carried with them from the *Massilia* — or contracted in New York. How could they imagine the revulsion and fear they would soon conjure in the eyes of many Americans? Unlike countless other steamships that transported destitute immigrants in their steerage, the *Massilia* Jews faced a far different fate. As the *New York Herald* later declared, "Death, disease and widespread trouble was the cargo the *Massilia* brought."[39]

The Typhus Ward

The journalist Jacob A. Riis, himself an immigrant from Denmark, graphically described the plight of New York City's urban poor in his 1890 best-selling book *How the Other Half Lives*. He characterized the Jewish Lower East Side in this exposé as "the typhus ward," a place where filth diseases "sprout naturally among the hordes that bring the germs with them from across the sea and whose first instinct is to hide their sick lest the authorities carry them off to be slaughtered."[40] This description appeared especially prescient during the 1892 typhus epidemic.

Abraham Cahan, then editor of the Yiddish American *Arbeiter Zeitung*, a socialist paper published by the United Hebrew Trade Union, presented a more poetic yet nevertheless distressing portrait of the crowded district in his 1896 novella *Yekl*:

> It is one of the most densely populated spots on the face of the earth — a seething human sea fed by streams, streamlets, and rills of immigration flowing from all the Yiddish-speaking centers of Europe. Hardly a block but shelters Jews from every nook and corner of Russia, Poland, Galicia, Hungary, Roumania; Lithuanian Jews, Volhynian Jews, South Russian Jews, Bessarabian Jews; Jews crowded out of the "pale of Jewish settlement"; Russified Jews expelled from Moscow, St. Petersburg, Kieff, or Saratoff; Jewish runaways from justice; Jewish refugees from crying

political and economical injustice; people torn from a hard-gained foothold in life and from deep-rooted attachments by the caprice of intolerance or the wiles of demagoguery—innocent scapegoats of a guilty Government for its blind fury.[41]

Situated almost on top of the other immigrant communities of Italian, Chinese, and Irish newcomers struggling to make their way in America, New York City's Tenth and Thirteenth Wards and portions of the Seventh and Eleventh Wards made up the crowded Jewish section described by Cahan. This small area, less than a half square mile in size, was "one of the [world's] most densely populated spots," with over 523 inhabitants per acre in some sections in 1890.[42] Bounded by the East River, the Bowery on the west, Monroe Street on the south, and Houston Street on the north (but already beginning to spill over as far north as Fourteenth Street), the Jewish Lower East Side was a district that inspired fascination from a few observers, worry from others, and intense concern on the part of most native-born Americans.

For example, a distinct affection for the Lower East Side was displayed by many literary luminaries of the Gilded Age. Lincoln Steffens, the well-known muckraking journalist, reported that as a teenager he was as "infatuated with the ghetto as Eastern boys were with the wild west."[43] Hutchins Hapgood spent years of his journalistic career writing sketches of ghetto life that romanticized the hard lives of the denizens of the Lower East Side.[44] Novelist William Dean Howells wrote sympathetically about the Russian Jewish ghetto-dwellers in 1896 as well as his avoidance of a quarantined "typhus quarter."[45] The fastidious Henry James noted in 1906 that the ghetto was a "crowded, hustled roadway where multiplication, multiplication of everything, was the dominant note, at the bottom of some vast sallow aquarium in which innumerable fish, of over-developed proboscis were to bump together, forever, amid heaped spoils of the sea."[46] British writer Arnold Bennett described the Lower East Side in 1912 as a region where "the architecture seemed to sweat humanity at every window and door."[47]

Many Americans familiar with life on the Lower East Side and other urban ghettos during the 1890s could not help but be concerned about the potential for illness to creep uptown. Even pro-immigrant groups during this era publicly worried about the health risks brewing on New York's Lower East Side. For example, during the mid-1880s, a group of prominent New Yorkers formed the Sanitary Aid Society of the Tenth Ward of New York City. Its membership included Kilean van Rensselaer, Theodore Roosevelt, Jesse Seligman, and former mayor of New York Abram Hewitt. Their mission was to improve health and sanitary conditions on New York's Lower East Side. Yet even this group, sympathetic enough toward the urban poor actually to do something about their squalor, revealed its revulsion for these immi-

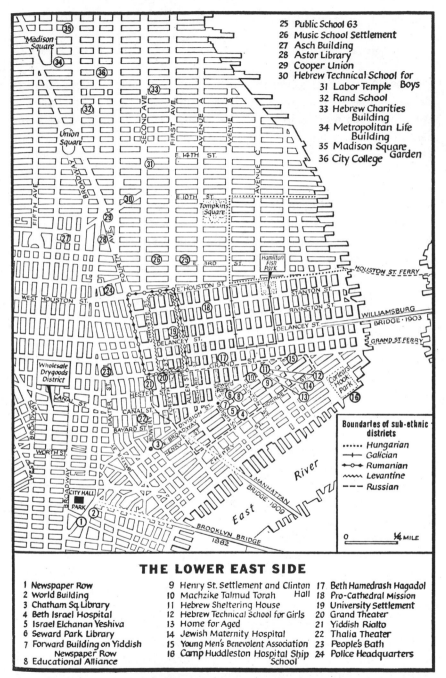

25 Public School 63
26 Music School Settlement
27 Asch Building
28 Astor Library
29 Cooper Union
30 Hebrew Technical School for
31 Labor Temple   Boys
32 Rand School
33 Hebrew Charities
      Building
34 Metropolitan Life
      Building
35 Madison Square Garden
36 City College

Boundaries of sub-ethnic
districts
······ Hungarian
——+—— Galician
—o—o— Rumanian
〜〜〜 Levantine
– – – Russian

0   ¼ MILE

THE LOWER EAST SIDE

1 Newspaper Row
2 World Building
3 Chatham Sq. Library
4 Beth Israel Hospital
5 Israel Elchanan Yeshiva
6 Seward Park Library
7 Forward Building on Yiddish
      Newspaper Row
8 Educational Alliance

9 Henry St. Settlement and Clinton
      Hall
10 Machzike Talmud Torah
11 Hebrew Sheltering House
12 Hebrew Technical School for Girls
13 Home for Aged
14 Jewish Maternity Hospital
15 Young Men's Benevolent Association
16 Camp Huddleston Hospital Ship
      School

17 Beth Hamedrash Hagadol
18 Pro-Cathedral Mission
19 University Settlement
20 Grand Theater
21 Yiddish Rialto
22 Thalia Theater
23 People's Bath
24 Police Headquarters

Figure 1.5. Map of the Lower East Side, New York City. From Moses Rischin, *The Promised City: New York's Jews, 1870–1914* (Cambridge, Mass.: Harvard University Press, 1962).

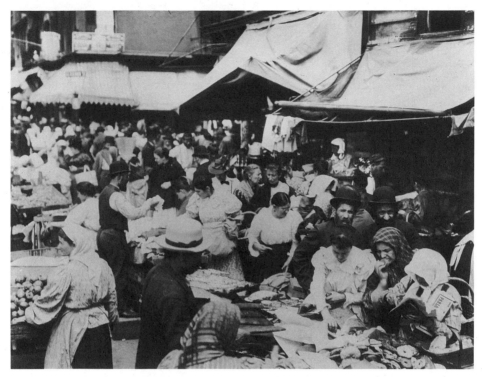

Figure 1.6. Hester Street vendors, circa 1895. Byron Collection, Museum of the City of New York.

grants as it described them in its annual reports. The Sanitary Aid Society routinely mixed their noblesse oblige with judgmental descriptions of the people they were trying to help. Their immigrant charges were routinely referred to as "human maggots" who led dismal lives consisting of "so much filth, so many filthy homes and pestilential rookeries, so many human beings with insufficient breathing space, bad ventilation, plumbing, [and] . . . festering masses." As the society's *Annual Report for 1890* concluded, without the society's guidance and aid, New York's immigrants were destined to lead lives of poverty, degradation, immorality, and crime.[48]

The Russian Jews' co-religionists, the well-assimilated German Jewish Americans, were both supportive and fearful of the consequences of the wave of East European Jewish immigration. In many respects, the German Jewish American community held the East European Jewish immigrants at a symbolic arm's length—helping them adjust to life in America through successful charitable enterprises while avoiding close physical or social contact with them. German Jewish patricians could be counted on for funding to address the refugee crisis, but they would not welcome a *grine kuzine* (green immigrant)[49] to Sabbath services at their Reform temple on Fifth Avenue. The most powerful symbol of this fear was, of course, New York's Lower East Side.

The editorial pages of the *Jewish Messenger,* a leading American German Jewish weekly based in New York, reflect this ambivalence. Most issues of the *Messenger* during the early 1890s covered some aspect of the cruel plight of Jewish brethren in Czarist Russia. During the fall of 1891, for example, one finds weekly updates on Czarist atrocities and anti-Semitic sanctions. Alongside these dispatches from Russia was a series of articles on public health conditions of those Russian Jews living on the Lower East Side. The articles are a sophisticated and thorough survey of the squalid living conditions and potential for disease among the newly arrived Russian Jews. The reporter clearly takes the side of the New York City Health Department, blaming much of the health conditions on the noncooperation of the "ignorant immigrant community." The articles nervously warned the paper's well-assimilated Jewish readers that "the surroundings of the Fiji Islander are more conducive to health than those that environ thousands of Israelites who continue to live in the slums of New York."[50]

The theme that rings loudest in contemporary accounts of life in this urban slum during the 1890s is that of overcrowding, dirt, foul odors, unsanitary living conditions, and noise. In our present era of an all but pious allegiance to personal hygiene (often manifesting itself in the form of frequent showers and use of deodorants, the advanced management of sewage, the pristine packaging of foodstuffs, and, for most Americans, decent living quarters), it is difficult to imagine fully the pervasive filth and dirt of life on the Lower East Side during this period.[51]

The average 25-foot by 25-foot cramped, airless tenement apartment housed four or more people to a room often without a window or, at best, with access to a stifling "airshaft." These airshafts were actually architectural loopholes in the New York City Housing Code and more typically served as makeshift garbage chutes than as a source of sunshine and ventilation. Most tenement apartments consisted of a front parlor that was 10.5 feet by 11 feet (usually the largest room of the flat), a tiny kitchen area, and one or two bedrooms about 7 feet by 8.5 feet.

More than half of the East European Jewish families living on the Lower East Side during this period were required to take in boarders simply to make ends meet. This only further crowded an already overcrowded flat. Some entrepreneurial "landlords" even rented out cots or couches precariously placed between the parlor and the kitchen on a shift basis. The tenement home also frequently served as either an extension or a primary site of the sweatshop where fathers, mothers, and children spent their hours at home sewing piecework for the city's burgeoning garment industry.[52] For the newly arrived immigrant who had not yet found a suitable place of his own, living conditions were even more objectionable. A common way for an unscrupulous tenement house landlord or "hotel keeper" to earn money was to lease one room to ten to twenty newly arrived immigrants "just off the boat."[53]

Matters of decent living were further constrained by a lack of toilet facilities in these tenement homes. There were two per floor among the very best and most recently built tenement houses. More commonly, tenements built before 1885 only provided outdoor privies for their tenants and these were sporadically emptied by the city's Sanitation Department or private "night soil" removal services. No matter how hard the classic "Yiddishe Mama" struggled to keep her home decent and clean for her family, it was always an uphill battle. Add to this the odor of rotting fish, meat, and vegetables sold on uncovered pushcarts, the immense amount of animal waste from horse-drawn wagons and trucks, dirty streets, and the stench of a crowded humanity where over 82,000 people lived, worked, and played within fifty square blocks. Dirt was "all-pervading" in the Lower East Side, as were its frequent companions: crime, prostitution, and vice.[54]

Even as late as 1892, there were some New Yorkers who believed in the miasma theory of disease, which postulated that malodorous, decaying organic matter — such as sewer gas, rotten fruits, vegetables, and meats, animal or human feces, and other common environmental features of the Lower East Side — could "infect" the air and yield an epidemic. If a modern-day reader can imagine the realities of life on the Lower East Side in an era when concepts of epidemics still held vestiges of miasma theory and when immigrants were the personification of dirt, filth, and disease, he or she can begin to understand some rationale behind the revulsion expressed by native-born Americans toward impoverished and unkempt immigrants. Instead of the fascination exhibited by Howells, Hutchins, or Steffens, most were content to read about immigrants in the comfort of their parlors and to avoid physical contact entirely.

What the American public read in *Scribner's Monthly*, the *Century*, *Harper's Weekly*, *Leslie's Illustrated Weekly*, and other popular magazines about East European Jews and the Lower East Side was rarely complimentary.[55] There were, of course, occasional authoritative reports of positive health conditions along the Lower East Side, such as one written by John Shaw Billings in 1890 revealing that immigrant Jews enjoyed the lowest rates of infant and adult mortality among immigrant populations in New York and the lowest rates of tuberculosis among all New York populations. Nevertheless, the popular perception among many native-born New Yorkers was that the Lower East Side was a "breeding ground for pestilential disease."[56]

The social quarantine informally imposed by native-born New Yorkers around the Jewish Quarter of the late nineteenth century was not lost on immigrant observers. Milton Reizenstein, the superintendent of the Hebrew Educational Society of Brooklyn, described imaginary "massive portals" separating the Lower East Side's Jewish Quarter from the "Non-Jewish districts of New York." Similarly, Abraham Cahan commented on the metaphorical social quarantine imposed on the Jewish ghetto of New York and its few "chances of contact with the English-speaking portion of the population."[57]

Using the terms of contagion and quarantine, perhaps no contemporary observer discusses this social separation more emphatically than Dr. George M. Price. Price, a Russian Jew who emigrated from Poltava in the Pale of Settlement to New York in 1882, graduated from the New York University Medical School in 1895. During the year 1891–92, Price contributed a series of articles to the Russian Jewish periodical *Voskhod* on the Russian Jews in America. His articles, although spiked with sarcasm, accurately record the struggles, tribulations, and achievements of East European Jewish immigrants in New York City during the early 1890s. His views on the public health of the Lower East Side are especially interesting since Price ultimately went on to a distinguished career as a physician, medical author, and inspector of tenement and factory health conditions for the New York City Health Department:

> A Jewish neighborhood grows in width, height, and depth, pushing out members of other nationalities, helping to build ten-story barracks, filling the attics, basements, and streets. These inhabitants — the poor, ignorant populace — are trying to eke out their daily bread, with from 100 to 200 families in one building or, as we might call them, penitentiaries. Can we, then, expect cleanliness, healthy air in these streets with their many buildings and large population? What then is the result? — A Jewish ghetto, filthy, odiferous and unsanitary. It is a ghetto where poverty, disease and epidemics prevail . . . [where] there is complete isolation from the American population.[58]

Adding to the difficulties in maintaining the public health in such an overcrowded area was the intense animosity between the immigrant communities and the city's Health and Police Departments. New Yorkers living on the Lower East Side frequently complained to the authorities about unscrupulous landlords, foul living conditions, and unclean streets. Their requests, however, were often ignored or denied by the Health Department unless it deemed the particular situation worthy of its attention.[59] Partly out of fear and partly out of retaliation, the Jewish immigrants on the Lower East Side, like other immigrant groups, responded as best they could in this hegemonic relationship: They avoided the Health Department at every opportunity. In

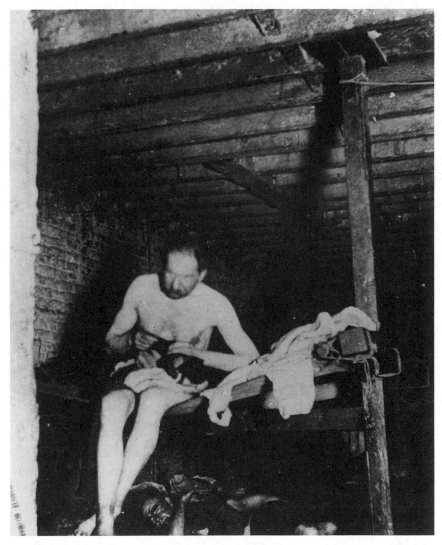

Figure 1.7. Lodger in a seven-cents-a-night lodging house on the Lower East Side, circa 1890. Jacob A. Riis Collection, Museum of the City of New York.

1890, Jacob Riis described a classic, yet all-too-typical confrontation between the Health Department and the Jews of the Lower East Side on market day:

> An English word falls upon the ear almost with a sense of shock, as something unexpected and strange. In the midst of it all there is a sudden wild scattering, a hustling of things from the street into dark cellars, into backyards and byways, a slamming and locking of doors under the improvised shelves and counters. The health officials' cart is coming down the street, preceded and followed by the stal-

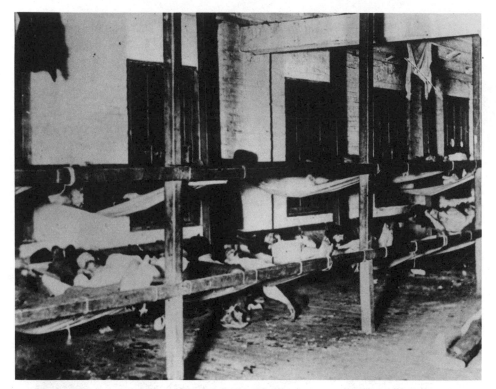

Figure 1.8. Interior, seven-cents-a-night lodging house in New York City. Jacob A. Riis Collection, Museum of the City of New York.

wart policemen who shovel up the eatables — musty bread, decayed fish and stale vegetables — indifferent to the curses that are showered on them from stoops and windows, and carry them off to the dump. In the wake of the wagon, as it makes its way to the East River after the raid, follow a line of despoiled hucksters shouting defiance from a safe distance.[60]

In the event of a "real" public health emergency, such as an epidemic, the orders of the Health Department doctors frequently came down with resounding force on the lives of the Russian Jews in the Lower East Side. For example, if a contagious disease was thought to be brewing in a lodging house for transient immigrants, the Health Department entered the home and evicted its lodgers. Unfortunately, few of these people had the means or support to find other lodging quickly and often found themselves temporarily homeless after a public health raid.

If a public health officer believed that an immigrant pushcart peddler was somehow violating the sanitary code of the city of New York, he had the power to destroy not only the goods on the pushcart but also the cart itself.

When one considers that this type of peddling was the slender financial support system of many immigrant families, one can understand the severe consequences of such an action. Similarly, kosher butchers and East European Jewish-run restaurants were favorite targets of the sanitary police and were not only closed during public health emergencies but were also frequently destroyed or burned down, preventing their reopening after the emergency had passed.

Lodgers or residents of private homes and tenement apartments discovered to have a contagious disease were escorted out of their homes by an armed sanitary policeman and taken to one of the city's public contagious disease hospitals. The public perception among most people of Gilded Age New York, across lines of class and ethnicity, was that those who were taken away to "public" hospitals were not likely to return home alive.[61]

Common among the experiences at a city quarantine island were harsh treatment, poor nutrition, inadequate facilities and health care, and, for some, death. The quarantine islands were well known and discussed among immigrant circles in New York. They were commonly described as places to avoid at all costs. For example, Dr. George Price recalled the "long routine under quarantine" he endured shortly after his arrival in the United States in 1882 before being set free and allowed "to breathe the air of the great republic." During a typhus fever epidemic that year, he and about five hundred immigrants were confined at Wards Island. The immigrants were isolated in a barracks building with cots arranged 125 to a row in four rows. Adding to the gross overcrowding was insensitive treatment at the hands of the assimilated East European Jewish immigrants hired by the Health Department to watch over the immigrants on the island:

> The Father, or manager and taskmaster over the immigrants, was an American Jew who looked down upon the earthly beings, as the immigrants were called and not in a friendly tone. His assistant, the Hungarian Jew, was a brazen scoundrel and treated the immigrants like cattle. The other Russian Jews, who through flattery managed to secure soft jobs, imitated them in behavior. The food fed to the immigrants was poor and spoiled. The fault was most probably the Father's who considered it more important to stuff his pockets than to care for the well-being of the victims entrusted to his charge. . . . [Meals consisted of] a sort of half-baked bread . . . a sort of liquid in which very often, instead of grains of cereal, there floated worms, and finally a slice of smelly meat. On holidays they added a plate of some sort of fruit dish, which they called *tzimes* [pudding] of a somewhat suspicious quality. . . . But the moral suffering from the stern and humiliating treatment of the officials was even worse than the material and physical privations. . . . After the exodus from Russia . . . they were suddenly exiled on an island, where they were confined in a prison and were treated like criminals.[62]

Another penalty for being associated with a contagious disease was the Health Department's publication of the names of the afflicted and their families, upon discovery. These families were subsequently stigmatized by prospective employers, neighbors, and others for long periods after the emergency passed. All of these public health measures, from mere harassment to physical removal, must have seemed to the Jewish immigrants uncomfortably reminiscent of their lives in the Pale of Settlement.

The Yiddish American *Arbeiter Zeitung* discussed the treatment received by East European Jewish immigrants at the whim of the Health Department and accused it of using public health issues as a veil for anti-Semitism. In a pointed editorial published in the early fall of 1892, the newspaper chastised the Health Department for showing concern over the abject poverty, unsanitary living conditions, and social problems of the poor *only* when epidemics threatened to "creep into the palaces of the rich. . . . Once everything passes over, the wealthy people's social awareness of such problems becomes dormant and it isn't until another extraordinary danger arises that fear and panic awaken the senses of the bourgeoisie again." [63]

Relations between New York's immigrant communities and uniformed New York City policemen, regardless of their assignment, were markedly worse than with the physicians working for the Health Department. The journalist Lincoln Steffens, recalling his police reporter days in New York in the early 1890s, detailed the activities of one typical New York cop referred to as "Clubber" Williams. Williams earned this sobriquet because of his habit of using a billy club to beat poor Jewish and Italian immigrants as retribution for petty crimes such as public assemblies or striking without a permit:

> The door opened, showed a row of bandaged Jews sitting against the wall in the inspector's office, and at his desk, Clubber Williams. "See the others. There's a strike on the East Side, and there are always clubbed strikers here in this office. I'll tell you what to do while you are learning our ways up here; you hang around this office every morning, watch the broken heads brought in, and as the prisoners are discharged, ask them for their stories. No paper will print them, but you yourself might as well see and hear how strikes are broken by the police." . . . Many a morning when I had nothing else to do I stood and saw the police bring in and kick out their bandaged, bloody prisoners, not only strikers and foreigners, but thieves, too, and others of the miserable, friendless, troublesome poor.[64]

Issues of control, violation of civil liberties, and the assumption that the Lower East Side immigrants were unlawful or diseased, combined with vast differences in cultural viewpoints, language, class, and experience, created an ambivalent relationship under the calmest of times between the municipal authorities and the immigrant communities of New York City. When tested by the stressors of a public health emergency, that relationship was frequently one of heated contention. Not surprisingly, when the Health Department swept a neighborhood looking for the contagious, a common response of the immigrants was simply to hide until the crisis, and the sanitary police, passed. In the event that a fugitive immigrant might actually harbor a contagious disease, the public health of the community was obviously compromised.

This, then, was the environment in which the *Massilia* Jews found themselves in early February 1892. After their landing, the United Hebrew Charities placed the 268 passengers in eight boarding houses located at 42 East Twelfth, 5 Essex, 49 Pike, 85 Monroe, 46 Delancey, 31 Monroe, 84 Norfolk, and 166 Division Streets—tenements scattered about the Jewish Quarter. Having settled in their temporary lodging homes on February 1, 1892, however, the *Massilia* Jews soon became the source of great panic across New York City and, indeed, throughout the nation.

CHAPTER 2

The City Responds to the Threat of Typhus

The Chief Inspector

By early 1892, thirty-five-year-old Cyrus Edson was an important figure in the New York City Health Department hierarchy. His position as chief inspector of contagious diseases, the largest division of the department, placed him in a subordinate position only to the sanitary superintendent W. A. Ewing (whose job Edson would occupy in a matter of months) and the commissioner of the board of health, the distinguished surgeon and physician Joseph D. Bryant. Edson's success at the Health Department was the result of sound family connections and political savvy combined with hard work as a public health physician.[1]

A tall man with a finely manicured beard and military bearing, Edson was a direct descendant of Roger Williams, the founder of Rhode Island, on his mother's side, and early settlers of the Massachusetts Bay Colony on his father's side. Young Cyrus was educated at the Albany and Throgs Neck Military Academies in New York, followed by travel to Europe and studies at Columbia College. He was also a star member of the Columbia varsity crew team that won the championship at Henley on the Thames in 1878. Edson subsequently entered medical school at the College of Physicians and Surgeons in New York, graduating in 1882.

In the spring of 1882, Edson's father, Franklin, strongly encouraged the newly minted medical doctor to accept his first professional post as a temporary summer sanitary inspector for the New York City Health Department. Not insignificantly, Franklin Edson was then mayor of New York City. The summer of 1882 was notable for a severe epidemic of smallpox. During those months Cyrus Edson worked assiduously to enact the rapid quarantine of New Yorkers infected with smallpox and the widespread vaccination of those who were susceptible. He participated in the exciting work of searching for and finding possible smallpox patients throughout the city, risking his own life, to the great acclaim of his superiors.

Edson was given a permanent position with the Health Department in the fall of 1882 on the recommendation of a health board commissioner appointed by his father. He rose steadily over the next ten years in a variety of positions, ranging from assistant sanitary inspector to food inspector, and, in 1892, to chief sanitary inspector. Edson impressed his colleagues with an astute ability to diagnose contagious diseases accurately based almost entirely upon a physical examination and observations.

Diagnosing contagious diseases in an era before culture methodology was routinely used to confirm or to deny their presence was no small matter. For example, when a physician today is entertaining the diagnosis of a bacterial infection such as cholera, he or she will obtain a stool sample from the patient and place it on a special agar-nutrient plate for culture and growth. Within forty-eight hours, if the patient is ill with cholera, the stool sample culture should reveal, upon microscopic or biochemical examination, recognizable colonies or clusters of the disease's causative organism. Depending on the bacterial disease in question and the type of human tissue an organism tends to attack, cultures of different body fluids or tissue samples help physicians determine with relative certainty what type of bacteria is infecting the patient.

Instead of a binary, deterministic "yes or no" question that is answered, or at least perceived to be answered, by current bacteriological culture methods, the diagnostician of the 1890s had to rely on empiric observations and broad experience. What did the patient look like? What was the exact symptom pattern? What was the extent and severity of the patient's fever and at what time of the day was the fever the highest? Were there any rashes associated with the fever? How did the disease appear to spread to others? These and similar "clinical" questions were essential to ask and to answer if one were to diagnose an infectious disease with any amount of confidence.[2]

Edson's abilities as a diagnostician of infectious diseases were so highly regarded because this branch of clinical medicine was still a difficult and poorly understood enterprise in New York during the early 1890s. Formal instruction on contagious diseases was rarely taught in the hospital wards to training physicians in medical schools, ironically, because of a lack of clinical material. Most of the major teaching hospitals in New York City, such as New York, Mount Sinai, Presbyterian, and Bellevue Hospitals, tended not to admit patients with contagious diseases if they could possibly avoid it. Instead, these patients were typically sent to the city's contagious disease hospitals that were operated by the Health Department. This was not a form of negligence but, instead, a means of controlling the potential spread of infection among the other hospitalized patients. In the event that these hospitals did admit patients with contagious diseases, the patients frequently died or were quickly removed to one of the contagious disease facilities, again as a means of disease containment, before budding student doctors had a chance to analyze and to examine the cases firsthand.

At one 1893 meeting of the New York Academy of Medicine, several promi-

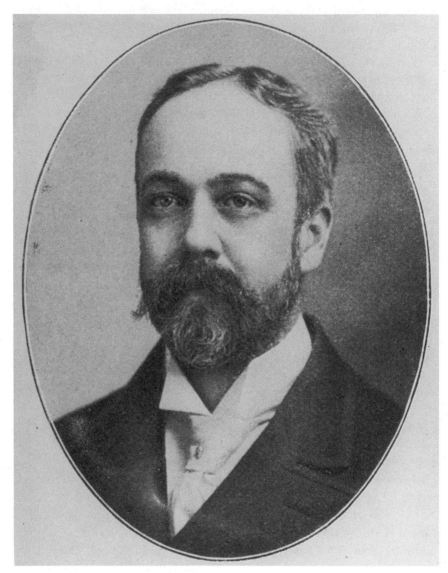

Figure 2.1. Cyrus Edson, M.D., circa 1896. From King's *Notable New Yorkers of 1896–1899.*

nent New York physicians, including Edson, lamented the dearth of clinical teaching on contagious diseases at New York City medical schools and hospitals. The New York physician and editor of the *Medical Record,* George Shrady, recalled that as a young practitioner with an excellent medical education he had so little experience in this branch of medicine that he could not recognize an early case of the measles, let alone cholera or typhus.[3]

Equally important to Edson's résumé and success as a New York City public health official was his active membership in the Society of Tammany and New York City Democratic Committee. Tammany Hall, under the iron-clad rule of Boss Richard Croker, controlled almost every aspect of New York City municipal government during this period, including its Health Department. Nominally employed as the mayor of New York City between 1888 and 1892, the Honorable Hugh Grant essentially did what Croker told him to do.[4]

Edson was both a prominent member of Tammany's twenty-fourth Assembly district and a long-time friend of many of those who were in a position to execute the patronage politics that was the trademark of Tammany Hall. Indeed, one example of Edson's political machinations was the promotion he sought and received shortly after the typhus fever epidemic. In June 1892, Edson was named the sanitary superintendent of the Health Department, a job similar in importance to that of managing editor of a newspaper or managing partner of a law firm. Unfortunately, Edson was promoted at the expense of the man who had already held that job with distinction for three years, Dr. W. A. Ewing. The obvious political maneuvering by health board president Charles G. Wilson (a Tammany appointee and friend of Cyrus's father, Franklin), Boss Richard Croker, and Mayor Hugh Grant in promoting Edson at another's expense was met with great hostility by the New York medical community. Three ex officio health board members, the well-respected New York physicians Abraham Jacobi, T. Mitchell Prudden, and E. G. Janeway, resigned from their honorary advisory posts with a mixture of outrage and disgust at Edson's appointment.[5]

The bulk of Cyrus Edson's professional responsibilities as chief inspector of contagious diseases was directed at the immigrant and impoverished populations of New York City. Edson made frequent rounds through the slums and immigrant quarters of New York City in order to ferret out disease. His office was situated on Mott Street, around the corner from the Police Department and "between the tabernacles of Jewry and the Shrines of the Bend."[6] The well-bred, patrician Dr. Edson was a striking contrast to the foreign-born, urban poor.

Just how disparate Edson's background, upbringing, and cultural values were from a major percentage of his patient population may be best documented by reviewing his published writings and interviews on the subjects of immigrants and immigrant health conditions. For example, in 1891 he referred to the inhabitants of countries where leprosy was still prevalent as "the shiftless, lazy and ignorant who live upon unwholesome food and who habitually violate moral and sanitary laws."[7]

The following year, while commenting on the typhus fever epidemic for the prominent monthly *North American Review,* Edson espoused a commitment to immigration restriction on the basis of safeguarding American public health: " 'Near is my coat, but nearer is my skin' runs the Spanish proverb, and while it may be our duty to welcome the oppressed, it is certainly true that our first duty is to our own people and our own homes . . . for with disease as an immigrant, it is true that forewarned is forearmed in this day and generation."[8] In the same article, Edson provides evidence that he used class lines to draw the boundaries of the typhus quarantine: "Respectable New Yorkers" exposed to typhus fever were allowed to remain at home, provided they underwent frequent medical examinations. The *Massilia* Jews and the urban poor who lived in cheap lodging houses, "taking their rooms by the night, here to-day, and there tomorrow," on the other hand, demanded an immediate quarantine.[9]

Most offensive to the East European Jewish, Italian, and other immigrant communities of New York City, however, were Edson's disparaging comments about their collective character in the New York press. For example, in a lengthy article Edson penned for the *New York Herald* in mid-March on the 1892 typhus epidemic, he described the "Russian Hebrews" as "phlegmatic, dull and stupid," a group so docile, oppressed, and "ground down" for generations that even the delirium of typhus fever failed to elicit an active response from them.[10] One offended Russian Jewish immigrant sarcastically rebuked Edson's comments on the pages of the *Yiddische Tageblatt:* "I did not know that a doctor of medicine can have such a deep outlook and an expansive soul. Every word of Edson's report is a slap in the face of our civilization and if Europe would be a cheek of that face, she would become wholly red from shame."[11]

Months later, as Edson heartily accepted the front-page congratulations of the *New York Times* for averting the typhus epidemic, the sanitary inspector delivered an even harsher indictment of the city's Italian and Jewish residents:

> Anybody who has ever tried to find out even the simplest things from the Italian or Jewish residents of the tenement districts can appreciate the difficulty of this work before the health department. They are sullen and suspicious and refuse all information asked by Americans on general principles. But when it comes to a question of disease, they will hide in closets, burrow in cellars, run away, do anything to avoid the visit of a physician and lie with the most magnificent elaboration as to all matters touching their own sickness or those of their neighbors. They throw every possible obstacle in the way of the Board of Health in its regu-

lar rounds of the inspection of the tenements where they live, and in the typhus emergency they followed out all their traditions.[12]

Like many of his contemporaries charged with providing medical care for New York's immigrants, Edson clearly displayed what historian Charles Rosenberg has called "a mixture of contempt and sympathy for the working poor."[13] But there was far more to Edson's contempt for the urban poor than the mere rude treatment of an immigrant patient at a free dispensary or the occasional racial slur in the press. As sanitary inspector, Edson could not only form and shape public health policy; he could enforce it without the interference of others.

New York City's Health Department had evolved into an extremely powerful and independent municipal department following its major restructuring with the 1866 Metropolitan Health Bill.[14] By 1892, it was a body with both executive and legislative powers. In other words, the Health Department had the power to enforce the sanitary code it created and, through a system of sanitary inspections, to impose fines for violations or health nuisances. The Health Department could also order the imprisonment of recalcitrant offenders and was backed up by its own police corps, the sanitary police, who had all the authority of the regular police squad but were assigned to the Health Department.

With the broad responsibilities of a mission that defined a public health nuisance as "anything that interferes with the proper enjoyment of man's health," the department inspected plumbing, faulty building construction, ventilation, living conditions, food, water supplies, restaurants, meat-handlers, and other potential hazards. Edson's Division of Contagious Diseases was responsible for all issues pertaining to the propagation of epidemic diseases. In such a capacity, the chief inspector conducted investigations on reports of contagious diseases in the city made by physicians or keepers of boarding houses and lodging houses. In addition, the division supervised the city's vaccination and ambulance corps.[15]

Cyrus Edson summarized his absolute power as chief sanitary inspector of New York City when he confidently declared to the U.S. Congress Joint Committee on Immigration that "if we see fit, we may take possession of the City Hall forcibly and turn it into a contagious disease hospital if in our opinion it is necessary to do so."[16] This authority, especially in the power of forcible removal and quarantine, combined with a less than tolerant attitude toward the immigrant community, proved to be a double-sided means of public health enforcement during the typhus epidemic. One side was success in terms of the isolation and confinement of typhus cases; the other was the huge personal trauma and travail of the *Massilia* passengers.

The Dragnet

Cyrus Edson began his day on February 11, 1892, as he began most workday mornings. After a hot breakfast prepared by his wife Mary at their town-house at 54 West Ninth Street, a phaeton drawn by two horses took him to his office downtown at 301 Mott Street. Edson's first course of official business, on behalf of the New York City Health Department, was to review the incoming correspondence pertaining to possible epidemic diseases brewing in the city. As required by municipal law, practicing physicians reported all persons to the chief inspector's office suspected of being ill with cholera, yellow fever, smallpox, diphtheria, typhus, typhoid fever, spotted fever, re-lapsing fever, scarlet fever, measles, and "any new disease of an infectious, contagious, or pestilential nature, and also any other disease publicly de-clared by this Board dangerous to the public health." [17]

In early 1892, there were three principal means of contacting Chief Inspec-tor Edson: telephone, telegraph, or postal card. Telegrams from practicing physicians were typically reserved for the most urgent situations whereas private telephones were still limited to the most wealthy practitioners. Post-cards were most often used, and on the morning of February 11, Edson found four of them on his desk from a Dr. Leo Dann of the United Hebrew Charities reporting several cases of typhoid fever in the same house, 42 East Twelfth Street.

An outbreak of typhoid fever limited to one house was an "exceedingly unusual fact," Edson later remarked to the New York press corps. Attribut-ing the possible spread to the "filthy living conditions" common along the Lower East Side, Edson called his best sanitary inspectors into his office and made the necessary assignments to investigate what had the potential to be-come a severe typhoid fever epidemic.

The team of physicians, inspectors, and sanitary policemen rushed to the scene in the black Health Department ambulances. Waiting on the steps of the tenement boarding house on East Twelfth Street was Dr. Leo Dann. The United Hebrew Charities physician explained to the Health Department offi-cials that the tenement house catered to newly arrived or transient Russian Jews and received a fee of forty-five cents per boarder per day for food and lodging from the United Hebrew Charities. Although the accommodations were far from plush, they were inspected daily by United Hebrew Charities agents for cleanliness.[18]

Dann was a Jewish physician practicing on the Lower East Side who, like many of his contemporaries, supplemented his income with contract work for Jewish benevolent or cooperative organizations such as the United Hebrew Charities. The general practitioner explained to Edson that he was called to the boarding house in question on Monday, February 8.[19] That night, Dann became particularly concerned about Henoch Griner, a twenty-year-old locksmith who complained of severe stomach pain and a fever of 105°F. Although Dann was unsure of the exact diagnosis, he worried that Griner's condition was "far more serious than the mere grippe." This concern was substantiated by Dr. Dann's documentation of similar symptoms among Henoch's five brothers, Binzivn (age 24), Rubin (age 22), Leon (age 18), Solomon (age 12), and Moses (age 6), as well as three other residents in the boarding house, Abram (age 20), David (age 18), and Samuel Dikar (age 11). When Dann returned to the boarding house on Wednesday the tenth, he was struck by the worsening condition of the nine original patients; they now exhibited a "curious red rash" all over their bodies. Dann noted similar symptoms of fevers, aches, and malaise among eleven other boarders, all of whom had close contact with the Griner and the Dikar families. It was at this point that Dr. Leo Dann notified the Health Department.[20]

Dr. Edson and his associates, Drs. Charles Roberts and Fred Dillingham, entered the boarding house over the fearful protests of its owner, Abram Jaffe. The three physicians began their inspection by checking for faulty plumbing and sources of food or water contamination that might explain an outbreak of typhoid fever. They found none. The house was judged to be fairly clean and in "surprisingly good order" for an "immigrant boarding house." When the physicians began examining the residents of the boarding house, a very different picture emerged. In one room alone, Edson reported finding fifteen immigrants prostrate with high fevers, delirium, excruciating headaches, pains, and the tell-tale mulberry rash of typhus, rather than typhoid, fever.[21] This was not a lightly made diagnosis; typhus fever was regarded in 1892 as "one of the most highly contagious of febrile affections."[22]

The celebrated German bacteriologist Robert Koch, when discussing the control of cholera almost a decade earlier, warned that sound public health regulations required "the most firmly grounded scientific foundation." This foundation, rooted in Koch's four postulates of germ theory, was difficult to apply to typhus fever because of the lack of clear evidence of a specific etiologic agent.[23] Plainly put, typhus fever was difficult to diagnose and even more difficult to trace from victim to victim since no one had a clear understanding of the disease's transmission.

For example, it is not surprising that Dr. Leo Dann had trouble distinguishing typhus from typhoid fever in the early cases he examined. As Dr. William Osler, physician-in-chief of the Johns Hopkins Hospital noted, "It is easy to put down on paper elaborate differential distinctions [between typhus and typhoid] which are practically useless at the bedside, particularly when the disease is not prevailing as an epidemic."[24]

An early case of typhus, even with the appearance of a rash, was easily confused with those rashes seen with typhoid fever, measles, and other infections that cause purpuric, petechial, or ecchymotic (bruise-like) lesions. It was not until a number of similar cases began to appear that the clinical picture became clearer and confidently diagnosed by late-nineteenth-century physicians. This, of course, was typically done after those most infectious had contact with other susceptible persons and the potential for an epidemic had already developed. More commonly than not, physicians with less than adequate training in the diagnosis of infectious diseases, or a hesitancy to diagnose such a malady, responded to typhus fever epidemics a step or two behind the marching organism.

Typhus fever's uncertain etiology also hindered the elaboration of public health safeguards against the 1892 typhus epidemic. The impulse for aggressive quarantine is, of course, greatest for those contagious diseases whose terms of transmission remain poorly understood. Any and all precautions against its spread seem reasonable during such crises. In 1890, for example, the journalist and champion of the urban poor, Jacob Riis, offered a theory of the transmission of typhus in a chapter of *How the Other Half Lives* entitled "Jewtown." Typhus fever epidemics in New York City, in Riis's estimation, almost always seemed to proliferate among the Jews of the Lower East Side through the common vector of clothing made in the Jewish sweatshops:

> It has happened more than once . . . that a typhus fever patient has been discovered in a room whence perhaps a hundred coats had been sent home that week, each one with the wearer's death warrant, unseen and unsuspected, basted in the lining.[25]

Chief Sanitary Inspector Cyrus Edson, on the other hand, elaborated a far more complicated theory of the etiology of typhus during the spring of 1892 that in a few paragraphs summarizes the history of ideas concerning contagion. Edson's explanation of the cause of typhus included elements of miasma, zymotic, ventilation, spontaneous generation, and germ theories:

> The typhus cases could have risen under the conditions such as existed on that ship; where the hatches have been battened down and the people were overcrowded and the conditions have been filthy, and they have breathed impure air for a certain length of time and had food which was not of a proper character to nourish them; these conditions would tend to breed typhus *de novo*.[26]

In almost the same breath, Edson further declared that typhus probably requires "the presence of a distinct poisonous germ" but in the case of a large number of "filthy persons," poisons emanate "and change chemically until they become exceedingly poisonous to other human beings."[27] Edson concluded that he "did not bother his brain" on whether typhus had developed de novo during the immigrants' ocean voyage or by other means. Instead, his focus—and that of the New York City Health Department—was on the fact that "all the cases have occurred among the Jewish people."[28]

It was not until 1909 that Charles Nicolle of the Institut Pasteur in Tunis demonstrated that the human body louse was the vector of typhus fever. The following year, American microbiologist Howard Taylor Ricketts described a new form of bacteria in the blood of typhus patients as well as the feces of infected body lice. Although Ricketts died (ironically of typhus fever) before he could confirm these findings, Henrique da Roche Lima of Brazil demonstrated the same organism in 1916. Da Roche Lima named it *Rickettsia prowazekii,* commemorating both the work of Howard Ricketts and Bohemian protozoologist Stanislaus Prowazek, who also succumbed to typhus in the line of scientific duty.[29]

A word or two of medical explanation is warranted. Physicians and epidemiologists refer to a disease transmitted between animals and humans as a zoonosis. The intermediary in the pathological relationship between humans and the germ that causes typhus fever, *Rickettsia prowazekii,* is the human body louse. People who live in impoverished, overcrowded conditions with no change of clothing and little access to soap, water, and other means of personal hygiene are at risk of becoming infected with the body louse, *Pediculus humanis corporis.* This parasite causes an especially contagious skin infestation and spends its entire life cycle in the clothing of the human victim. Four to six times a day, the body louse bites the human host in order to consume its only food, human blood. The louse also spends a good deal of its time reproducing and laying its eggs in the seams of the host's garments; underwear is a particularly favored spot. When the lice are infected with the typhus fever germ, what under normal circumstances is an annoying skin rash becomes the multiplier of a deadly epidemic. As the body louse ingests the human host's blood, it deposits fecal material loaded with rickettsia. The human host typically scratches the itchy feeding site of the louse and the rickettsial-laden feces find their way into the human bloodstream. The results are the clinical manifestations and high fever of typhus. Body lice leave human bodies that are feverish or dead in search of new hosts to infest, which increases the spread of typhus fever.

In 1892, of course, none of this epidemiologic evidence had yet been uncovered, despite Riis's fascinating "sweatshop transmission" theory. The threat of a disease that appeared out of nowhere and could spread rapidly justified, to many New Yorkers, the massive quarantine efforts and other strong-arm tactics directed at the Russian Jewish immigrants that winter.

Consequently, Cyrus Edson was required to act, and act quickly, if he had any chance of containing a potentially devastating epidemic to as small an area and to as few New Yorkers as possible. Not knowing the exact source of typhus or even how it might have spread within the city certainly placed Edson and his staff at a distinct disadvantage. This epidemic, Edson admitted to a reporter for the *New York Sun,* was "the worst outbreak of a contagious disease that we have had in New York for many years. I would rather handle four times as many cases of small-pox. Typhus is malignant and very contagious." The tenor of urgency was increased when a representative of Henry Rice, the president of the United Hebrew Charities of New York, informed Edson that the boarders of the Twelfth Street tenement house and several other lodging houses on the Lower East Side were all Russian Jewish passengers from one ship: the SS *Massilia.*[30]

The epidemiological convenience of the situation is difficult to deny: one dreaded disease, one social scapegoat, one neighborhood, even one ship that brought the "vectors of disease" from the Old World to the New. And while there were no official proclamations of anti-Semitism emanating from the Health Department offices, their strategies and actions differed decidedly when dealing with someone within this particular circle of disease causation.

Edson ordered an immediate dragnet of the boarding homes listed by the United Hebrew Charities in order to find "every single Russian Jewish passenger of the *Massilia.*" His staff of eighteen physicians then set out to inspect every resident of every boarding house, accompanied by armed, uniformed sanitary policemen and ambulances waiting at the curbside to escort the afflicted away. A contemporary account of the scene, as recorded in Joseph Pulitzer's *New York World,* captures the intensity of social upheaval and the fear of disease:

> [The health inspectors, accompanied by a Yiddish-speaking agent of the United Hebrew Charities,] climbed the rickety steps of the houses, penetrated the stifling rooms, questioned in their own rasping patois men toiling over sewing machines, women stitching to keep body and soul together and black-eyed children even; critically examined everybody and with the most peculiar care those whom they found abed; carried away women while their husbands tore their hair and their children wept in frightened ignorance. It was a dreadful task, for all of the patients were ignorant and already cowed by oppression. They were being hurried to execution for all they knew.[31]

The roundup of the Russian Jews extended beyond the United Hebrew Charities boarding houses to other areas the *Massilia* Jews were reported to have frequented. These included the nearby "pig market" on Hester near Ludlow where, ironically, "everything but pig could be bought off pushcarts . . . and where greenhorns would bunch up in the morning to wait for employers looking for cheap labor."[32] The inspectors proceeded to synagogues,

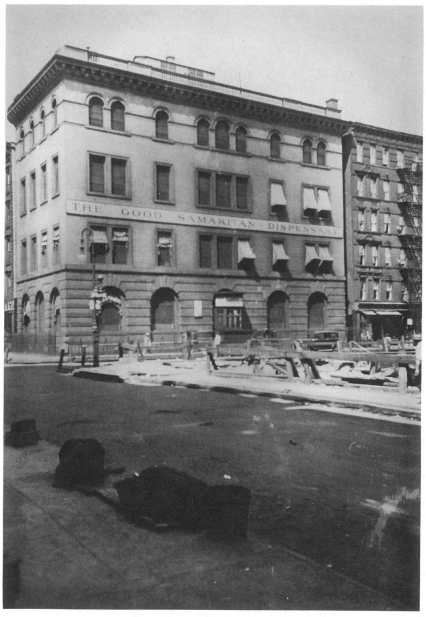

Figure 2.2. The Good Samaritan Dispensary on Essex and Broome Streets, undated. Courtesy United States History, Local History, and Genealogy Division, the New York Public Library, Astor, Lenox, and Tilden Foundations.

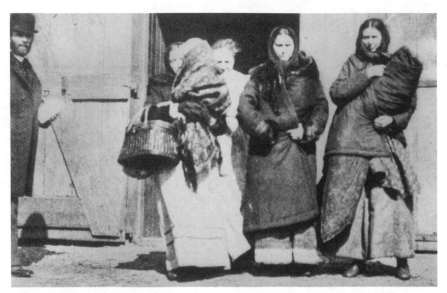

Figure 2.3. Patients from the quarantined SS *Massilia* being turned over to the receiving hospital. *Frank Leslie's Illustrated Weekly* 74 (1892).

restaurants, and even public steam bathhouses, or *shvitzes*.[33] At the Good Samaritan Dispensary on Broome and Essex Streets, two Russian Jewish children were diagnosed with typhus fever by the pediatrician and soon-to-be describer of the pathognomonic sign for measles, Henry Koplik.[34] Although the two children were immediately removed to the city's quarantine hospital on North Brother Island, the front page of the *New York Sun* worried about the Good Samaritan Dispensary as a potential source of typhus fever since it was not known how many people the children had come in contact with.[35]

The *Arbeiter Zeitung* recorded the events during the typhus dragnet as an incarnation of the immigrant's worst nightmare:

> The sick alone were crazed with fever and made terrible noises and crazed movements. Their relatives and parents, also green Jews, alas who didn't understand what was going on here, made alarming screams and outcries as if their children and relatives were being taken to the slaughterhouse.[36]

The typhus fever victims in the Twelfth Street boarding house were immediately removed to the contagious disease lazaretto. Just as important to the quarantine process, however, was the isolation and subsequent removal of the many more healthy *Massilia* passengers and their contacts who might yet come down with typhus fever. These Russian Jewish immigrants, too, were forcibly removed from their various boarding houses and consolidated under "rigid quarantine" at 42 East Twelfth Street and 5 Essex Street, which were the largest of the eight "typhus houses" under the guard of the New York City sanitary police.

The Italian passengers of the *Massilia* were more difficult to track down since most had dispersed widely, beyond the metropolitan New York City area. A few Italian passengers were quarantined in the coming weeks for possible typhus fever in locales such as Trenton, New Jersey; Baltimore, Maryland; Kinderhook and Newburgh, New York, but there were not many actual cases of disease among them. For example, two Italian immigrants who traveled on the *Massilia* were rounded up by health officials in Trenton, New Jersey, and delivered in a cattle car to Edson's office in New York on the evening of February 16. Edson was outraged by the "criminal behavior" of the Trenton authorities, but placed the two Italian men under temporary quarantine in the ambulance stables for the night. They were found to be healthy and were released the following day. Representatives of the Febre line insisted the next day that the Italian passengers were not as great a health risk since "they had little contact with the Jewish passengers aboard the *Massilia*."[37]

The *Massilia* Jews, however, were forced to wait, for the eventual fact, as Dr. Cyrus Edson explained to the press, that all of those quarantined would

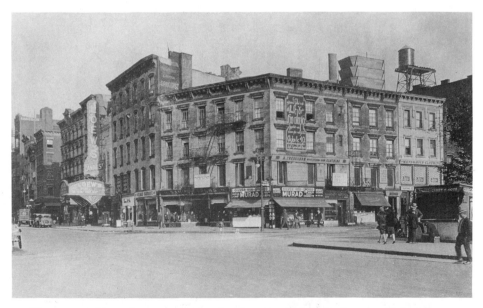

Figure 2.4. 5 Essex Street, late 1920s (*rowhouse at far right*). Courtesy United States History, Local History, and Genealogy Division, the New York Public Library, Astor, Lenox, and Tilden Foundations.

inevitably become infected with typhus fever. As Edson telegraphed Surgeon General Walter Wyman on February 17, "All exposed Hebrews [have been] rigidly quarantined."[38] Indeed, so many of the Russian Jews quarantined at the Essex and Twelfth Streets lodging houses developed typhus over the next weeks, that by February 23 Edson ordered still another consolidation of the *Massilia* passengers to the Essex Street house in order to contain the epidemic among that group.[39]

Using a similar public health strategy, Edson ordered the mass inspection of all "cheap lodging houses" on the Lower East Side and the Bowery that were frequented by impoverished Russian Jewish immigrants. These transients paid between seven and ten cents a night to sleep in a filthy barracks with hammocks stretched across two tiers of wood. The sanitary police hunted through over 125 lodging houses in their dragnet. The lodgers were roused out of their sleep in the early morning hours and forced to undergo smallpox vaccinations and a cursory medical examination for evidence of typhus.[40] Suspicious lodgers were immediately removed to North Brother Island.

Despite the intensive efforts to contain the epidemic, new cases continued to appear not only among those quarantined at 5 Essex Street but also among some Russian Jewish boarders of the Phoenix Lodging House on the Bowery. There were also reports of inmates of the "quarantine house," especially children, breaking quarantine regulations by climbing out of the home's windows to walk about or to play in the streets. One child, a twelve-year-old Russian Jewish girl named Eva Chittel whose father owned one of the boarding houses that held the *Massilia* Jews, may have contributed unknowingly to the typhus fever epidemic in this manner.[41]

Not surprisingly, there were vigorous requests from neighbors of the Essex Street "typhus house" to remove the quarantined immigrants to another location. Even their healthy East European Jewish brethren wanted nothing to do with the "diseased" *Massilia* Jews. As February drew to a close, Edson realized his strategy was not doing enough to stem the tide of the typhus epidemic. The knot of public health control was tightened once again when Edson declared on February 28 that every "Russian Hebrew" passenger of the *Massilia* and all of their contacts should be considered to have typhus fever. Shortly after this declaration, Edson ordered all of the healthy contacts to be forcibly evacuated to the lazaretto, Riverside Hospital, on North Brother Island.[42]

The recently arrived émigrés had been stigmatized on many levels over the preceding year. They were initially separated in the Pale of Settlement by their religious beliefs, the Czarist anti-Semitic edicts, persecution, and famine. Following their expulsion from Russia and the nomadic trek across the

Atlantic, the layers of separation only increased for these travelers upon their arrival in the land of "Kolumbus."[43] Socially isolated in the Jewish ghetto and now targeted as importers of a deadly epidemic, they were dragged out of their homes in the middle of the winter by the sanitary police and subsequently isolated on an island far away from their only link to the New World—their Yiddish-speaking co-religionists. Their fate was that of quarantine, physically, spiritually, and emotionally. And as the preceding scenario suggests, the level of distress among the quarantined Jews as they were, quite literally, sent up the river was intense.

The Lazaretto

Five miles up the East River, approximately 1,500 feet east of 140th Street in the South Bronx and, on a bad day, downwind from the city's garbage dump at Riker's Island, was the city lazaretto, Riverside Hospital on North Brother Island. Even a century later, when one stands on the rocky shoals of the island, peering into the distance, the city seems remote and inaccessible. The sense of loneliness on North Brother Island is almost palpable.

The site had been used as a small hospital for the poor afflicted with contagious diseases since the 1850s when it was operated by the Sisters of Charity Hall. The 16.5-acre island was incorporated into the city of New York in 1880 as a solution to the overcrowded city hospital on Blackwell Island and as a means of "isolating and treating those with contagious diseases."[44]

Administered by the board of health, the Riverside and Willard Parker Hospitals (adjoining Reception Hospital at East Sixteenth Street) comprised the contagious disease in-patient service of the New York City Health Department. Its board of directors consisted of prominent New York City physicians appointed by the commissioner of the board of health, Dr. Joseph D. Bryant. These physicians met monthly to discuss administrative and medical issues in addition to individually serving as attending physicians and instructors, on a rotating basis, for the interns and residents assigned to the hospitals.[45]

In its long career as an agent of quarantine, North Brother Island deserves mention as the enforced residence of New York City cook Mary Mallon, best known to medical historians as "Typhoid Mary." Typhoid Mary was responsible for infecting numerous people over the years with *Salmonella typhosa*, the causative organism of typhoid fever. She also helped physicians begin to understand the concept of carrier status, whereby seemingly healthy people can spread typhoid fever because they harbor the disease-producing bacilli in their bodies without apparent harm to themselves.

Tracked down by the New York City Health Department in 1907 and

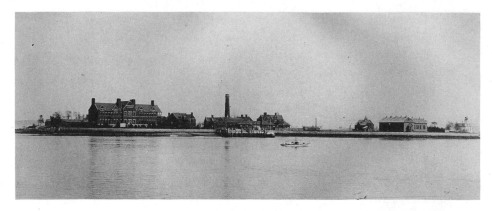

Figure 2.5. Riverside Hospital, North Brother Island, New York City, undated, probably after 1920. Collection of the New-York Historical Society.

forcibly removed from her home, Mary Mallon was discovered to be "crawling with typhoid bugs." She was given an ultimatum by the Health Department physicians: Submit to an operation to remove her gall bladder (the site where carriers harbor the germ of typhoid fever) or be imprisoned at the lazaretto. She refused the then risky and not always successful surgical procedure and was removed to Riverside Hospital for three years. Mallon was released in 1910 after a lengthy court battle. Typhoid Mary, of course, continued to ply her trade and spread typhoid fever. The cook and infamous vector of disease was again hunted down by the Health Department. She was returned to North Brother Island in 1915 and there she remained, in her own small frame house on the island, until her death in 1938.[46]

In 1892 Riverside Hospital on North Brother Island was just as undesirable a place to be sent as it would be for "Typhoid Mary" in the early twentieth century.[47] The facilities lacked space, financial resources, adequate medical equipment, and nursing personnel. As late as 1894 there were no telephone or telegraph lines connecting the remote island to the city, which could only be reached via ferry.[48]

The hospital's on-site medical staff consisted of two rotating resident physicians assigned to the lazaretto for four-and-a-half-month periods. Attending physicians with experience in practice and diagnosis rarely made visits to the island during their assigned month of duty. Training physicians assigned to Riverside frequently complained about the lack of instruction or therapeutic direction from the senior attending physicians, the paucity of ward rounds, an "epidemic of incomplete patient records," and the inhumane overcrowding of patients. Indeed, the risk of furthering the spread of a contagious disease at the lazaretto due to insufficient means of isolating the ill from the healthy was a common concern of many New York City physicians during the 1890s.[49]

Sanitary technique, at least that required to prevent the spread of contagious disease among the quarantined inmates, was rarely practiced at Riverside. For example, as late as 1902, instruments such as tongue depressors were in such short supply that they were not routinely cleaned or sterilized between use on individual patients. The lazaretto's facilities for personal hygiene were hardly better: Outhouse privies were rarely cleaned and the inmates had limited access to soap and running water unless they waded in the East River.

The chronic overcrowding of patients made contagious disease control on the island extremely difficult. Even during the periods when the hospital was not beset by an emergent epidemic, Riverside interns complained that the beds in the wooden, almost shack-like, pavilions were so close together that it was "difficult for the physicians to pass between them in the examination of patients."[50] Bed space was at such a premium during the 1892 epidemic that many patients were put up in tents. These flimsy forms of shelter against the New York winter were heated with wood-burning radiators precariously placed on wooden platforms that served as the tent's floor. Six of the tents erupted in flames on February 13 but, fortunately, no one was hurt.[51]

The loneliness experienced by resident physicians assigned to the remote lazaretto was an ongoing complaint and probably affected how they interacted with patients. Although the one-year appointment was considered a valuable stepping-stone in a young physician's successful career path in urban medicine during the 1890s, the glow of pleasure over the appointment soon wore off when strictly confined to Riverside Hospital for four and a half months followed by a similar stint at Willard Parker Hospital. Even the exciting city ambulance service that rounded out the internship year prevented any type of personal or social life for these predominantly young men.[52]

Also stationed full-time at the lazaretto were a matron of nurses, ten nurses, twelve ward helpers, one general helper, ten clerical orderlies, five kitchen staff workers, five maids or laundresses, and twelve nautical workers. Occasionally, by chance or design, one of the attendants spoke Yiddish, Italian, or another foreign language by virtue of his or her own immigrant roots.[53]

In short, a trip to the lazaretto was justly perceived as one to be avoided at all costs. The *Massilia* Jews and their contacts, of course, had no such option. The roundup had only one objective: the rigid isolation of the unfortunate immigrants. The scenes of removal were heartbreaking and filled with the anxious screams of fear, protectiveness, and fever-induced mania. If children were discovered to be ill with typhus, a healthy adult—almost

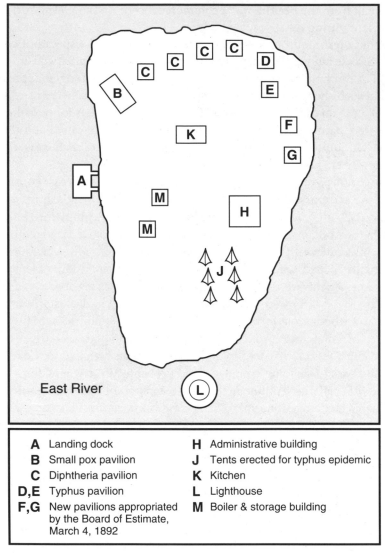

Figure 2.6. Diagram of Riverside Hospital, 1892. Adapted from the *New York Herald*, February 15, 1892.

exclusively the mother—was allowed to accompany them. These frightened immigrant mothers held on to their sick babies with fierce maternal governance and unknowingly placed themselves at high risk for developing typhus. Those less cooperative were exposed to more forceful methods. The sickest of the typhus victims were carried out of the United Hebrew Charities boarding homes immobilized in special rubber bags with a drawstring at the neck. Both the ill and those who had close contact with them were then driven at rapid speed, by the horse-driven, black-wagoned Health Department ambulances through the snow- and manure-covered streets of Lower Manhattan up to Willard Parker Hospital on East Sixteenth Street. At the time of the typhus epidemic, the weather in New York City became suddenly bitter cold, with temperatures in the teens and daily rain or snow storms, making the trip even more difficult.[54] From Willard Parker Hospital, the ill boarded the New York City Health Department tugboat, ironically named for Cyrus Edson's father Franklin. The tugboat then transported its "pestilential cargo" up the ice-cold East River to the quarantine island.

Between February 12 and April 1, 1892, about 1,200 people, mostly Russian Jews, were quarantined on North Brother Island. The overwhelming majority, about 1,150, were healthy people who had the bad luck to live near the original *Massilia* passengers who developed typhus. Edson's "wholesale removal of Russian Hebrew Refugees to North Brother Island" was announced to be in effect for a period of twenty-one days or "after the last case had developed among them," whichever came first.[55]

Such a huge demand of quarantine and medical care quickly exhausted the resources of the lazaretto and its staff. By February 16, only one week into the epidemic, the board of health had spent all of the financial resources it was allotted for epidemic control and applied for a special appropriation from the New York City boards of aldermen and estimate and apportionment. Board of health secretary Emmons Clark reported to the aldermen that "the number of the afflicted has been such as to fill up completely the present accommodations on the island."[56] The New York City municipal government begrudgingly agreed to appropriate $12,000 to erect new pavilions and to pay the salaries of two more doctors, fifteen nurses, fifteen helpers, six laundresses, and four orderlies. Ten extra physicians to complete the "house to house inspection of the Italian and Hebrew quarters" of New York City for contacts of the *Massilia* Jews were also budgeted.[57] Unfortunately, the improvements to be afforded by the appropriation were not completed in time to affect the care of the majority of those quarantined. The money was not made available to the Health Department until March 6, 1892; by that time, the epidemic appeared to be already on the wane.

CHAPTER 3

The Results of the Quarantine

The typhus epidemic was essentially conquered by the Health Department by April 1892. No new cases were being discovered on the Lower East Side by the Health Department's surveillance team. The quarantined East European Jews who recovered from typhus or did not develop it after three weeks of observation were released from North Brother Island throughout late March and early April.[1] By spring, life on the Lower East Side and uptown returned to its daily routines, inequities, and pleasures.

At the close of the 1892 typhus fever epidemic, scores of native-born Americans and institutions applauded the efforts of the New York City Health Department. The *New York Times,* for example, commended Cyrus Edson and the Health Department for "averting a pestilence" with "fearless promptitude of action, an efficient system of search and discovery in suspected places combined with the unsparing use of money to carry out the most approved modern ideas." According to the *New York Tribune,* it was "the isolation of all Jewish suspects and their stringent quarantine that was responsible for the success."[2] Similar laudatory remarks appeared in the native-born American press, the German Jewish press, and the municipal accounts of the events. With historical perspective, however, the management of the epidemic seems somewhat less exemplary.

In the strict terms of disease containment — the number of cases and fatalities — the public health efforts to keep typhus restricted to the Lower East Side were successful. Actual cases of typhus were kept to a minimum and, for the most part, the disease did not spread outside the Lower East Side. Success, however, is a relative term. How successful the efforts were depends largely upon one's perspective. For the native New Yorker living outside the immigrant districts, the board of health performed a magnificent job of disease control. If, on the other hand, one was unfortunate enough to have been a passenger on the *Massilia,* there was a huge price to pay in the form of violated civil liberties, cultural insensitivities, inadequate financial or physical resources devoted to their medical care, and the macabre fate of quarantine and possible death.[3]

Different People, Different Quarantine

The success of the 1892 quarantine cannot be judged only in terms of the numbers of new cases over time. No matter how well contained an epidemic, those quarantined always undergo some type of stigmatization. Understandably, even the most carefully thought out and administered policy of disease separation can be extremely dangerous if an individual or group happens to fit the criteria for isolation and is quarantined under less than perfect conditions.[4] Quarantine is simultaneously a protective social or public health policy and, for the victims, a plan of medical treatment. On the broadest level, a quarantine's primary aim is to prevent germs from infecting the healthy community; unfortunately, these germs happen to reside in human beings. This equation of human pathology and society encapsulates the classic public health paradigm of protecting both the needs of the individual and those of the public at large. A critical question to ask, then, in assessing the success or failure of the quarantine is: What were the experiences of those isolated on North Brother Island that winter of 1892?

One example of the intensely personal wreckage of Dr. Edson's quarantine was the Mermer family. Fayer (age 40) and her husband Isaac (age 48) had been living with their five children in America for less than two weeks when disaster struck with a force strong enough to make their earlier hardships on the *Massilia* seem like minor annoyances. On February 12, Fayer Mermer was dragged out of her temporary lodgings at 5 Essex Street, in the heart of the Lower East Side, kicking and screaming, partially out of fear at the actions of the armed sanitary police and partially out of a typhus-induced delirium, in full view of her husband, children, and neighbors. Matriarch Fayer Mermer's worst fears, whether generated by the infection or previous episodes of persecution, would come true; the immigrant woman died only six days later, on North Brother Island, never to see her family again and becoming the first to die in the epidemic.[5]

Another poignant case was that of Rebecca Leboff, a thirty-five-year-old woman who was eight months pregnant when she was noted to be suffering with typhus fever in a February 14 raid on the Essex Street boarding house affectionately referred to in the press as the "Hotel de Russia." Leboff gave birth to her infant on North Brother Island while in the throes of a typhus-induced delirium. Her pitiful situation and difficult delivery even evoked a bit of sympathy in the rabidly immigration-restrictionist *New York Press:* "The poor little thing only opened its eyes to close them again and that probably forever. The mother knew nothing of her babe. It is probable that she, too, will die." The *Press* actually carried its sympathy a step too far since both mother and infant survived their ordeal of illness and delivery.[6]

On the morning of February 11, Celia (age 22) and her eighteen-month-old daughter Etta Hotch were removed from the Hotel de Russia during a Health Department roundup of typhus victims. The child, reported the *New York Sun,* was staring "wonderingly at the driver as he carried her out of the house and placed her in the ambulance and seemed delighted when she found that she was going to have a ride." At the same time, Etta's mother sat "huddled in a corner of the wagon holding her head and moaning in Hebrew and German that it was 'bursting, bursting.'" Both mother and daughter would die of typhus fever in a matter of weeks.[7]

Late on the evening of February 14, the sanitary police were called to a second-floor tenement apartment at 32 Hester Street. At the scene was a bewildered and frightened peddler named Hayim Solomon. In the back room of the apartment were two small children, Gerschan (age 3) and Milia (age 7) Galinsky, in different stages of typhus fever-induced madness. The Galinsky family had recently arrived in New York on a ship other than the *Massilia* and were, unluckily, assigned by a United Hebrew Charities agent to board at the "typhus house" at 5 Essex Street. Responding to the stories and rumors surrounding the typhus houses on the Lower East Side, Mr. and Mrs. Galinsky arranged to secret the children, most likely for an exorbitant fee, at the Solomon flat while they looked for housing outside the metropolitan New York area. The little ones were stricken with typhus fever only a few days later. The sanitary police rushed the children by ambulance to the Gouverneur Hospital at Gouverneur Slip along the East River, but the admitting surgeon there refused to accept them.[8] The board of health was notified and Assistant Sanitary Inspector Alonzo Blauvelt, M.D., arranged for their immediate transfer to Willard Parker Hospital on East Sixteenth Street. The two children survived, but they were never reunited with their fleeing parents. Their voyage took them from immigrant ship to quarantine island to orphanage.[9]

While it is important to note that the Health Department was acting responsibly and with authority in its focused case-tracing among the Jewish and Italian neighborhoods, it is equally important to note that it applied different regimens of prevention to different groups of people. Often these class-based distinctions were in violation of contemporary principles and understanding of contagious diseases and epidemics. For example, a nine-year-old girl named Belle Devlin and her three-year-old sister Ellen somehow contracted what several qualified physicians diagnosed as typhus fever on March 7. They lived on West 136th Street in Harlem with two other sisters and their parents, Edward, a blacksmith, and Sarah, a homemaker. The family, of Irish Catholic heritage, were native-born New Yorkers.

Although Belle's case was reported to the Health Department by her physicians, the doctors at the Health Department refused to accept the diagnosis of typhus. Dr. Fred Dillingham, an assistant sanitary inspector, steadfastly asserted that such a diagnosis was "impossible" given that the child had had no contact with the *Massilia* passengers or residents of the Lower East Side.[10] As Cyrus Edson had announced only days before, the focus of all case-tracing was exclusively on the Russian Jewish immigrant community: "We will thoroughly sift the Russian Hebrew quarters and inspect every person in the district east of the Bowery and south of Second Street to the Bridge" (i.e., the Jewish Lower East Side).[11] The notion that typhus fever, no stranger to New York City, might have been imported by a group other than the Russian Hebrews or simply developed on American soil and then casually spread, did not seem to be a consideration for the Health Department efforts.

No quarantine was established over the apartment house where the Devlins lived, nor were Belle's family members removed to North Brother Island. Edward, Sara, Josephine, and Kathleen Devlin were allowed to remain living on West 136th Street without interruption. In contrast, the sporadic cases that occurred on New York's Lower East Side in early March were quickly sent off to the lazaretto. For example, the day before Belle Devlin's case of typhus was reported in the press (March 6, 1892), Abram Jaffe, the proprietor of the East Twelfth Street boarding house, was removed to North Brother Island because his ten-year-old son, Isaac, was discovered to be ill with typhus.[12] Both Abram and Isaac were quickly escorted out of the boarding house to an ambulance that would begin their journey to the lazaretto. The neighbors living on Twelfth Street watched from a distance with wide eyes and covered mouths, hoping to protect themselves from the seeds of contagion.

Another point of preferential treatment had to do with the burial of people who died of typhus fever. The New York City sanitary code for 1892 provided explicit regulations on the postmortem handling of contagious disease victims. The code required a formal autopsy by Health Department pathologists, followed by rapid cremation or interment in a metal casket. The day after Belle and Ellen Devlin died, they were buried in a regular cemetery under the rites of their church without any of the sanitary precautions prescribed by municipal law. This was in definite contradiction of the New York City sanitary code.[13]

The issue of being able to bury one's dead according to one's religious beliefs was not inconsequential to the East European Jewish community. In addition to the obvious sensibilities of such a request, Jewish ritual law stipulates burial regulations that are among the most strict in the Five Books of Moses. Cremation, burial delays, performing an autopsy on the body, and selecting an inappropriate coffin, such as any box not made simply and of

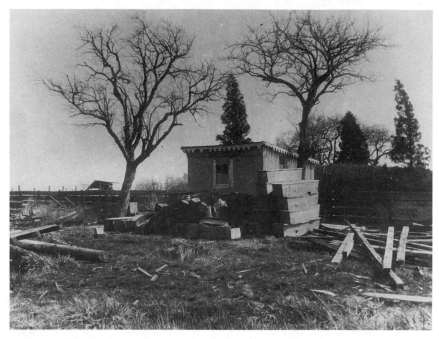

Figure 3.1. "Coffin Corner" on North Brother Island, circa 1890. Jacob A. Riis Collection, Museum of the City of New York.

pine, are forbidden and believed by Orthodox Jews to have serious consequences in the afterlife. All initial pleas by the Jewish community for exceptions to the code in an effort to respect the religious beliefs of the typhus victims were initially denied by Cyrus Edson and the Sanitary Division.

Rabbi Jacob Joseph, the "Chief Rabbi of New York's Lower East Side," an unofficial title that sounds far more important than any role he ever played in the daily life of the Jewish Quarter, beseeched the city coroner, a Tammany Democrat and German Jew named Ferdinand Levy, to intervene on the *Massilia* Jews' behalf. Joining forces with the Hebrew Benevolent Burial Society, an arm of the United Hebrew Charities that offered to pay for all expenses incurred, Levy convinced Edson and the board of health to compromise: The Jewish patients who died of typhus would not be autopsied, embalmed, or cremated, but, instead, would be placed in metal caskets with appropriate markers on Potter's Field, Hart Island, until the epidemic was over. At that point, gravediggers hired by the Hebrew Benevolent Society would exhume the dead and inter them in full accordance "with Jewish rites."[14]

Another significant cultural hardship endured by the quarantined Jews that adversely affected the medical care they received at Riverside had to do with the authorities' failure to provide them with kosher food. The immigrants were a devoutly religious lot; many were certain that their voyage and quarantine represented some form of divine punishment. Not willing to incur further divine wrath by breaking the strict dietary codes of Judaism, several of the inmates refused any form of nourishment during the quarantine. One woman detained at Riverside Hospital became so debilitated from her refusal of food that her doctors knocked out her front teeth and injected liquid with a "squirt gun." After lengthy appeals to the Health Department by the East European Jewish American community and established American German Jews, kosher cooks and provisions made available through the United Hebrew Charities were finally provided for the quarantined victims on March 1, 1892. At the food's arrival, even the once-healthy detainees were "so weak [from hunger] that they fell over each other when they tried to walk about."[15]

The native American newspapers, including the distinguished *New York Herald,* characterized the requests for kosher food as "unworthy" complaints and paternalistically commented that "two months ago they were homeless wanderers in Europe and since their arrival in New York they have been pen-

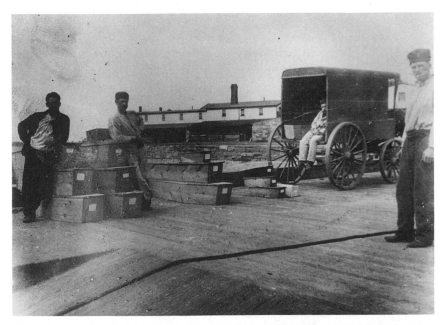

Figure 3.2. Undertakers at the docks arranging to take coffins from North Brother Island to Potter's Field on Hart's Island, circa 1890. Jacob A. Riis Collection, Museum of the City of New York.

sioners on the bounty of the United Hebrew Charities but yesterday they were ready to kick the pavilions down for coffee three times a day howling and demanding to live off the fat of the land."[16] Similarly, the *New York Times* reported, in an insidious dispatch that melded the myths of Jewish penury and the immigrant's social irresponsibility, that the United Hebrew Charities had to be "induced" by Cyrus Edson to donate any money to support the *Massilia* Jews. The reality was that the Charities gladly contributed to the cause, as they typically did whenever the board of health asked them to contribute to their immigrant brethren's health needs.[17] The International Order of B'nai B'rith's monthly magazine, *The Menorah,* responded angrily to the Health Department's clumsy handling of the kosher food issue and the American press's callous dismissal of Jewish doctrine:

> They [the *Massilia* Jews] preferred to starve rather than do violence to their religious conscience. People with a character so unyielding in its strength to temptation should form a welcome addition to the population of any community.[18]

Another symptom of preferential treatment for the "American" victims of the typhus fever epidemic was reflected in the descriptions of the epidemic offered by the daily, native-born American press. It was far more sympathetic to the Devlins and the few other nonimmigrant victims than to their isolated Russian Jewish counterparts. Edward Devlin was routinely described as an "honest, hardworking" artisan and family man. The cause of this American family's tragedy was hypothesized to be a result of the "immigrant threat" of typhus as opposed to unsanitary living conditions. The Devlins were, as the *New York Herald* reported, "the victims of infection by a half dozen Hungarian Jews" whom Samuel Joseph, the Devlins' landlord and himself a Jew, hired to make repairs in the house three weeks before the illness struck.[19]

Similarly, sanitary policeman Edward Whalen, who died of typhus on March 1, was described in *New York Commercial Advertiser* as "one of those martyrs to duty who risked his health and life in the attempt to stay the progress of the scourge . . . [and] contracted the disease by going into the house at No. 42 East 12th Street to quell a disturbance among some of the Russian Hebrews under quarantine there."[20] Whalen was canonized by the other daily New York newspapers in even more obsequious phrases.[21]

The specific distinctions drawn between "innocent victims," such as police officer Whalen and the Devlin family, and the pestilence-importing hordes of East European Jews had an influence far wider than the municipal district of New York City. It had the potential to become a sentinel call for immigration restriction. As the *New York Times* declared on its editorial page of February 13, 1892, there was a clear equation between typhus and immigra-

Table 3.1 *Typhus Fever Epidemic in New York City, February 1–April 1, 1892*[*]

Patient Type	No. of Cases	No. of Deaths	Mortality Rate (%)
Massilia typhus victims	138	13	9.4
New York City residents[*]	49	6	12.2
Policemen	2	1	50
Nurses/helpers	11	4	36.4
Total	200	24	12

Sources: "Supplement B: Report on Typhus Fever in New York, 1892," *Ann. Rep. N.Y.C. Health Dept.*, 122–42; R. Lubove, *Progressives and the Slums*, 262; J. Riis, *How the Other Half Lives*, 82–93; *New York Herald*, February 24, 1892, 3:6.
[*]In addition to the two hundred typhus victims placed under quarantine by the New York City Health Department, approximately one hundred additional *Massilia* passengers, five hundred United Hebrew Charities boarding house lodgers, and four hundred "cheap lodging house" lodgers were also quarantined.

tion: "Such immigrants are not wanted either in this city or any other part of the United States. They should be excluded. The doors should be shut against them."[22]

The preferential quarantine effort was most adversely experienced by the typhus victims or the healthy immigrants who were isolated for being "contacts" of the typhus patients but not yet ill themselves. Because of Cyrus Edson's premature and public prediction that all of the *Massilia* Jews and their contacts would inevitably develop typhus fever,[23] no precautions were taken on the island itself to halt the spread of the disease from the typhus victims to the healthy inmates. The interminable waiting and fear of contracting the disease the healthy suspects endured at Riverside must be considered one of the most egregious aspects of Edson's quarantine effort. Approximately 1,200 people were quarantined in close proximity, first on the Lower East Side, and subsequently, on North Brother Island between early February and April 1, 1892. Of these, forty-nine developed typhus fever and six died (Table 3.1).[24]

One brave, or at least ambitious, reporter for the *New York Commercial Advertiser*, Frederick Hamilton, smuggled himself into the quarantine house on Essex Street and, a week later, visited the *Massilia* Jews on North Brother Island. Although Hamilton succumbed to typhus fever within two weeks of filing his remarkable story, he left behind a chilling record of the detained *Massilia* Jews:

Pallid bearded men with startled faces gathered in groups of three and four gesticulating, wringing their hands, and all speaking at once in a strange language.

Their gestures, however, were translatable enough. They wanted to get out. A scared hunted look bespoke their wonder at being held prisoner in this fashion in a strange land.[25]

The East European Jewish community on New York's Lower East Side, obviously, had deep feelings and resentments concerning the epidemic. Indeed, the strongest objections to the 1892 typhus quarantine appeared in the Yiddish American press. These documents are a vital source in interpreting the cultural history of this immigrant community. As Irving Howe characterized these rich repositories of a life now gone, the Yiddish newspapers were less "ventures in journalism than . . . outpourings of collective sentiment. They were deeply 'internal' papers serving as voices in a communal dialogue — equivalent to immigrant gatherings, over tea in the kitchen where people 'talked things over.' "[26] The surviving remarks of the Yiddish reporters who observed the quarantine efforts of 1892 articulate a profound and devastating experience of social isolation.

There was one daily Yiddish paper published in New York City in 1892 (the *Yiddishe Tageblatt*) and three weeklies (the *Yiddishe Gazetten,* a weekly collection of *Tageblatt* articles and pieces from some of the smaller Yiddish newspapers that appeared elsewhere in the United States; the socialist *Arbeiter Zeitung,* which was published by the Hebrew Trade Union; and the occasionally published anarchist broadsheet, *Freie Arbeiter Shtime*). During the typhus epidemic and its aftermath, the first three of these Yiddish papers were filled with outrage as they reported the inequities of Cyrus Edson's quarantine against the Russian Jews.[27]

Abraham Cahan was unarguably the most prominent of the Yiddish American journalists of the late nineteenth and twentieth centuries. In 1892, he still supplemented his income with money he earned teaching greenhorn immigrants how to speak English and he was enjoying some success in selling a few pieces on ghetto life to the native-born American press. Cahan was also an active member of the Socialist Party, an organizer of labor unions and socialist groups, and even conducted a literary correspondence with Friedrich Engels. Although Cahan's greatest fame was yet to come with his editorship of the *New York Daily Forward* and a distinguished career as a novelist of the Jewish American immigrant experience, he was already a well-known commentator in Yiddish American circles in the 1890s.

Cahan's major journalistic efforts in 1892 were devoted to serving as editor of the New York *Arbeiter Zeitung,* a journal devoted to the principles of socialism. In any given issue, Cahan played many different roles in the rush to fill four to eight pages with copy each week, ranging from "poet, feutilletonist, popular-science writer, socialist theoretician, story teller, [and] re-

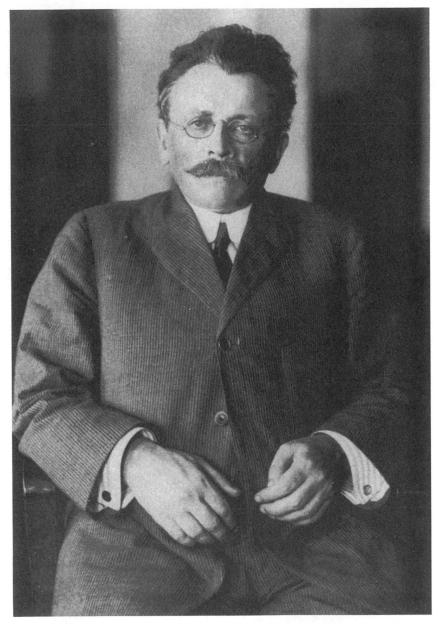

Figure 3.3. Abraham Cahan. Brown Brothers.

porter." [28] In an essay entitled "The Sickness Without an End," published in the February 26 issue of the *Arbeiter Zeitung,* Cahan pointed his vitriolic pen at the inconsistencies of public health authorities and the medical establishment:

> There was a small storm in America with the typhus epidemic which Russian Jewish immigrants from the *S.S. Massilia* have dragged here with them. The truth is that this is no laughing matter. The American community's "authorities" do not need any more reasons to strike out against Jews and such an occurrence doesn't help. The authorities are making this small occurrence one thousand times worse than it is. Their outcry is a thousand times worse than it should be and the alarm is worse than the actual threat. Because of this story, 'the typhus epidemic,' the Health Board created so many difficulties for so many of our people, that anyone can see that their actions were far more than necessary. The Health men imprisoned healthy Jews on the ships coming into New York and on the island. They packed them together and dragged them, quarantined them — *Nu?* — so? These poor Jews could have become sick simply from being lumped together with the true typhus patients. The health inspectors burned the poor people's belongings, they emptied out houses and ran around sending alarming telegrams — in short it was a good business for the spoon-people (*lefl-leit*).[29]

The politically conservative New York *Yiddishe Tageblatt,* published by the pioneering Yiddish American journalist Kasriel Sarasohn, appealed to the older Russian Jewish immigrants on the Lower East Side. *Tageblatt* readers were typically Orthodox Jewish men, redolent of the Old World shtetl but eager to prove allegiance to their adopted country. The newspaper often hesitated to disagree with the American government out of the newcomer's sense of both respect and fear.[30] Yet its pages during the typhus epidemic reveal an even greater sense of outrage at the goings-on at North Brother Island than does its socialist competitor. This campaign was principally waged by the *Tageblatt's* chief columnist, Getsl Zelikowitch, who signed his pieces with the nom de plume the *"Litvak Philosophe"* (the Lithuanian Philosopher).

Zelikowitch was a former *yeshiva bucher* (rabbinical student) in Lithuania. He was influenced by the *Haskalah* movement of secular thought at the age of sixteen and gave up the Talmud for study in Paris at the Sorbonne in 1879. He was a scholar of Sanskrit, Arabic, and English in addition to his facility with Yiddish, Hebrew, and Russian. In 1887 he was called to America as professor of Egyptology at the University of Pennsylvania but left the faculty the following year "because of intrigues." He then began a long career as a journalist for a number of Yiddish newspapers and as a penny-novelist.[31]

In March 1892, Zelikowitch devoted his columns to a discussion of what he considered to be a far more serious epidemic than the one imported by the

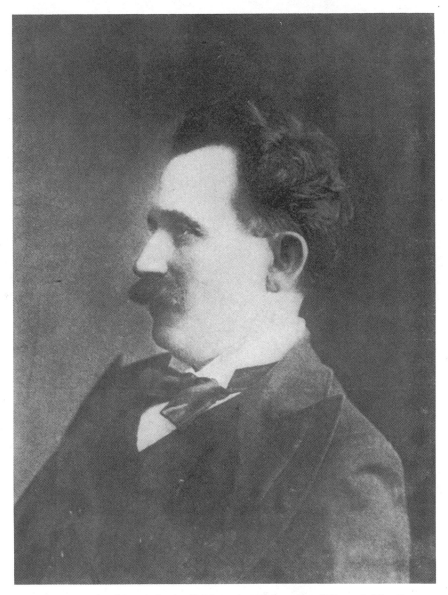

Figure 3.4. Getsl Zelikowitch, the "Lithuanian Philosopher." From *Jubilee Program Honoring Professor Getsl Zelikowitch*, 1913, in author's possession.

Massilia: "the typhus of the soul which is called anti-Semitism." Alluding to the problems that might arise from the popular perception that Russian Jews were importers of epidemics, Zelikowitch asked his readers, "Do you know where the real pest is living? Anti-Semitism is her nest." The Lithuanian Philosopher underestimates the numbers of the *Massilia* typhus victims in his columns, but he does provide the reader with a savvy understanding of immigration politics and epidemiologic case-tracing:

> It is because of typhus, we are told, that we must no longer allow Jews to enter this country in order to guard the American public from a terrible disease. The truth is that they simply don't want us because we are Jews. . . . Blaming these sick Russian Jews, fifty of them who came here in a sickly state, for bringing the scourge is a patriotic lie, ragged and tattered to its very construction. Listen, in the last two years more than 150,000 Russian Jews have arrived in the United States and from this amount only fifty, last month, brought the typhus. And of these, five sick ones were on the steamer *Massilia* which came to New York from the Mediterranean Sea, from Marseilles, and Constantinople.[32]

In distinct contrast to the Yiddish responses to the aggressive features of the quarantine, of course, was the native-born, and frequently nativist, American popular press. In 1892, especially for those who did not live in the largest East Coast cities such as New York, many Americans could honestly say they never actually saw a Jew except, perhaps, an actor portraying one in a popular production of Shakespeare's *The Merchant of Venice*.[33] Indeed, in 1892, Jewish Americans made up less than one percent of the entire U.S. population.[34] But despite America's lack of firsthand experience with Russian Jews, East European Jews were all-too-commonly described in the popular press as dangerous. The addition of a deadly and contagious disease to the equation only magnified the potential for dehumanizing responses from the healthy society at large. For some Gilded Age Americans, the problems of the ill-fated *Massilia* Jews had the potential to lead to a much broader conclusion: Russian Jews posed a threat to the public health of the United States and the problem required immediate action.

For example, one anonymous anti-Semitic pamphleteer from New York City not only accused the Jews of "crimes" such as "controlling the currency, fixing public opinion, overthrowing government, driving working men into useless strikes, poisoning whisky, and crushing out Christianity," he also insisted that they were responsible for spreading typhus and cholera in the United States.[35] Similarly, physicians in the town of Plainfield, Connecticut, attributed epidemics of scarlet fever and diphtheria to "filthy" Hebrew pack peddlers reputed to be *Massilia* passengers. The peddlers were accused by the Plainfield board of health of forcing or threatening their way into homes. The "wily" Hebrew peddlers then enticed local housewives into buying their wares while leaving behind the "seeds of the diseases."[36] There were similar panics over the possible arrival of *Massilia* Jews or simply other Russian Jews in Newburgh, New York; New Castle, Pennsylvania; Oakdale, Massachusetts; Baltimore, Maryland; and Valatie, New York.[37]

Many American newspapers seized the theme of Russian Jews as diseased scapegoats and published articles and cartoons that graphically depicted them as the vectors of typhus fever to the United States. The *New York Press,* long targeted by the Yiddish press as hostile toward Russian Jews, published cartoons on its front page representing both Russia and Italy as sources of disease. Their captions called for a total ban on immigration so that the United States did not "become the dumping ground of the diseased and depraved of all nations."[38] On February 18, 1892, for example, the *New York Press*'s front page featured a cartoon of a throng of Russian Jews knocking at the door of the U.S. commissioner of immigration. Above the door is a sign reading "The Law forbids the landing of immigrants likely to become a public charge." The cartoon's caption reads: "And yet the door is thrown wide open for the sick, destitute and disease bearing throng from European shores."[39] Similar cartoons appeared in former Hungarian immigrant Joseph Pulitzer's *New York World,* showing Europe as a giant skull sending forth immigrant ships labeled "Hunger Typhus," "Diphtheria," "Yellow Fever," and the like with the caption: "Even McKinley Could Not Tax These Imports Too High" — slyly combining the issues of immigration restriction and tariff policy.[40]

Readers of the daily newspapers were also anxious to make their opinions heard. Soon dozens of "letters to the editor," similar to the one presented below, began to appear in the daily New York City newspapers:

> We do not want and we ought to refuse to land all or any of these unclean Italians or Russian Hebrews. We have enough dirt, misery, crime, sickness and death of our own without permitting any more to be thrust upon us by any of the foreign powers and it is only such that they are desirous of getting rid of and send to us.[41]

Even the staid *Boston Medical and Surgical Journal* editorialized negatively on the event: "We open our doors to squalor and filth and misery—which means typhus fever."[42]

These complaints and racist rantings were not without effect. The fears expressed by native-born Americans were folded into the public health policies of jurisdictions wider than the New York City Health Department. On February 13, 1892, Dr. William Jenkins, the health officer of the Port of New York, announced a strict policy detaining and quarantining *all* East European Jews coming through New York Harbor, regardless of their port of embarkation. The quarantine ordered by Jenkins was informed by neither common sanitary practices imposed against "infected ports" (i.e., areas where specific contagious diseases were reported to exist) nor isolation techniques advocated by public health officials in 1892. The net was specifically cast for East European Jews. Only ships carrying these immigrants "would be detained and inspected for typhus."[43]

An example of the "quarantine by ethnicity" occurred the following day, February 14, 1892. After inspecting the SS *Nevada,* Dr. Jenkins announced that he did not have the "slightest suspicion" that typhus was on board but, nevertheless, detained thirty Russian Jews who arrived from the relatively disease-free Port of Liverpool. When it came to the inspection of East European Jewish immigrants, Jenkins declared that he could not afford to "take any chances." The ninety-three Scandinavian passengers who were also traveling in the *Nevada*'s steerage compartments were, on the other hand, allowed to land without delay.[44]

The following day, Jenkins quarantined 1,400 Russian Jews traveling in the steerage of the transatlantic steamers *City of Berlin, Belgenland,* and *Russia.* Again, passengers traveling cabin class or originating from non-Russian ports were immediately released. The Russian Jews who were quarantined on Hoffman Island presented no signs of illness or contagion but because they were "of the impoverished, unkempt class that usually comes from that land, and of the kind that such a scourge as typhus would be likely to mark as its own," Jenkins ordered their detainment. The reasoning was clear, if misguided, when one considers 1892 concepts of bacteriology and maritime quarantine. The *Massilia* carried Russian Jews, some of whom developed typhus fever; therefore, all subsequent Russian Jews arriving in the United States were considered by Dr. Jenkins likely to do the same, requiring "careful scrutiny before [their] being allowed to land."[45]

Jenkins' quarantine policy persisted well into April 1892, leading to a striking decrease in the transportation of Russian Jews to New York City. He rescinded his selective order once the Health Department announced the epidemic was over. Nor would it be Dr. Jenkins' last foray into quarantine policy for East European Jewish immigrants; in a matter of months, Jenkins was to control the quarantine of the Port of New York against the threat of cholera that was linked to Jewish immigrants. Several other quarantine stations along the eastern seaboard also detained Russian Jews as a typhus preventive during March and April 1892. The steamship companies, under the Immigration Act of March 3, 1891, were required to return all medically rejected immigrants at their own expense. This risk, exacerbated by the huge expense of transatlantic steamers being detained in Quarantine for three or more weeks, made such steerage service too expensive to bear. In response to these regulations, the Red Star, Hamburg-American, and North German Lloyd steamship lines announced a temporary cessation of Russian Jewish, but not other immigrant, traffic. This action was essentially a death sentence for many Russian Jews trying to escape the tyranny of Czar Alexander III.[46] None of these policies were long-lived, however, and immigration traffic returned to its pre-typhus epidemic rates by late April 1892.

Perhaps the most problematic aspect of these quarantine policies was the denial or ignorance of the fact that the *Massilia* passengers spent a considerable time, three months, in Constantinople, where typhus was known to be a problem. Typhus fever is an acute and sudden illness with a relatively brief dormant or prodromal phase (one to three days). Given the natural history of typhus, there is little likelihood that some of the *Massilia* Jews contracted typhus in Odessa, remained healthy for over ninety days in Turkey and then developed symptoms several weeks later in New York. Dr. Jenkins openly acknowledged to Congress that the *Massilia* passengers had had no contact with Russia since October 1891.[47] Nevertheless, both Jenkins and the supervising surgeon general of the U.S. Marine Health Service, Walter Wyman, declared Russian ports rather than Turkish ones to be the source of typhus and arranged their quarantine policies accordingly.[48] In fact, typhus fever was far more prevalent in Switzerland (148 deaths), Germany (116 deaths), the Netherlands (107 deaths), Italy (99 deaths), Brazil (93 deaths), and Japan (89 deaths) between January 1891 and March 1892 than it was in Russia (50 deaths).[49]

No policy of quarantine was established for people originating from these other ports by the state of New York or the federal health authorities. Moreover, none of the American health officials guiding the quarantine efforts, from the local to the federal levels, acknowledged the distinct possibility that the seeds of infection could have originated during the passengers' temporary exile in Constantinople or, worse yet, from the boarding houses on the Lower East Side of New York.

Quarantines and Immigrants: The View from Washington

The appropriation of the 1892 typhus epidemic as a rationale for restricting the entry of East European Jews and other new immigrants was led by Senator William Chandler of New Hampshire, chairman of the U.S. Senate Committee on Immigration. Early during the events, Chandler saw the potential political power of an epidemic tied to undesirable immigrants. Brandishing a number of newspaper clippings covering the *Massilia* episode on the floor of the U.S. Senate, Chandler declared on February 15 that the *Massilia* Jews and others like them should "not have been allowed to land," adding that "self protection was the first law of nature."[50]

Like the tempest raised by the newspapers, however, the public's conflation of disease with restricting the immigration of Russian Jews was not much more long-lived than the typhus epidemic itself. Interest in and reaction to the typhus fever epidemic, the *Massilia* passengers, and the efforts of New York City's Health Department were fading fast as fewer cases began to be reported in mid-March 1892. Nevertheless, Chandler's attempt to conflate issues of imported contagion with both the federal quarantine and the immigration laws marked a momentous and early attempt at justifying immigration restriction policies with the language of public health.

Nicknamed the "stormy petrel," after the seabird that sailors regarded as a harbinger of trouble or strife, William Eaton Chandler was one of the most powerful men in the federal government. A Harvard-educated lawyer-turned-journalist, Chandler was a lithe, compact man with a manicured goatee, pince-nez glasses, and a forceful way with words. He was first elected to the New Hampshire legislature in 1863 and became a strong supporter of Abraham Lincoln, gaining prominence among the "War Republicans." During Lincoln's second term, Chandler was appointed to the post of solicitor and judge-advocate of the Navy. He was subsequently promoted to assistant secretary of the treasury during Andrew Johnson's presidency in 1865 but returned to the practice of law and publishing his newspaper, the *Concord Monitor and Statesman,* in 1867. Remaining active in the Republican National Committee for a number of years, Chandler returned to Washington as secretary of the navy under President Chester Arthur in 1882. He was elected to the U.S. Senate in 1887, a post he held until 1901.[51]

In 1892, one of William Chandler's principal interests was the "alarm and danger" of immigration. An avowed nativist and immigration restrictionist as well as a professional politician, Chandler knew that a controversial measure such as an immigration restriction bill had little chance of passage during the Fifty-second Congress with a Democratic House and a Republican Senate. On a pragmatic level many senators and representatives from the Midwest and West supported open immigration because their states required additional population and laborers for development; other representatives, especially Democrats along the eastern seaboard, were hesitant to infuriate the naturalized immigrants among their constituents by supporting a restriction bill. Nevertheless, Chandler proposed passage of several federal immigration restrictions that year. His bill required immigrants to pass literacy tests if they were over the age of twelve years, to possess financial assets of at least $100.00 for the head of the family and $25.00 for each subsequent family member, and certification of an immigrant's physical and moral fitness to enter a country. Furthermore, he would have placed extensive bans on what he called "certain obviously undesirable classes."

In an article Chandler penned for the popular monthly *The Forum* in March 1892, he explained exactly what he meant by these "undesirable classes" and identified them more specifically as "southern Italians and Russian, Polish, or Hungarian Jews":

> The alarm springs from the constantly increasing influx within our borders of classes of immigrants of a most undesirable character. The danger is the reduction of wages to the injury of the American workman, and of his home and family, the debasement of the suffrage, and wide contamination of society.[52]

Despite his active role in the passage of the Immigration Act of March 3, 1891—a law historian Thomas Archdeacon labeled the "linchpin" of federal control over immigration[53]—Chandler remained far from satisfied with the government's power to restrict the immigration of these "undesirable classes." He later called the 1891 law "little more than the re-enactment of the act of 1882."[54] Actually, it was far more. It gave the federal government sole authority over immigration, instead of the unsatisfactory partnership that had previously existed with the various state authorities; reenforced the responsibility of steamship companies to return, at their cost, all immigrants rejected by U.S. inspectors, including those who became public charges within one year of landing; broadened the categories of those deemed inadmissible for landing; and attempted to improve immigrant ship manifests and bills of health record keeping (although a stricter and international means of inspecting and certifying ships was yet to be developed). Chandler was unsatisfied with these regulations and insisted, instead, that wider-sweeping restrictions, such as literacy requirements and various forms of "head taxes," were essential to safeguard the United States against the dangerous foreign hordes.[55]

The literacy restriction was an especially potent and cynical means of restricting the immigration of Russian Jews in the 1890s. Clearly few of them knew English but even if the laws were written so that they were required to be literate in the language of their native land, Russia, still fewer would be allowed to enter. Russian Jews, as it may be recalled, were forbidden to obtain an education under Czarist rule and consequently many did not speak or read Russian fluently. The overwhelming majority were literate in Yiddish, but this language was still regarded, by German Jews and Gentiles alike, as jargon rather than a full-fledged language. Yiddish fluency, not surprisingly, did not satisfy Chandler's proposed literacy requirements.

One person who tried to explain the unfairness of a literacy test applied to Russian Hebrews was the Louisville lawyer, politician, and Orthodox Jew Lewis Naphtali Dembitz. The five-foot-tall scholar, whom we remember today as the maternal uncle and role model of Supreme Court Justice Louis

Dembitz Brandeis, was "a balding man who peered intensely at the world through rimless glasses that perched on his nose and barely corrected his vision."[56] Surviving in the many bound volumes that comprise Chandler's papers and correspondence at the Library of Congress is a three-page, hand-written letter from Dembitz explaining why the Jews from Russia were not illiterate and why such a law would be an unfair criterion for restriction. Dembitz also listed the admirable qualities the Russian Jewish immigrants brought to America's shores. Unfortunately, Dembitz's letter relied heavily on the stereotyping and social scapegoating of *other* immigrant groups as he made a plea to Chandler for the continued immigration of Russian Jews:

> They are very anxious to become Anglicized and Americanized. . . . Unlike the Irish, they carry no foreign politics with them to the country of their adoption. They easily abjure all faith and allegiance to the Czar, but their hatred with which they regard him, can in no way disturb their position as American citizens as the Irish hatred of England does. They fall naturally into Republican life. The idea of the sovereignty of the people is inborn to the Jew. In fact, its first and strongest ex-pression is in the Old Testament. . . . They are law abiding. There is no fear of their founding a branch of the Mafia in New York like the Sicilians did in New Orleans. Their intense love for wife and children keep them from becoming rioters or strikers. They are not apt, like the Chinese, or the Cosacks from North Hungary to depress the labor market. For they have the keen Jewish love for wealth, and as soon as they have saved enough out of their tailor's or cigarmaker's wages, will go into trade, or set up a shop of their own. . . . To these considerations should be added that among all the immigrants of our time the Russian Jew is the only one who is driven to our shores to avoid a decree of starvation: for all the exceptional decrees of Alexander III against the Jews amount to this and nothing more. To drive them back from our shore would be nothing less than becoming accessory to the Czar's murderous cruelty.[57]

Another effective halt to immigration from Eastern and Southern Europe was the proposed "head tax" or, in more bureaucratic language, "asset re-quirements." Migrating Russian Jews and Southern Italians of the late nine-teenth century were overwhelmingly from the impoverished classes; fre-quently, travel plans went awry to deplete even the well-situated immigrant's bankroll, as we saw with some of the *Massilia* passengers. Not surprisingly, there were great overlaps between the poorest immigrants and those emi-grating from the most "undesirable" places. A head tax of $100 (which was seven to ten times more than a steerage transatlantic steamship ticket) would significantly restrict the entry of the target group. Yet these proposals held little appeal for many Gilded Age Americans, who felt uncomfortable linking financial worth or literacy in English on arrival to eligibility for American citizenship, and they never had a serious chance of passing during the Fifty-second Congress. As immigration historian John Higham noted, because of the wide-based opposition to such measures, particularly in the House of Representatives, Chandler and his immigration committee would have to resort to other "schemes for restriction."[58]

The *Massilia* affair proved to be an excellent albeit temporary means of promoting Chandler's restrictionist cause between February and March 1892. Armed with letters from citizens calling for the restriction of all "disease carrying" immigrants from Russia and Italy, Chandler argued that the time to investigate the U.S. immigration laws was at hand. A particular focus of his committee's investigation, Chandler declared, would be the "recent admission of . . . pauper Russian Hebrews [who] in contravention and disobedience of our laws . . . have been distributed from one end of the Eastern states to the other, perhaps to infect whole communities with typhus fever . . . when they should have been excluded by the immigration commissioner of New York City."[59]

With approval from both the House of Representatives and the Senate, Chandler brought the Senate Committee on Immigration and the House Committee on Immigration and Naturalization to New York City during the weekend of March 5–6, 1892. Alternating between testimonies from all the officials who played a role in either admitting the *Massilia* passengers or fighting the typhus epidemic, Senator Chandler hoped to establish once and for all the dangers of admitting paupers who were both "likely to become a public charge" and "likely to import an epidemic scourge."[60] This task proved difficult even for a seasoned politician like Chandler.

The Joint Committee on Immigration began its inquiry on the typhus epidemic with the testimony of Immigration Commissioner John C. Weber. In a goading manner, Chandler recalled Weber's humanitarian work on behalf of the destitute Russian Jews and accused him of letting his "sympathies" for these "pauper Russian Hebrews" get in the way of performing his job at Ellis Island. Chandler insisted that since the *Massilia* passengers were "clearly paupers likely to become a public charge" they should never have been admitted in the first place. Chandler worried aloud how the Ellis Island inspectors could be trusted with the nation's public health if they could not protect the nation's economic health by identifying obvious paupers. Self-protection and stronger immigration restriction laws, rather than excessive sympathy, Chandler insisted, would have avoided the epidemic altogether.

Weber, a former congressman and able debater himself, strongly disagreed with Chandler. The commissioner explained that the *Massilia* immigrants were not paupers when they originally fled Russia; it was the unusual circumstances of their lengthy voyage that used up all their funds:

These people have landed here who had means when they started and were, by reason of brutalities and inhuman persecutions reduced temporarily to a condition that has appealed to the benevolence of their co-religionists and by reason of that they have assisted them. I do not regard such a person as a pauper.[61]

Chandler countered Weber's statement with charges that *any* immigrant assisted by a benevolent society, such as the United Hebrew Charities or the Baron de Hirsch Fund, should be considered a pauper. Chandler insisted that these "Russian Hebrews may excite our sympathies but nevertheless they are paupers" and, consequently, should have been excluded.

Carrying on the stalemate, Weber presented data that showed that the Russian Jews who were assisted by the United Hebrew Charities or Baron de Hirsch Fund were not only well cared for, educated, and given employment; they also, to his knowledge, "almost never become public charges." The matter remained hanging unpleasantly in the air as Weber pointedly called the senator to task for his nativist beliefs and the convenience of restrictions based on labels:

We can exclude anybody we want; bald-headed men or one legged men or anybody we choose; Jews or Italians or anybody else. Russia claims to exclude these people because they are usurers and shylocks, and other countries refuse to receive them because they are paupers.[62]

The level of ambiguity only increased as Senator Chandler and his colleagues examined the health officers of the New York quarantine station, Ellis Island, and the *Massilia*. Not a single health officer was found responsible for failing to diagnose immigrants with an incubating case of typhus *before* any physical manifestations were present. One by one, each medical inspector was exonerated.[63] Nor did the congressmen investigating the epidemic find fault with the inspection procedures, bills of health, or other practical matters concerning the flow of immigration into the United States despite the glaring inadequacies in the medical inspection of the *Massilia*.

Equally confusing was the disagreement among the various physicians interviewed, including Cyrus Edson, Hermann Biggs, William Jenkins, and former health officer William Smith over the actual source of the infection and the etiology, transmission, and incubation period of typhus fever, all critical issues for elaborating bacteriologically informed policies of medical inspection and quarantine.

There were three points the physicians could agree on: the great difficulty they had in diagnosing typhus; its rapid spread from the sick to the healthy; and its frequent confusion with other diseases that resembled it.[64] Yet actually proving the exact origins of the epidemic—whether imported in the clothing of an impoverished Russian Jewish immigrant or a natural reoccurrence of the disease in New York's poorest districts — was quite impossible. And so the hearings went through May of that year at the favored address of New York Republicans, the Fifth Avenue Hotel. Side trips to the quarantine hospitals at North Brother, Ellis, and Hoffman Islands and interviews with seamen aboard the *Massilia,* shipping agents, and immigration experts failed to add new information on exactly how and where the typhus epidemic began.

Despite Chandler's desire to link the danger of epidemic disease to immigrant Russian Jews in order to enact stronger immigration restriction laws, the ambiguity surrounding his investigation and the lack of public interest in epidemics once they have been tamed thwarted his desire to "shut the gates" to "undesirables such as southern Italians and Russian, Polish, or Hungarian Jews."[65] The Senate and House were about to recess for the summer and Chandler's dream of enacting an immigration restriction bill would have to wait until the next session in the fall.

But Chandler did learn a valuable lesson: the powerful message of an undesirable social group linked to a deadly illness that could easily spread throughout the population at large. He quickly realized that epidemic diseases often inspired quarantines and quarantines might be used as a means of restricting immigration if enough Americans could be convinced that "new immigrants" were bringing such scourges with them. With the typhus epidemic of 1892 reduced to a whimper well before his committee had a chance to act with a bill, he was not successful in such a move that winter. Instead, he bided his time for what the *New York Commercial Advertiser* deemed inevitable — another immigrant-imported epidemic: "Without present facilities for collecting and admitting the pestilences of all creation, we ought to have cholera, yellow fever and the Black Death on hand in large quantities before the year ends."[66] Senator Chandler would not have to wait very long.

PART II

"CHOLERA MAY KNOCK, BUT IT WON'T GET IN"

Cholera, Class, and Quarantine in New York Harbor

A history of the affair would furnish an excellent illustration of nearly everything that is bad in the social and political life of this city.

—*E. L. Godkin, writing James Bryce about the cholera epidemic, October 16, 1892*

CHAPTER 4

Awaiting the Cholera:
"Choleria!"

Although the New York City Health Department successfully contained the typhus epidemic by mid-April and the congressional hearings on the epidemic's cause drew to a close without any action in early May 1892, many Americans continued to worry about the public health risks of unrestricted immigration, particularly from the undesirable locales of Eastern Europe and southern Italy. In Washington, D.C., for example, members of the Fifty-second Congress were inundated with a "flood of petitions" advocating immigration restriction on the grounds of public health. The petitions represented Americans from over twenty-three states, numerous labor unions, brotherhoods, church groups, and social clubs.[1]

One outcome of the anti-immigrant fervor during the first half of 1892 was the passage of the Chinese Exclusion Act of May 5, 1892 (27 Stat. 25). This law extended existing restrictions against the Chinese and other Asians hoping to settle in the United States for another ten years and established special registration for all Chinese laborers residing in the United States (endorsed by "at least one credible white witness") as well as stricter deportation regulations.[2] Although their concept of race was markedly different from present-day definitions, many Gilded Age Americans had a far easier time supporting legislation that halted Chinese and Asian immigration than they would limiting European immigration, perhaps because they believed that the racial separateness between whites and Asians could never be blurred no matter how many coats of Americanization were painted on them.[3]

During the spring and summer, labor unrest across the nation resulted in a number of disputes and violent strikes. Charismatic, and frequently foreign, labor union leaders were branded as "charlatans" and "poisonous agitators." Strikes broke out among steel workers in Pennsylvania, miners in Wyoming and Idaho, and textile workers in Tennessee. Nowhere was the relationship between labor and capital more savage than in Homestead, Pennsylvania, just six miles upstream the Monongahela River from Pittsburgh, where workers of the Carnegie Homestead Steel Works were locked out in a labor dispute on June 29. Bloody battles between three hundred armed Pinkerton guards and the steel workers resulted in ten deaths (seven workers, three guards) before Robert E. Pattison, the governor of Pennsylvania, and President Benjamin Harrison ordered 8,500 state militiamen and

National Guardsmen to seize both the steel mill and the town. One now forgotten historical actor in the Homestead debacle, Alexander Berkman, seems in retrospect an almost too convenient symbol of the menacing triad of labor unions, socialism-anarchism, and foreign influences in America. Berkman, the "Russian Hebrew nihilist," attempted to murder Carnegie's chief of operations at Homestead, Henry Clay Frick, with a pistol and a knife. Berkman was wrestled to the ground by the seriously wounded Frick and his associate, J. G. A. Leishman, before being hauled away to jail by the National Guardsmen.[4] As historian Matthew Josephson noted, "the light wounds of Frick, 'intrepid and lion-like,' brought him glory and hardened the resistance of the steel masters until they had won the day."[5]

In Chicago that summer, architects, builders, and laborers were busy shaping the strange concoction of plaster of Paris and horsehair onto steel frameworks for the magnificent beaux arts "White City" of the 1893 Columbian Exposition and World's Fair, scheduled to open that October. Over $22 million was appropriated by the U.S. Congress to build the 644-acre fairgrounds that featured exhibits of the world's finest arts, industries, and products as well as the "Ferris Wheel" designed by Pittsburgh inventor George Washington Gale Ferris.[6] Far more than a mere exhibition, the upcoming Chicago World's Fair was, as Henry Adams wrote, "the first step in the concept of America as unity." Anxious Chicagoans, and others across the nation involved in preparing the event, began to wonder if the potential health risks of unrestricted immigration might ruin the fair.[7]

As the summer progressed and the presidential election contest between incumbent Republican Benjamin Harrison and former Democratic president Grover Cleveland heated up, immigration continued to be discussed as a potential threat to the United States for reasons of economic strength, social stability, and public health. Presidential platforms written on behalf of the Republican, Democratic, Prohibition, Populist, and Socialist Labor Parties all called for some form of legislation that restricted immigration as a means of protection from "undesirable immigration."[8]

No event more clearly embodied American misgivings about unrestricted European immigration than the severe epidemic of cholera raging in the Middle East, Russia, and parts of continental Europe that summer. Daily dispatches in American newspapers reported on the huge loss of life and the rapid westward spread of the epidemic. By mid-June, cholera became especially rampant in famine-stricken Russia. Precise figures for the 1892 cholera epidemic in Russia are difficult to ascertain, but the best estimates suggest that there were about 620,000 cases of cholera that year and over 300,000 deaths resulting from the epidemic. To make matters worse, public health efforts were frequently thwarted by suspicions and superstitions of the peasant class against the Russian medical community; by panic, riots, and unrest; and by a poorly organized health care delivery system.[9] As the cholera epidemic appeared to gain ground in continental Europe, Americans became more and more concerned about the possibility of cholera reaching their shores.

Cholera has been described as "the classic epidemic disease of the nineteenth century."[10] It was also the era's most highly feared epidemic disease. During the first two-thirds of that century, American experiences with cholera were devastating. Severe epidemics were imported from Europe, the Middle East, and India to the eastern seaboard states in 1832, 1845, and 1866. Many Americans reading about the possibility of another visitation that fall had had firsthand experience with these public health crises. By 1892, the means of preventing a cholera epidemic were better understood by most physicians and sanitarians, yet the popular perception of cholera as a rapidly spreading and certain agent of death persisted. More than any other serious epidemic disease of that era, cholera was considered by most Americans to be an exclusively "foreign" disease that required one's most vigilant guard.

There was good reason to avoid this horrifying disorder of the gastrointestinal tract. The onset of cholera typically begins with the victim's nonspecific sense of simply not feeling well. Soon after this intuition of illness, perhaps only a matter of hours, comes a violent wave of vomiting and diarrhea. So forceful are the choleraic propulsions, from both ends of the gut, that the victim experiences intense, painful spasms of the abdominal muscles. The relentless diarrhea soon gives way to dehydration and shock. The victim's face appears blue and tight; the eyes are deeply sunken; the mouth and lips are parched and cracked. The cholera victim's vitality wanes as the diarrhea increases, accompanied by a clouded sense of reality, painful muscle spasms, seizures, and coma. Between 30 percent and 80 percent of all cases of cholera during this period resulted in death.[11]

Observers of cholera have likened the victim's massive evacuation of diarrheal stools to "rice water" because of their distinct appearance of dirty water studded with flecks of grey-white matter (damaged and shedded intestinal mucosal lining). So copious is the loss of fluid by diarrhea that physicians employed a special "cholera bed," which was little more than a canvas cot with a hole cut in its center and a large bedpan placed directly below it. In an era where the act (and place) of defecation was becoming increasingly sanitized and domesticized, a disease like cholera inspired intense anxiety among Gilded Age Americans.[12] As historian Richard Evans has written about this psychologically "unmanageable" disease as it was experienced in nineteenth-century Germany, cholera "was felt to be a vulgar and demeaning disease. Its reputation as a disease of the poor only strengthened its repulsiveness."[13]

Fueling American fears of a potential cholera epidemic was the news of a mass exodus of Jews escaping the famine and cholera-ravaged provinces of Russia for America. The major travel path from Russia to America during this period was through Hamburg. Memories of the recent typhus epidemic among Russian Jews in New York City undoubtedly contributed to the public's concern. The lead article of the *New York Times* on August 29, 1892, ominously warned its readers about the entwined risks of undesirable immigration and cholera:

> With the danger of cholera in question, it is plain to see that the United States would be better off if ignorant Russian Jews and Hungarians were denied refuge here. . . . These people are offensive enough at best; under the present circumstances, they are a positive menace to the health of the country. Even should they pass the Quarantine officials, their mode of life, when they settle down makes them always a source of danger. Cholera, it must be remembered, originates in the homes of this human riff-raff.[14]

After much delay and attempts at concealment, Hamburg officials finally admitted on August 23, 1892, that they were dealing with a devastating and ongoing cholera epidemic in their city. The shipping records of the Hamburg-American Steamship Company demonstrate that it, in collaboration with the Hamburg government, was anxious to rid the city of the accepted vector of cholera, East European immigrants, even if it required mistruths and concealment. Steamship traffic, carrying a large cargo of steerage immigrants, continued their daily schedules out of Hamburg for several days *after* Hamburg health officials finally admitted that the cholera epidemic existed.[15] Such a policy, of course, had worldwide ramifications. As the largest port in the world, Hamburg sent off dozens of steamships each day — and many sailed to American ports such as New York.[16]

During the late spring and summer, immigration steamship routes were expanded and the human river of East European and southern Italian immigrants once again flowed through the Ellis Island immigration center. Russian Jews were especially anxious to escape Europe because of Czarist persecution and harsh living conditions. In 1892, they comprised 10.4 percent of total immigration to the United States. The continuous flow of Russian Jewish immigrants was described by *Harper's Weekly* as "the scum of invalided Europe."[17] Nativist and labor groups as well as newspapers representing a wide variety of political views and readership sounded vigorous calls for the restriction of "the filthiest and most objectional class" of immigrants as a means of preventing the entrance of the cholera germ into the United States.[18] Despite occasional warnings against making "the unlucky steerage passenger the scapegoat for every evil that may menace these shores,"[19] the

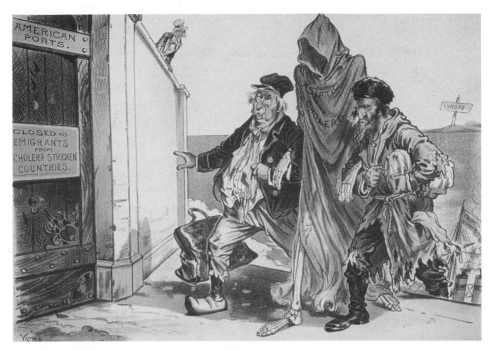

Figure 4.1. "They Come Arm in Arm." *Judge* 23 (1892).

most frequently singled out vector of cholera that year were the Russian Jews. Recalling the 1892 typhus fever epidemic and its association with Russian Jews, the *New York Herald* suggested that there was a clear equation of danger: Immigrant Russian Jews equaled cholera.[20] The *New York Times* not only warned its readers about the danger of "ignorant Russian Jews"; it also called for an absolute prohibition on their immigration.[21] In a similar vein, *Judge* magazine published a cartoon depicting a Russian Jew, complete with a hooked nose, fur-lined cap (*strimle*), forelocks (*payess*), and beard, and a German immigrant walking into the U.S. Immigration Office, arm in arm with a shrouded skeleton labeled "Cholera."[22]

Calls for suspending immigration as a cholera preventive were voiced not only by journalists, immigration restrictionists, and working-class Americans fearful of losing their jobs to the new wave of immigrants; public health and medical experts such as Drs. William Osler, Howard Kelly, and Henry Hurd of the Johns Hopkins Hospital, U.S. Surgeon General Walter Wyman, New York City Chief Sanitary Inspector Cyrus Edson, and Dr. E. O. Shakespeare of Philadelphia were all strongly in favor of "shutting the gates" to immigrants.[23]

Awaiting the "cholera ships" sent from Hamburg and headed toward New York Harbor in late August were the Tammany Hall-appointed health officer of the Port of New York, members of the New York City board of health, and physicians from the U.S. Marine Hospital Service. What ensued was a political struggle among federal, state, and local public health officials, all of whom wanted control over managing the public's health. At the center of this event was the imposition of a strict quarantine over the Port of New York, a measure that among other things resulted in the confinement of thousands of healthy people on steamships and isolated islands; the harsh treatment of immigrants; the detention of prominent New Yorkers who had the misfortune of traveling on the same boats; and the involvement of President Benjamin Harrison, who for the first time in American history issued an executive order that brought immigration almost to a halt for a period of five months.

Cholera at the Gate

As health officer of the Port of New York and chief of the quarantine station, Dr. William T. Jenkins faced a daunting task in the late summer of 1892. Even as early as mid-August, Jenkins appeared destined to have public scorn thrust upon him no matter how he handled the coming cholera epidemic. If he was too strict in halting the flow of commerce and immigration to America's busiest port, the business and immigrant communities would voice vigorous complaints; on the other hand, if even one case of cholera passed through his carefully guarded gate, there was the risk that panic would erupt in New York City and Jenkins would be named the culprit. As the eminent New York surgeon and health commissioner Joseph D. Bryant noted, Jenkins' abilities were "the key to the situation." [24] In the midst of his difficulties in administering the quarantine of New York Harbor, Dr. Jenkins later admitted to the press that he often wished he had refused the job of health officer, a position he accepted in order "to be rid of the dreary lot" of being deputy coroner and "to devote more time to home interests and to the education of his children." [25]

Born in Holly Springs, Mississippi, on October 25, 1855, Jenkins earned a bachelor's degree from the University of Mississippi in 1877 and an M.D. degree from the University of Virginia in 1879. Following a few months in private practice in Oxford, Mississippi, Jenkins enrolled in the postgraduate course at the Bellevue Medical School in New York, where he studied clinical, hospital, and dispensary treatment for eighteen months. Jenkins' most important career move had little to do with his medical studies. Instead, it was his marriage in March 1881 to Elizabeth Roberts Croker, the sister of Tammany Hall Boss Richard Croker, which was most responsible for his subsequent success in obtaining professional employment. In the beginning of the new year, 1882, Jenkins' powerful brother-in-law presented the young physician with an appropriate Tammany wedding gift: a position as deputy physician in the New York City Coroner's Office, an important entry-level professional post in the control of patronage politics.[26]

Jenkins served in the Coroner's Office for almost a decade, where he worked as an anatomist and autopsy pathologist.[27] In 1891, after a Democratic sweep in the state elections, Boss Croker pulled more strings to appoint Jenkins to the far more lucrative and powerful position of health officer of the Port of New York, a job that offered an annual salary of $12,500 plus a spacious home on Staten Island. Members of Tammany Hall were overjoyed at the summary dismissal of the previous health officer, Dr. William Smith, a former Republican state assemblyman.[28] Other New Yorkers were not nearly as enthralled with Croker's patronage appointment. As E. L. Godkin pointed out from his editorial pulpit in *The Nation*, the appointment of Jenkins as health officer was motivated by nepotism and machine politics rather than professional qualifications. Jenkins may have developed into a fine anatomic pathologist during his ten years as deputy coroner, but his training, which was distinctly lacking in any expertise in sanitation, public health, daily clinical practice, hospital administration, maritime health, or bacteriology, was not consistent with the qualifications necessary to be health officer of a busy American port in 1892.[29]

Jenkins' tenure as health officer, it may be recalled, began rather badly. Confirmed for the position by the New York State Senate on January 30, 1892, he began his responsibilities on February, 3, 1892. One week later, the typhus fever epidemic broke out on the Lower East Side. Although Jenkins was eventually cleared of any responsibility for the epidemic — the immigrants actually landed three days before he took office — many New Yorkers, infuriated at the nepotism displayed in his appointment, directed their scorn at him. Resolving not to let any more scandal taint his office, Jenkins immediately instituted a two-month policy of extensive inspection and disinfection of all Russian Jews entering the Port of New York.[30]

Between August 31 and October 14, some 997 vessels, 80,777 passengers, and thousands of tons of baggage and cargo were inspected by the quarantine staff.[31] Each morning that fall, as Jenkins walked across the grounds of the quarantine station from his home to his office, he was followed by a legion of newspaper reporters shouting questions, accusations, and catcalls at him while he tried to perform his difficult duties. Pledging to "deal with

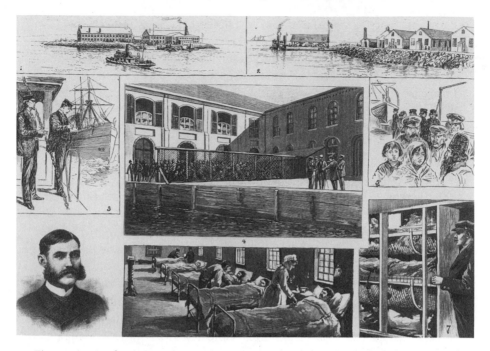

Figure 4.2. At the quarantine station, New York Harbor (including a portrait of William Jenkins, M.D. [*lower left*]). *Key: 1,* Hoffman Island; *2,* Swinburne Island; *3,* on board the doctor boat; *4,* consultation of the doctors on Hoffman Island; *5,* immigrants on the SS *Moravia; 6,* hospital, Swinburne Island; *7,* disinfection room, Hoffman Island. *Harper's Weekly* 36 (1892).

every vessel as its condition warranted without discrimination," Jenkins also vowed "no chances would be taken, no matter who the passenger was or how he traveled." [32]

In reality, at the New York quarantine station there was a distinctly different means of handling the steerage-class immigrants and the first- or second-class cabin passengers, who for the most part were wealthy Americans returning home from summer travel abroad on the same ships departing from the same infected ports. On August 30, 1892, the health officer announced that only steerage passengers would be inspected, disinfected (with both steam and bichloride of mercury solution), and detained for approximately five days for observation. Jenkins' policy allowed cabin-class passengers to have their baggage fumigated on board ship, be briefly medically examined, and then be allowed to land without delay via steamer to the various line piers. [33] In a similar acceptance of the belief that the real public health danger to New York was the flow of East European immigrants, the U.S. Treasury Department's Immigration Bureau continued to allow transatlantic traffic from the acknowledged cholera-infected port of Hamburg after August 26 provided that the steamship companies placed steerage passengers in slow-moving older vessels and cabin-class passengers in the faster, newer ships. This segregation by vessel allowed the rapid passage and inspection of the cabin class at their final destination and, in the event of a cholera outbreak on a particular steerage steamer, the immediate detention of immigrant passengers aboard the slower ships.[34]

The first "pest ship" to arrive in New York from Hamburg was the aging, slow-moving steerage steamer, the SS *Moravia*.[35] After only two days at sea, several passengers, mostly Russian or Polish Jews and a small group of German and French immigrants, developed the hallmark symptoms of cholera: sudden cramping, vomiting, and violent diarrhea, progressing rapidly to dehydration, coma, and death. Between August 19 and 29, twenty-two passengers died; two passengers were acutely ill when the ship arrived in New York Harbor late on the evening of August 30, 1892. Twenty Russian Jewish children under the age of ten years were among the twenty-two deceased.[36] A correspondent for the *Yiddishe Tageblatt* reported that during the voyage the dead, along with their few possessions, had been hastily wrapped in canvas and urgently thrown overboard "as if they were dead birds or garbage" in the presence of their horrified, grieving parents. The reporter concluded

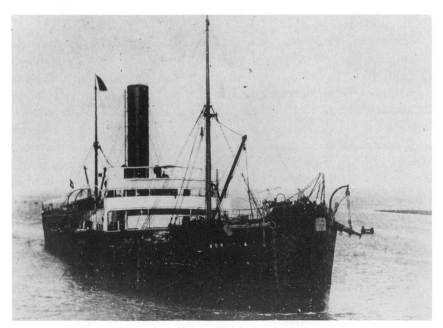

Figure 4.3. SS *Moravia*. From Steamship Historical Association of America, University of Baltimore.

that the gruesome story of the *Moravia* passengers locked up on board with the *szvartzer immigrantka* (the black immigrant of death) — cholera — "makes your hair stand on end." [37]

The *Moravia* dropped anchor at the New York quarantine station late Tuesday night, August 30, but was not boarded for inspection by Jenkins' deputy health officer, Dr. A. T. Tallmadge, until midmorning on August 31. Tallmadge was reported as being "almost taken off his feet" when the ship's surgeon, Dr. David Israel, informed him of the illness and death that had taken place during the voyage.[38] The deputy health officer ordered the ship to moor at Gravesend Bay and sped to Quarantine to inform his chief that cholera had just arrived in the bay.[39] Later that afternoon, when Jenkins boarded the vessel to investigate the situation, Dr. Israel insisted that the illness aboard the ship was not due to Asiatic cholera but the more benign "cholerine," brought on by the immigrants' debilitating "long railway trips" to Hamburg.[40] Dr. Jenkins found a far more compelling explanation for the alarmingly high death rate of 91 percent among the "cholerine victims": The ship's log stated that the water drunk by the passengers during the voyage had been drawn directly from Hamburg's Elbe River — which, by the time of the *Moravia*'s landing, was admitted by Hamburg officials to be heavily contaminated with the *Vibrio cholerae*.[41] Jenkins quickly ordered the strict quarantine of all the *Moravia*'s passengers, regardless of health status, for as long a period as necessary.

Only a few miles from the quarantined Russian Jews, journalist Abraham Cahan sat in the *Arbeiter Zeitung* newsroom on Ludlow Street on the Lower East Side. He was spending the evening translating the American newspaper dispatches of the cholera epidemic into Yiddish. Cahan became troubled by the consequences of conflating East European Jewish immigration with the importation of a deadly epidemic. The young journalist pushed aside his translation work and began to compose a pointed editorial that described his fears of being forcibly removed from his home and quarantined simply because he was a Russian Jew who was experiencing a mild case of diarrhea during a cholera epidemic:

> Believe me, my dear readers, that as I sit and write these words I have thoughts that you or any good person should not know. You see, I am suffering at present from a terrible headache and a ripping pain in my *kishkas* (gut). And while I believe that the cholera cases being reported in the daily newspapers are only fabrications, I know that I am quite lucky that these newspapers or the lying doctors do not know about my complaints. If they did, I can imagine the result: headlines saying "A case of cholera has shown itself in New York" would be trumpeted around the world. And who knows what they would do to me; they might send me away to a lazaretto, or choke me for several days in the smoke of fumigants,

in order to disinfect me as they refer to it in the scientific language, or they might burn all of my belongings and clothes—so that I have none to wear for a holiday—all that cholera might not spread itself.[42]

The President and the Health Officer

President Benjamin Harrison was once described by his commissioner of civil service, Theodore Roosevelt, as a "prejudiced, obstinate, timid, old, psalm-singing Indianapolis politician." Chauncey DePew, the former U.S. senator and president of the New York Central Railway, called him "the finest legal mind in the history of the White House." The chief executive, more often referred to behind his back as "the White House Iceberg," was spending the summer months of 1892 at Loon Lake, New York, when the news of the *Moravia*'s arrival broke.[43] Preoccupied with his wife's precarious health brought on by the end stages of pulmonary tuberculosis and by what would prove to be an unsuccessful presidential reelection bid that November against Grover Cleveland, Harrison initially hoped to let the local and state authorities in New York handle the matter as quietly and quickly as possible.[44]

Benjamin Harrison was long a proponent of "restricting the immigration of Russian Hebrews" and stated so emphatically in his final two annual addresses to the U.S. Congress.[45] But despite this decidedly nativistic viewpoint, Harrison announced from his cottage on Loon Lake in late August that his presidential powers were extremely limited in terms of halting immigration as he had been repeatedly asked to do over the last days of August in order to resolve the cholera problem in New York Harbor.

The president communicated frequently via telegraph with Secretary of the Treasury Charles Foster, U.S. Attorney General William H. Miller, and Supervising Surgeon General of the Marine Health Service Walter Wyman, consulting them on the issue of immigration restriction as a cholera preventive. The president's men suggested that the key to federal intervention for the prevention of cholera's entry was not in the language of immigration per se. Instead, it rested in the existing federal statutes pertaining to the regulation and administration of quarantine.

The U.S. Congress had passed quarantine legislation as early as 1796, but the first real attempt to create a national system of quarantine regulations was enacted on April 29, 1878, in response to a yellow fever epidemic. The law empowered, first, the National Board of Health and then, from 1883, the supervising surgeon general of the Marine Hospital Service to prevent ships with infected immigrants or those vessels originating out of infected ports from landing at American ports without a medical inspection and, if nec-

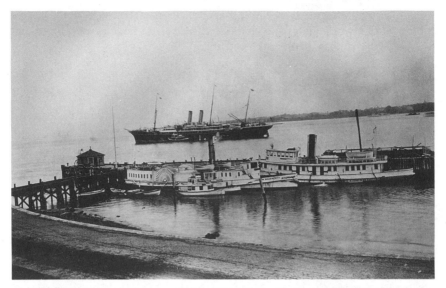

Figure 4.4. Ships in quarantine, Port of New York. Courtesy United States History, Local History, and Genealogy Division, the New York Public Library, Astor, Lenox, and Tilden Foundations.

essary, a period of quarantine. The act weakened the federal government's authority, however, by stipulating that the federal regulations enacted could not "conflict with or impair any sanitary or quarantine laws or regulations of any state or municipal authorities." Issues of public health and quarantine, consequently, remained largely a municipal or state responsibility for most of the nation during the nineteenth century. Attorney General Miller offered an alternative interpretation of the last clause of the 1878 act as meaning that the federal government could, in the case of an emergency, add additional quarantine restrictions to a specific port provided it did not interfere with the original length of quarantine imposed at the local or state level.[46]

Late on the evening of August 30, while dining at the Westchester County, New York, estate of his vice presidential running mate Whitlaw Reid, Harrison received a telegram from Attorney General Miller. Describing the situation in New York City as a potential crisis, Miller urged the president to return to Washington immediately. Harrison complained to Reid about the rigors of the presidency and instructed him to arrange the fastest possible transportation to the capital.

Reid's best surrey, horses, and driver were quickly enlisted to take the president to the White Plains station, where a train would take him to New York City and thence to Washington. The coachman decided to take a short-cut through Reid's estate, a road described by one reporter as "hilly, wooded, dark and dangerous." At a particularly steep hill, one of the horses suddenly shied and the coach veered off the road, throwing the president in "a heap from the wagon."[47] Slightly shaken, bruised, and soiled, Harrison leaped back into the vehicle and urged the driver to continue. A special train sped the bedraggled president from White Plains to New York City's Grand Central Station at a speed of a "mile a minute." There, the determined chief executive boarded his special railway car, the *Nimrod,* which left the station for Washington at 12:30 A.M. on September 1.

That morning, Harrison called his cabinet to the White House to discuss the matter. After lengthy discussion, the Harrison administration elected to circumvent the politically sensitive issues of immigration restriction and state rights by encouraging individual states to agree to quarantine all immigrant ships for a period long enough to make their transport too expensive for the shipping companies to bear. Such a move would force the shippers into discontinuing steerage passages. If this were not possible, it would be followed with an executive order mandating a national twenty-day quarantine rule based on Attorney General Miller's interpretation of the existing federal quarantine law.[48] The originator of this roundabout method of quarantine was the surgeon general, Walter Wyman. Wyman had long hoped to control quarantine policy on a federal rather than local level in order to achieve more uniformity in regulations across the nation. Wyman's critics, on the other hand, such as former supervising surgeon general of the U.S. Marine Hospital Service and then professor of medicine at Rush Medical College, John Hamilton, accused him of simply using the epidemic to increase his jurisdictional powers as surgeon general. The impending cholera epidemic would give Wyman such a chance.

Only hours before President Harrison returned to Washington to endorse his plan, Wyman sent a "confidential telegram" on September 1 ordering a junior Marine Hospital Service officer, W. A. Wheeler, stationed at Ellis Island, "unofficially" to call on the New York City board of health president Charles G. Wilson. The objective of the visit was to encourage the local authorities to impose a twenty-day quarantine on all vessels entering New York as an economic "method of stopping immigration during the cholera epidemic."[49] Ironically, Wyman directed his junior officer to contact the wrong bureaucrat. The president of the New York City board of health had no jurisdiction over maritime quarantine or other health matters of the port. Municipal health officials could only become involved if cholera appeared in the city itself or if invited by the health officer of the port.

After meeting with his cabinet and the surgeon general on the morning of September 1, President Harrison endorsed Wyman's Marine Hospital Service circular establishing quarantine restrictions on immigration as a means

of preventing cholera's entry into the United States.[50] The circular characterized immigrants and the ships carrying them as "a direct menace to the
public health" and ordered a twenty-day quarantine on all such ships. The
twenty-day period applied only to steerage immigrant passengers and not
to cabin passengers, even if they originated from the same infected port,
such as Hamburg, and had nothing to do with bacteriological concepts of
cholera culture diagnosis or incubation periods. It was explicitly conceived
as a financial brake to halt steerage immigration.[51] Simply put, no steamship
line could afford the huge costs of having its vessels docked in Quarantine
for a period of three or more weeks at the expense of $5,000 or more per
ship per day in lost income and fees to care for the detained passengers as
mandated by federal law. Consequently, the steamship companies would be
forced to halt all steerage transportation in order to avert an economic disaster.[52] The document attempted to smooth over potential concerns about the
state rights issue by allowing individual states to impose a longer quarantine
period if they considered it necessary. Finally, the circular gently suggested
that the aid of the U.S. Marine Hospital Service would be speedily and generously provided, if requested.

The federal government's preferential treatment of cabin-class passengers originating from infected ports elicited relatively few complaints in the
native-born American press. One lone editorial writer for the New York Tribune, however, did express his dismay at the "quarantine by class": "The
mere fact that a traveler is able to pay for a cabin passage should be held to
indicate that he has a charmed life and is incapable of transmitting contagious diseases passes comprehension."[53] Overall the public response to the
quarantine circular was supportive. Indeed, many local boards of health and
nativist groups around the country magnified the order with subsequent attempts to construct quarantines around Russian Jewish immigrants.

A common quarantine effort mounted by local health officials in Baltimore, Boston, Chicago, Cleveland, Detroit, Port Huron, and Montreal was
the police blockade of railroad stations or ports of entry to all "Russian
Hebrews."[54] Similarly, the New York City Health Department instituted
daily inspections of the neighborhoods where Russian Jews lived or worked.
Among the most prominent cholera dragnets during this period were the
sanitary police raids and closure of several kosher chicken slaughterhouses
on the Lower East Side.[55] The New York Tribune warned its readers that New
York City was practically inviting a visitation of cholera in the form of immigrants: "The people in the Hebrew, Italian, and Chinese Quarters . . . cause
the Health and Street Cleaning Departments more trouble than any other
class of people in the city."[56]

In contrast to the wide support by the American public accorded the Harrison quarantine circular and its primary target, steerage-class immigrants, the health officer of the Port of New York reacted to the president's order with great hostility and a bellow that could be heard from "Quarantine to the Battery."[57] Jenkins' first point of contention had to do with the state rights issue: Who had domain over safeguarding public health in New York Harbor? The health officer was quick to insist that the existing laws clearly stated that he held supreme control over *all* health issues in the Port of New York, but especially in terms of setting the length of quarantine for cholera suspects, which many medical experts estimated at about five to eight days rather than the twenty-day figure selected by Surgeon General Wyman.[58] A second reason had to do with the age-old issue of local "turf" and patronage. At the close of the nineteenth century, local or state government remained in control of public health matters. The strains of this shifting outlook of public health from local to national were showing themselves in New York Harbor that fall. Tammany Hall and the Democratic Party of New York were in control of the quarantine station in 1892, a source of great power and influence over the commerce of the Port of New York. Boss Croker instructed Jenkins to resist every attempt by the federal government to erode Tammany's stronghold over the port.[59] Finally, there was the issue of personal pride. Since his assumption of power, Jenkins, perhaps unfairly, had been ridiculed by the press as the beneficiary of nepotism, "incompetent," "inexperienced," and unfit for his position. Consequently, he was anxious to prove his critics wrong and emerge as a successful and respected health officer.[60]

Jenkins challenged the president's intrusion into his jurisdiction with great vigor. Armed with an opinion by the New York state attorney general, S. W. Rosendale, that completely denied the federal government's claim to applying any quarantine regulations in New York Harbor, Jenkins insisted that he alone had "the power to release vessels and passengers whenever he thought it proper."[61] The day after Harrison's quarantine circular was announced, Jenkins was asked to inspect the SS *City of Berlin,* which carried steerage passengers as well as cabin-class passengers. The ship originated from Antwerp, where cholera was not considered to be a problem. After the inspection, Jenkins declared all the passengers to be healthy and gave the ship clearance to land, completely disregarding the president's twenty-day quarantine order. The U.S. collector of the Port of New York, the stalwart Republican and Harrison appointee Francis Hendricks,[62] refused to allow the ship to land and sent her back to Quarantine. Jenkins, in turn, gave the ship clearance.

This dramatic illustration of the confrontation between state and federal rights culminated in an almost comic sending of the unfortunate steamship up and down the bay between the quarantine station and the port collector's cutter, as each official refused to recognize the authority of the other.

The situation was finally resolved by the end of the day when Secretary of the Treasury Charles Foster, Surgeon General Wyman, and a hostile press urged the health officer to back down and cooperate fully with the federal effort to contain cholera. Perhaps more convincing was the midnight meeting Jenkins had with Boss Richard Croker, who ordered Jenkins to give in to the Harrison order since it was "neither wise judgment nor good politics" to fight with the president of the United States.[63]

Although a temporary accord was achieved between the federal government and Dr. Jenkins, largely through the conciliatory efforts of the Treasury Department, many federal officials privately wondered what was motivating Jenkins' angry and confrontational behavior during the public health emergency.[64] Specifically, the accord gave Jenkins complete control over those vessels that left their ports on or before September 1, 1892, while all vessels leaving after that date would be handled by the Marine Hospital Service. Federal assistance, in the form of personnel and disinfecting equipment, Foster delicately hinted in his public statements, would be provided for Jenkins' efforts, if the health officer would only cooperate with the federal health agency.

CHAPTER 5

"Knocking Out
the Cholera!"

At the Quarantine Station

September 3, 1892, was a difficult day for Dr. Jenkins and his small staff. Jenkins had at his command two experienced physician-inspectors routinely assigned to the station and two inexperienced ones he had hired five days earlier in anticipation of the cholera epidemic. The remaining workers at Quarantine consisted of two doctors (one a training or resident physician) at each of the contagious disease hospitals on Swinburne and Hoffman Islands, two disinfectors, ten nurses, and a number of aides and laborers.[1] In addition to supervision of the inspections of twenty incoming vessels, the annoyance of "yellow journalists" anxious to make their deadlines, visits from politicians and physicians advising and often criticizing Jenkins on quarantine matters, and an exhausting work schedule of twenty-four-hour shifts, Jenkins' meager resources would be further tested with the arrival of more unwanted cargo in the form of cholera. Entering the port that day were two ships that left Hamburg after German officials finally acknowledged cholera to be at large in that city.[2] The first steamship to arrive on the morning of the 3rd was the *Rugia*, an antiquated steamer carrying 436 immigrant passengers in her steerage and 91 first-class cabin passengers. During the voyage five adults in steerage died of cholera and another four steerage passengers (three adults and one eight-year-old boy) were acutely ill on arrival. As Jenkins and his assistant were examining the passengers of the *Rugia*, news came from another deputy health officer, Dr. Frank Sanborn, that more cases of cholera were breaking out among those detained aboard the *Moravia*.[3]

The fire of cholera in the harbor was fanned with the afternoon arrival of the *Normannia*. The *Normannia* was the pride of steamship magnate Albert Ballin's Hamburg-American fleet. Built in 1890, the twin-screwed, 8,242-ton, five-hundred-foot-long, sleek steamship could sail across the Atlantic in only six and a half days.[4] On this voyage, the ship carried 300 crew members and 482 immigrants assigned to "the cramped, airless steerage."[5] Four decks above, in first- and second-class cabins, were 573 passengers, including Lottie Collins, the British music hall star about to make her American debut singing the international hit song, "Ta-ra-ra Boom-de-ay," the eminent editor E. L. Godkin, U.S. Senator John McPherson of New Jersey, Mr. and

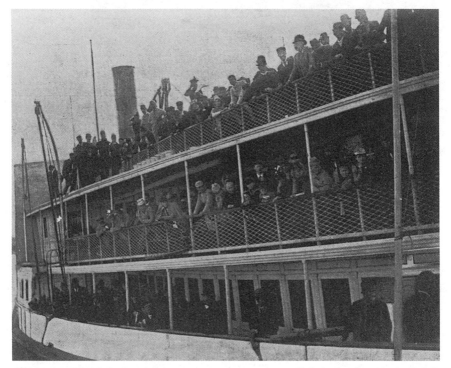

Figure 5.1. The imprisoned *Normannia* passengers off the wharf at Fire Island. *Harper's Weekly* 36 (1892).

Mrs. Courtland S. Van Rensselaer, and theatrical manager A. M. Palmer. At Quarantine, the *Normannia*'s captain announced there were four ill steerage passengers in the sick bay suffering from copious diarrhea, five deaths in the steerage, and, most significantly, a death each among the first- and second-class compartments during the voyage; the likely cause was cholera. Jenkins, unimpressed by the celebrities and socialites aboard the *Normannia*, vituperously announced that he had little choice but to quarantine the entire vessel, including the cabin class, given the failure of the cholera to obey President Harrison's circular and restrict itself "solely to the steerage compartment."[6]

The *Normannia*'s first cholera death was a fifty-seven-year-old German named Carl Hegert traveling in a second-class cabin for a visit to relatives in the United States. Stricken with diarrhea and vomiting on August 28, Hegert was dead by August 29 after a twenty-four-hour period of "great agony." The passenger was thrown overboard before "the body turned cold," along with his personal effects. Despite the urgency to rid the ship of the patient and the speed with which his rather specific symptom pattern brought about his demise, the cause of his death was vaguely listed as "bronchitis and diarrhea" instead of admitting to a cholera case in the second-class compartment.

Perhaps more gruesome was the experience of the Hornishes, a family of Russian Jews fleeing Odessa. The family was temporarily detained in a Hamburg boarding house where they might have contracted cholera before obtaining steerage passage on the *Normannia*:

> Little Ottlie Hornish died the day after Hegert, and the distracted parents, after watching her tiny body sink in the waves, had to hurry back to their other two children, Willie and Selma, three and five years old respectively. Both were looking very white and were beginning to complain.[7]

Five other deaths were reported to Jenkins during the declaration. Four were Russian Jewish children traveling in the steerage compartment. Of more concern to Jenkins was the death of Jacob Heynemann, a forty-five-year-old German, first-class passenger with diabetes who developed symptoms of vomiting and "copious diarrhea" followed by a rapid death on August 31. His condition was diagnosed as a diabetic coma despite the ship physician's open admission that Heynemann's symptoms were far more consistent with cholera than end-stage diabetes and its metabolic complications.[8] As health officer, Jenkins could not afford to take the chance of ignoring the distinct possibility that cholera had appeared in the cabin class, and he ordered an unspecified detention for all passengers. Before the ship's release almost two weeks later, fifty-three more people succumbed to cholera; meanwhile, the other 1,300 healthy passengers and crew members were imprisoned aboard the same five-hundred-foot-long ship.[9]

How cholera traversed the rather strict lines of class aboard the *Normannia* is not readily obvious. First- and second-class passengers were relatively free of physical contact with the steerage-class immigrants, who were not allowed out of their restricted squalor during the voyage. There were, however, common denominators that could facilitate the appearance of cholera across class lines. Some of the older ships that carried exclusively or primarily steerage passengers, such as the *Moravia,* had only one source of water supply; if the ship's drinking water was contaminated with the cholera germ, presumably all who drank from that source had a good chance of contracting the disease. Such a scenario probably explains the high rate of cholera among the steerage passengers aboard the *Moravia.*

The situation on board the *Normannia,* whose water supply was recorded as not originating from the Elbe River, may have had a different origin. On this vessel, cholera attacked only a few people in the cabin class, several members of the crew, and even more steerage passengers some three to five days after leaving Hamburg. This time frame suggests the possibility that many of the victims consumed cholera-tainted water drawn from the Elbe River in Hamburg *before* embarking for America. Socioeconomic conclusions from Richard Evans' study of the 1892 cholera epidemic in Hamburg suggest that the poorer the traveler, the more likely he or she was to lodge temporarily in a boarding house in Hamburg that had both inadequate sanitary facilities and contaminated water supplies.[10] Such a finding would explain the higher rate of "susceptibility" to cholera seen among the immigrants. Varying rates of disease distribution on the different decks of the ship can also be explained by the levels of sanitation, private toilet facilities, and personal hygiene. The greatest rates of morbidity and mortality were seen among the steerage immigrants and the crewmen, while the disease was well contained among the cabin class where sanitary conditions were markedly better than those available for the crew and steerage passengers.

What can the historian use to reconstruct a physician's understanding of cholera more than a hundred years ago? Almost certainly Jenkins had read the standard textbooks of medicine, such as William Osler's *Principles and Practice of Medicine,* although we have no proof of this. Periodicals that the quarantine officer received and, we assume, read, such as the *Weekly Sanitary Report of the U.S. Supervising Surgeon General* and the New York City Health Department periodicals, might also be used as evidence. Perhaps more useful is Jenkins' own *1892 Annual Report of the Health Officer,* in which he discusses cholera as he understood it during the fall of 1892. Jenkins' report includes a well-written summary of cholera's bacterial etiology (*Vibrio cholerae),* mode of transmission (hand-to-mouth contact with the excreta of those infected via food, water, or fomites), and its incubation period (two to five days).[11] Further, Jenkins discussed the futility of imposing arbitrary periods of quarantine, such as the Harrison twenty-day order, since different infectious diseases had markedly different time courses of incubation and contagiousness. Twenty days, he reasoned, would be both an individual and economic hardship not mandated by the relatively brief incubation and active period of cholera. Jenkins also made a point of reminding the public about the germ's egalitarian willingness to infect anyone who did not take proper sanitary precautions against it.[12]

But it was not Jenkins' (or any other health official's) scientific understanding of cholera that would primarily guide the management of the epidemic. Bacteriological knowledge had far less to do with the proceedings of the 1892 epidemic than politics and nativistic sentiments. Public health, after all, begins with the public, and issues that concern large numbers of people's health become political almost by definition. There remained, therefore, a striking tension in Jenkins' management of the quarantine throughout the epidemic between the modern science of bacteriology and the politics of nativism.[13]

As a public show of the type of "scientific management" he employed at Quarantine, Jenkins sought the advice of four of the most eminent bacteriologists in the nation. He first consulted with the New York physicians and bacteriologists T. Mitchell Prudden and Hermann M. Biggs on September 2. Prudden was professor of pathology and director of the bacteriological laboratory at the College of Physicians and Surgeons, Columbia University. As Robert Koch's first American student in 1885, he was also widely regarded as the man who brought bacteriological methods to the United States. In his consultation with Jenkins, Prudden prescribed rather liberal policies, including isolation of only those who were actually ill with cholera and paying more attention to rigorous medical inspection and the disinfection of baggage than a mass quarantine of immigrants. Jenkins, perhaps fearful of associating with the anti-Tammany bacteriologist and worried that the passage of one cholera-infected immigrant on his watch would result in his dismissal, alienated Prudden by ignoring his advice. At the same meeting, Hermann Biggs, the bacteriologist and pathologist to the city of New York Health Department and a pioneer in employing cholera culture techiques at maritime quarantine stations, offered Jenkins the use of his scientific advice and laboratory staff. But Dr. Jenkins declined these generous offers and offended Biggs as well.[14]

The following afternoon, Jenkins invited the noted pathologist and bacteriologist William Henry Welch of the Johns Hopkins Hospital for a visit to Quarantine. The rotund Professor Welch arrived for a brief visit on September 3, before catching "the 3:50 P.M. train for Norfolk (Connecticut)." Welch, like Prudden, was a vociferous opponent of quarantine and the enforced isolation of immigrants for cholera. Welch advised Jenkins to cooperate with the federal public health authorities, Prudden, Biggs, and the others, in order to pool all the best resources into one concerted effort. Perhaps more of an imposition for Dr. Welch were Jenkins' frequent statements to the press that he was following the advice of Welch. In reality, Jenkins' policy contradicted Welch's by attempting to maintain supreme control over the port with the limited involvement of the U.S. Marine Hospital Service or the municipal Health Department. Also disconcerting to Welch was being cited as Jenkins' authoritative source on quarantine policy in the daily press accounts of the epidemic. In a private letter to Prudden, Welch angrily described Jenkins' actions "as a spectacle of inhumanity without parallel in civilized lands in modern times."[15] Welch was so angry about being misquoted by Jenkins that he sat for two interviews in Baltimore with a "personal representative of Mr. E. L. Godkin" for the *New York Evening Post*. In the interviews, Welch denied any association of his theories on quarantine with the practices of the health officer of the Port of New York.[16]

Another advisor Jenkins publicly consulted on quarantine matters during the epidemic was Lieutenant Colonel (U.S. Army Medical Corps) George M. Sternberg, M.D. Few men were more qualified to be a scientific advisor on quarantine, disinfection, and cholera prevention in 1892 than Sternberg. A career soldier and physician in the U.S. Army, Sternberg found a way to indulge his scientific curiosity by conducting numerous experiments in bacteriology and by writing the *Manual of Bacteriology*, the first American textbook of its kind.[17] During the 1892 cholera epidemic, Lt. Col. Sternberg found himself temporarily stationed in Brooklyn as attending physician and examiner of recruits. Sternberg was also moonlighting as the director of the Hoagland Laboratory, which was affiliated with the Long Island College Hospital in Brooklyn and housed one of the premier bacteriology laboratories in the nation.[18]

Well-versed in almost all aspects of bacteriology of the 1890s, Sternberg had studied yellow fever and malaria epidemics for the army, discovered the most common causative organism of bacterial pneumonia (*Streptococcus pneumoccus*), advanced the technique of producing photomicrographs of bacteria including the tubercle bacillus, and addressed a number of other important issues in experimental methodology and immunity.[19] At the Hoagland, in 1892, Sternberg turned his attention to the practical matter of disinfecting passengers, ships, and cargos for cholera.[20]

In a lecture given before the Medico-Legal Society of New York on April 12, 1893, about six months after the epidemic, Sternberg addressed the significant and wide-reaching question, "How can we prevent cholera?" Most of Sternberg's lecture discussed the readily available and effective measures of preventing cholera's entry by means of chemical disinfection, careful medical inspection, and bacteriological cultures of the feces of those stricken with cholera. He asserted that such methods were ultimately responsible for defeating the cholera in New York during the 1892 epidemic. Yet his lecture included a few subtle jibes against William Jenkins' administration of the quarantine and a rather paternalistic, if not nativist, view of immigrants:

> In the present state of scientific knowledge relating to the prevention of this and other infectious diseases, someone is always responsible for the introduction and spread of such diseases. . . . It seems that there should be some legal responsibility and some punishment for neglect of duty on the part of public officials entrusted with these important public interests. Under certain circumstances ignorance is a crime. We cannot hold the immigrant criminally responsible for the injury he

ignorantly inflicts upon us when he lands upon our shores and sows cholera germs contained in his intestinal evacuations; but we must protect ourselves from this danger, and those who are charged with the duty of guarding the public health should be held to a strict accountability for any unjustifiable ignorance or neglect.[21]

What is so striking about the statements made by those involved in managing the 1892 cholera epidemic is the singular faith they shared in modern sanitary science and bacteriology to save the day. The precepts of public health as informed by germ theory were heralded by Jenkins and many other public health officials, politicians, and newspapers to be the modern savior of New York City from the scourge. Similarly, secondary historical accounts of the events emphasize the vital role bacteriology played in the successful control of the 1892 epidemic.[22] But despite declaring that he was being advised by the most prominent bacteriologists in the country, Jenkins rarely followed their scientific or practical advice let alone the widely published sanitary precautions against the spread of cholera he often cited in his statements to the press. Instead, Jenkins' quarantine in New York Harbor seemed more in keeping with traditional responses to the diseased: a scapegoating of those afflicted or perceived to be at risk of disease, namely, East European immigrants.

Yet even if Jenkins had wanted to follow all of the arduous public health precautions he quoted, he could not have done so; there were simply too many immigrants passing through a too poorly manned and outfitted quarantine station in too brief a time. For example, the medical inspection of immigrants and cabin-class passengers was probably too cursory throughout the crisis, relying on physical appearance rather than culture or laboratory diagnosis. In the sixty seconds of scrutiny allotted to each passenger by an overworked health officer, without the use of routine stool cultures, it was entirely possible for a passenger incubating cholera to pass inspection. Moreover, even though Jenkins hired bacteriologist John M. Byron for the epidemic, the other duties concurrently assigned to Byron as physician on Swinburne Island made it impossible for him to perform a systematic culture analysis of the thousands of passengers arriving daily. Both the Marine Hospital Service and the New York City Health Department offered their finest bacteriologists to assist in such an analysis at Quarantine, including Hermann Biggs, Edward K. Dunham, T. Mitchell Prudden, and Joseph Kinyoun, but Jenkins continued to refuse their help. Nor is it likely, even if their help had been accepted, that it would have made a huge difference in the events. Given the level of technical skill necessary to cultivate bacteriologic cultures in 1892, the lack of a large corps of highly trained bacteriolo-

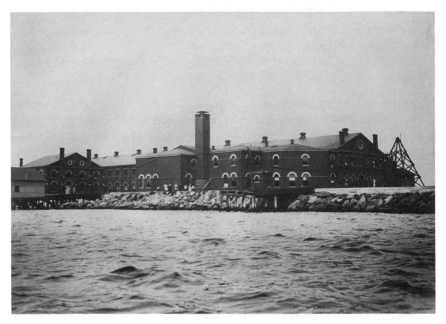

Figure 5.2. Quarantine station, Hoffman Island. Courtesy United States History, Local History, and Genealogy Division, the New York Public Library, Astor, Lenox, and Tilden Foundations.

gists, and the sheer volume of clinical material to be analyzed, it is doubtful that cholera culture diagnosis would have played a significant role at Quarantine in the fall of 1892.[23]

Perhaps the greatest obstacle to effective disease control among the detained immigrants was the acute lack of hospital and detention facilities at Quarantine. By September 3, three days into the epidemic, all nine hundred beds at Quarantine's two lazaretto islands, Hoffman and Swinburne, were filled with suspect immigrants who had already arrived, and Jenkins had not yet even inspected all the entering ships for that day. Worse still was the forced lumping together of cholera victims and suspects, in close proximity, on the same islands—without the proper sanitary precautions to ensure that cholera did not spread. Overcrowded Hoffman and Swinburne Islands with their paltry laundry, sleeping, and dining room facilities were excellent breeding grounds for a secondary cholera epidemic. The water supply for the immigrants detained was unprotected and was not monitored with cholera cultures, making it a ready source of contamination throughout the epidemic. The privies were filthy and contaminated with feces. Another problem was the sanitary habits of the immigrants themselves. The Special Physicians' Advisory Committee on Quarantine for the State of New York

Chamber of Commerce was outraged during its inspection of the quarantine facilities as it witnessed several immigrants defecating from the vantage point of a cliff onto other immigrants washing their clothing on the shore directly below—a novel but definite risk for the spread of cholera and other gastrointestinal infections. Jenkins, too, openly admitted to the press that the overcrowding on Hoffman and Swinburne Islands and the possibility of an outbreak of cholera among the detained immigrants were major hindrances to his administration of the quarantine.[24]

As often occurred in nineteenth-century America, the necessary facilities and organization to handle epidemics were inadequately provided for before the fact.[25] The administration of the quarantine station of the state of New York during the Gilded Age well mirrors this pattern of benign neglect. Almost the exact same committee of eminent New York City physicians asked by the same Chamber of Commerce in 1888 to evaluate the quarantine station warned about every deficiency that subsequently became a problem in epidemic management in 1892.[26]

By September 5, only five days into the epidemic, Jenkins became so desperate for bed space that he wired the Chamber of Commerce repeatedly for assistance. With the very real possibility of cholera crossing decks during

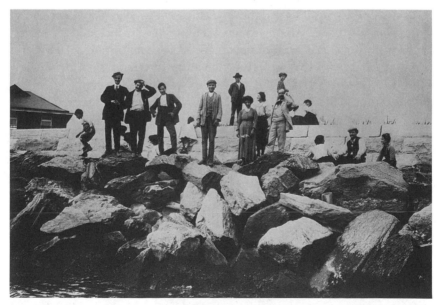

Figure 5.3. Immigrants at the New York quarantine station on Hoffman Island during the 1892 epidemic. Courtesy United States History, Local History, and Genealogy Division, the New York Public Library, Astor, Lenox, and Tilden Foundations.

the voyage of other incoming ships, the health officer was forced to make another unpopular executive decision: All detained passengers, irrespective of class, would remain on board the ships they came in on until it was certain that the cholera had died out.[27]

This was an undesirable solution for many reasons. Most obviously it held the risk — though small if proper sanitary precautions could be insured — of exposing even more healthy people to cholera. The *New York Herald* articulated this worry in a miasmatic editorial on the risks of combining all the passengers, steerage and cabin, together "to breathe the same air."[28] But even if the cholera sanitary codes as they existed in 1892 were strictly adhered to — which they were not — the psychological effects of being quarantined on a ship moored out in the middle of the vast New York Harbor, exacerbated by the fear of contracting cholera, could hardly have been borne well by the passengers aboard these ships or their waiting families and friends. In fact, the emotional torture of the enforced wait for freedom or for signs and symptoms of cholera was one of most frequently voiced recollections of those quarantined passengers who wrote letters to the editors of many of the New York City newspapers during the epidemic.[29]

Redoubling his efforts in response to the widespread criticism of his performance and his open antagonism toward President Harrison, Jenkins divided his attention between administrating a complex quarantine in the world's second largest port and the distracting circus of activities occurring daily in the Lower Bay. Among some of Jenkins' orders included the steam disinfection of all mail from the quarantined passengers and a New York City police harbor patrol to prevent the entry of quarantined passengers who might jump overboard and attempt to swim into the city. One of the oddest victims of Jenkins' quarantine regulations was a statue of Christopher Columbus that arrived on the Italian cargo ship *Garigliano*. A gift from Italian Americans to the city of New York in commemoration of the four hundredth anniversary of the "discovery of America," the statue spent a night quarantined on Hoffman Island before its final delivery at the head of Eighth Avenue, Columbus Circle.[30]

Perhaps Jenkins' most trying adversary was not the cholera itself, but the press. In a reverse of Shakespeare's axiom about those fortunate in having "greatness" thrust upon them, Jenkins seems, with hindsight, almost destined to have been steamrolled by failure and ignominy. In search of the journalistic "scoop," hundreds of reporters descended upon New York Harbor and the quarantine station in tenacious droves. Day and night, dozens of tugboats bearing the banners of the morning and afternoon dailies, filled stem to stern with newspapermen, circled the quarantined ships and shouted questions at the passengers hanging over the rails. There were wide-

spread rumors of the yellow journalists going so far as to smuggle themselves on board the quarantined ships. In response to these rumors, Jenkins
threatened to "shoot at sight" any reporter who attempted to have contact,
including verbal exchanges, with those on the quarantine ships. Jenkins'
vituperous personality combined with his controversial management of the
epidemic made him an especially easy target for the New York City reporters. Consequently, his public image, as a result of what became worldwide
newspaper coverage, was that of a bumbling, hot-headed incompetent.

"Ta-ra-ra Boom-de-ay"

It was the cabin passengers of the *Normannia* who captured the attention of
the press covering the event. For millions of readers throughout the nation,
these wealthy, socially prominent passengers came to symbolize the cholera
epidemic and the quarantine as both *Harper's Weekly* and *Frank Leslie's Illustrated Weekly* scrambled to feature them on their covers. Their detention and
treatment soon became a spectacle described around the world.[31] Perhaps
the angriest diatribes, directed at both the act of being quarantined and the
man who ordered the detention, emanated from the pen of E. L. Godkin.
Firmly established as an important political commentator, journalist, and
editor, Godkin served the dual role of founding editor of *The Nation* and
managing editor of the *New York Evening Post*. Never one to mince words
during his professional career, Godkin was an ardent critic of Boss Croker
and Tammany Hall domination over New York City government.[32]

From his first-class stateroom aboard the *Normannia*, Godkin composed a
series of scathing articles entitled "Letters from the *Normannia*," which were
published in newspapers across the country. Among other things, Godkin
ridiculed Jenkins for not knowing that cholera "is exceedingly rare among
the well-clothed, well-fed and cleanly class in any country." The editor's outraged invective quickly deteriorated into a vendetta against the health officer.
In one "letter" Godkin accused Jenkins of fabricating a diagnosis of cholera
among the cabin passengers as a means asserting his power. In another dispatch, he charged Jenkins with failing to provide adequate food, water, and
medical care, and neglecting to remove dead bodies from the ships for periods greater than twenty-four hours. On September 12, Godkin complained
about the "wretched table service" aboard the ship, which completely ruined
one of the few pleasures he managed to find in Quarantine: sitting down to
a rare beefsteak. Perhaps the most acute sign of Godkin's perception of his
quarantine was an article he penned for the *North American Review* entitled
"A Month of Quarantine." In real time, Godkin and the other *Normannia*
passengers were quarantined for thirteen days.[33]

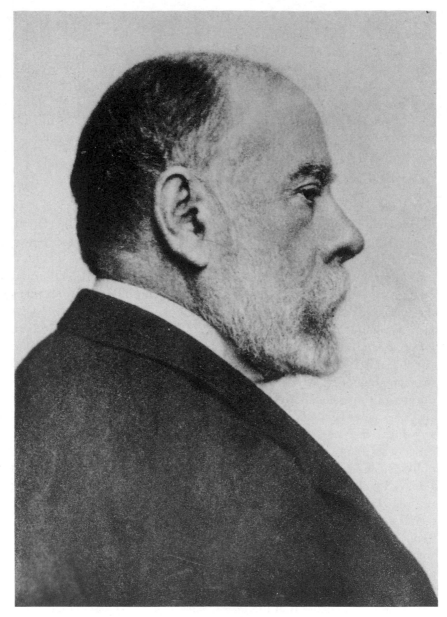

Figure 5.4. E. L. Godkin, editor of the *Nation*. Brown Brothers.

Lottie Collins was another prominent passenger on board the quarantined *Normannia*. The British music hall performer was scheduled to make her American debut at the Standard Theatre in New York for a three-month engagement beginning September 1 at $1,200 per week. Her fame was largely dependent on her charming stage presence, her vigorous dancing, and her association with the song "Ta-ra-ra Boom-de-ay!"[34] Collins, like her shipmate Godkin, was particularly adept at self-promotion during the cholera epidemic. She shouted out a series of interviews, over the side of the ship, that were featured on the front page of the *New York World* and quoted in many others. But E. L. Godkin and Lottie Collins were just a few of many cooperative sources for the press. Indeed, the vocally strident *Normannia* passengers were so cooperative in yelling interviews to the floating mob of media journalists that the newspaper reporters nicknamed them the "Kickers" after the trademark "high-kicking dance step" of Lottie Collins.[35]

The needs and concerns of the quarantined immigrants, when compared to the cabin-class passengers, were of less concern to most New Yorkers. Yet there were voices of opposition. Columbia University president Seth Low was so outraged by this negligence that he reminded his colleagues at the New York State Chamber of Commerce that the quarantine efforts must pay attention to those traveling in steerage as well as cabin class.[36] The East European Jewish community of New York City expressed their outrage over poor sanitary conditions and inadequate medical attention for the immigrants in Quarantine most loudly in the Yiddish press, where it had little impact outside its readership circle primarily because it was written in Yiddish, a language not understood by most Americans. For example, Abraham Cahan's *Arbeiter Zeitung* for September 9, 1892, angrily accused Jenkins of subjecting immigrants to "murderous injustice and inequalities" that were only augmented by language and cultural differences between the fearful foreign patient and the overworked physician.[37]

As an additional source of aggravation for Jenkins, the federal government maintained an active presence in the bay. A report of the illegal entry of ships around Long Island, via the Sound and exiting through Hell Gate to the Hudson River piers, prompted the secretary of the treasury Charles Foster to order U.S. Navy vessels to patrol all possible points of entry to New York—in defiance of Jenkins' objections to federal interference.[38] The federal government also began the construction of a "national quarantine station" on September 9 to be located at Sandy Hook, New Jersey, a foot of land projecting out into the head of the Lower Bay. Jenkins, still bristling at the presidential quarantine circular, angrily interpreted these actions as a message that the federal government might usurp his authority. Nevertheless,

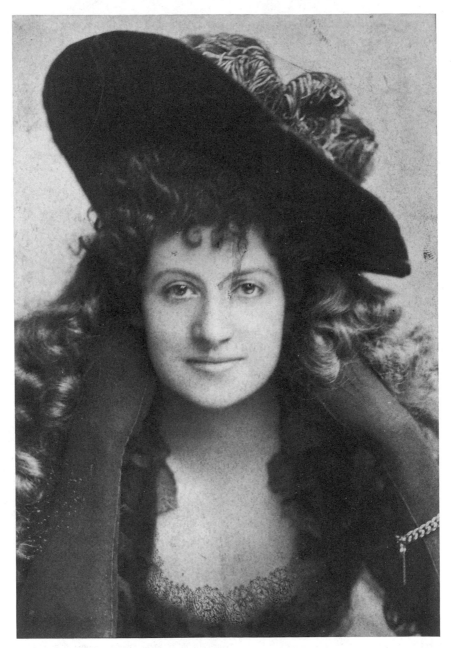

Figure 5.5. Lottie Collins. Courtesy Billy Rose Theatre Collection, New York Public Library for the Performing Arts, Astor, Lenox, and Tilden Foundations.

when he was questioned about these developments by the press, Jenkins insisted that he was cooperating fully with the Treasury Department.[39]

As more and more ships stacked up in Quarantine over the next few days, Jenkins and his staff had even less success in attempting to maintain healthful sanitary conditions. Nor was Jenkins successful in checking the progress of cholera in the steerage compartments of the *Normannia, Rugia,* and *Moravia,* and two newly arrived ships, the *Scandia* from Hamburg and the *Wyoming* from Liverpool.[40] Responding to the mounting cholera statistics and a critical press, who charged that Jenkins was leaving people to die aboard ships, the beleaguered Jenkins again reversed his decision and announced he was moving the healthy *Normannia* cabin-class passengers to more suitable detention quarters, while their steerage counterparts would be isolated and observed on the overcrowded Hoffman Island. But instead of waiting to take the federal government's offer to transfer the cabin-class passengers to the nearby, newly built facility at Sandy Hook, which would be ready for occupancy on September 20 (the following week), Jenkins hastily arranged for the purchase of a hotel on distant Fire Island, thirty miles from the eastern border of New York City.[41]

The purchase of the Surf Hotel on Fire Island as a temporary quarantine station by the state of New York has the whiff of Tammany patronage. The hotel's owner, David S. Sammis, negotiated the deal through Boss Richard Croker and Long Island businessman and Tammanyite Edward S. Stokes, who is best known to American historians as the murderer of the notorious Gilded Age financier, James Fisk Jr. Stokes arranged to be the Surf Hotel's caterer during the stay of the quarantined passengers as part of the deal. The hotel was purchased by the state of New York, on the personal check of Governor Roswell Flower, another Tammany member, for $210,000, some $100,000 more than the property was worth in 1892. At an interest rate of 6 percent, Governor Flower succeeded in simultaneously playing the hero and making a buck out of the transaction.

Again, we rely on the pen of Yiddish journalist Abraham Cahan for a description of Jenkins' class-oriented quarantine as the health officer prepared to transport the 1,300 cabin-class passengers and immigrants to, potentially, markedly different fates, let alone accommodations:

> The wealthy gentlemen, poor things . . . raised such a cry about the 'unpleasantness' which they had to undergo, that the entire wealthy class took to weeping and wailing over their plight. From all sides came the cry to have mercy on the poor rich people, and provide more conveniences for them in Quarantine. When rich people scream, there is, of course, an immediate response. . . . For the rich first class passengers they bought a fine hotel, and for the paupers, they put up military tents on a field in which they set up beds.[42]

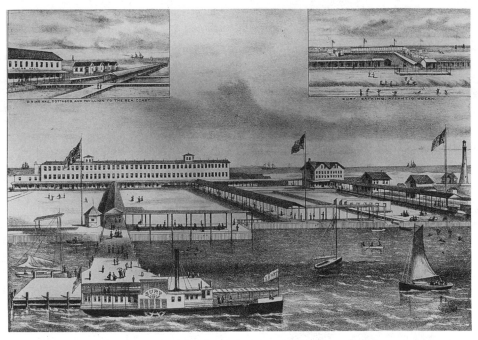

Figure 5.6. Surf Hotel, Fire Island Beach, D. S. S. Samis and Sons Proprietors,"
ca. 1882. From *The History of Suffolk County, New York* (New York: W. W. Munsell,
1882), pl. opp. p. 23 of the section entitled "The Town of Babylon." Collection of the
New-York Historical Society.

Jenkins arranged for the Kickers to be placed aboard a pleasure boat without sleeping facilities, the *Cepheus,* to be taken up the harbor to Fire Island
just off the Long Island shore of Islip. Stormy weather resulting in treacher-
ous conditions, which some wags ultimately blamed on Jenkins,[43] prevented
the transfer of the Kickers to Fire Island on the evening of September 11
and resulted in a twenty-four-hour delay aboard the *Cepheus.* The following morning, when the weather cleared, the sleep-deprived passengers were
finally taken to Fire Island.

Waiting for them at the docks was an enraged mob of several hundred
residents from Islip armed with muskets, guns, rifles, and "anything that
could be charged with powder in any expectation that it would explode."
This "seething throng" was prepared to repel the "pest ship's" passengers
from landing using any means necessary.[44] The Islip residents, referred to as
the "Clam Diggers" in the press, were described by Robert A. Caro as dis-
trustful of anyone "from away"—particularly New York: "Many boasted that
they had never been [to New York]—they feared that its 'foreigners,' hordes
of long-haired Slavs, hook-nosed Jews, and unwashed Irishmen, would de-

scend on and befoul their beautiful beaches at the first slackening in their vigilance."[45] Consequently, the Clam Diggers, aided by the Islip board of health, the sheriff of Islip, and an injunction from a local judge, were prepared to prevent the landing of any person from a cholera-infected ship on Fire Island.[46] The grounds of the court injunction, in an ironic twist of Jenkins' complaints about federal government interference, were based upon the rights of a local government to control issues of public health within its

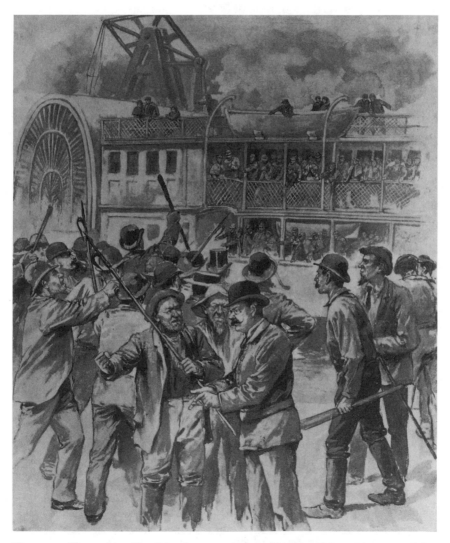

Figure 5.7. The mob at Fire Island preventing the landing of the passengers of the *Normannia* from the steamboat *Cepheus. Frank Leslie's Illustrated Weekly* 75 (1892).

own boundaries. The residents, fearing both the proximity to cholera suspects and cholera's possible effect on the local fishing industry, flatly rejected the pleas of Governor Roswell Flower and a number of other officials, reminding them that there were plenty of areas in New York City that could be used as a "quarantine station."[47]

The Kickers were forced to stay aboard the *Cepheus* two more days, without food, water, or comfort, anchored in Great South Bay opposite the Fire Island docks where the Clam Diggers stood guard. The less than stoic passengers, angry enough from nine days of detention aboard the *Normannia,* complained that they suffered "every imaginable horror" at the hands of the health officers and the Clam Diggers. Despite impassioned appeals for mercy and understanding by Senator John McPherson (R-N.J.) from the bow of the pleasure boat, the armed Clam Diggers only howled and jeered in return. Later that evening, some of the Clam Diggers attempted to burn down the Surf Hotel and destroy the telegraphic lines. Comparing the mob to "Ku-Kluxers," one correspondent for the *New York Herald* could "hardly believe" that such a spectacle of "lawlessness calling the law to its assistance" was occurring in the Empire State.[48] On September 13, New York Governor Roswell Flower, refusing to obey the local district judge's injunction, ordered two regiments each of the National Guard and the Naval Reserve to assure the safe landing of the Kickers. The Clam Diggers backed down with the organized show of force and within a matter of hours the *Normannia* passengers were comfortably checked into the hotel as the ship's band of German stewards played "Columbia, the Gem of the Ocean." When asked how she survived the threat of mob rule over the two days, Lottie Collins stiffly replied: "When I think of those ruffians, I long for a pistol."[49] The *Normannia*'s cabin-class passengers were finally released by Jenkins on September 14; their suites at the Surf Hotel were quickly filled with first-class passengers from the other detained ships.

The landing of the Kickers did little to ease Jenkins' overwhelming responsibilities or the widespread scorn directed at him. The daily arrival of new ships, more cases of cholera breaking out among steerage passengers aboard the Hamburg-American steamers *Scandia* and *Wyoming,* and Jenkins' desperate search for more beds were among the many issues the health officer juggled.[50] Insults, demands for his removal, and harsh criticism no matter what plan he adopted became the prevailing response to Jenkins' efforts. For example, as a result of the stresses of his job, even the state of Jenkins' mental health began to be reported in the daily press. He was described by the *New York Herald* as "a bitter, broken, crying, sobbing, prostrated man."[51] Jenkins was retrospectively diagnosed by one of the premier specialists in the treatment of mental illness in Gilded Age America, Dr. Allan McLane Hamilton, as suffering from "nervous demoralization."[52] As late as Christmas of 1892, Jenkins' troubled "state of mind" was discussed in the *New York Tribune*:

> Disquieting rumors come from quarantine every day now about Dr. Jenkins and his state of mind. Yesterday it was said that he has committed to memory the line "where the wicked cease from troubling and the weary are at rest," and that he repeats it over and over again, sadly, as he stands on the wintry shore amid dead leaves and blighted golden rod with the leaden sky above him. Not even the memory of the autumn's cholera days when he was a monarch absolute, and by his majestic bearing struck terror into the hearts of the bold seamen, can cheer him now.[53]

Cholera in the City

As cholera raged in the harbor during the first two weeks of September, the level of panic among New Yorkers intensified. Daily newspapers and popular magazines devoted almost entire issues to the coverage of the epidemic and filled additional space with articles on cholera panaceas and the recollections of past epidemics in New York City.

A number of widely publicized announcements were made by the New York City Health Department with conscious effort to allay the public's fear. A comic example of this public relations campaign came in response to the rumor that fish caught in New York Harbor or near the quarantined ships were tainted with cholera. The city's fishmongers soon saw their sales plummet. The business-minded Tammany health board president Charles G. Wilson dismissed the rumors as false and announced to the press that he had absolutely no intention of banishing fish from his dinner table. Wilson did add, however, that proper cooking was necessary in order to ensure that the fish was completely safe for consumption.[54]

The Health Department made ample use of the advance warnings they received throughout August of cholera's likely path to the United States. Unlike the public health officials in Hamburg, who failed to act quickly and competently, the health officials in New York City were, at least, one step ahead of the epidemic in terms of public health education efforts.[55] The New York City board of estimate and apportionment granted an additional $10,000 to increase the woefully inadequate facilities of its contagious disease hospitals. Further funding was allotted to outfit a floating barge cholera hospital, employ additional sanitary inspectors and policemen, and create one of the world's first municipal diagnostic bacteriological laboratories under the helm of the newly appointed city pathologist and bacteriologist, Hermann M. Biggs.[56] City merchants and citizens contributed an additional $200,000 to an Epidemic Fund organized by the New York State Chamber of

Table 5.1 Cases of Asiatic Cholera in New York City, 1892

Case No.	Date of Report	Name	Age	Sex	Race	Marital Status	Land of Nativity
1	Sept. 6	Charles McAvoy	32	M	W	Single	Ireland
2	Sept. 10	Peter Callahan	30	M	W	Single	Ireland
3	Sept. 11	William Wiegmann	52	M	W	Married	Germany
4	Sept. 11	Sophia Wiegmann	63	F	W	Married	Germany
5	Sept. 12	Minnie Levinger	20 mo.	F	W	Single	U.S.
6	Sept. 12	Adolph Levinger	42	M	W	Married	Hungary
7	Sept. 13	Charles Beck	35	M	W	Married	Germany
8	Sept. 13	Charlotte Beck	31	F	W	Married	Germany
9	Sept. 18	John Knox	31	M	W	Married	Ireland
10	Sept. 19	Lewis Weinhagen	56	M	W	Married	Germany
11	Sept. 29	Joseph Miller	45	M	W	Married	Germany
12	Sept. 18	**		M			

Source: Ann. Rep. N.Y.C. Health Dept., 111–21, 179–80.

*All cases, except for nos. 2, 6, and 7 were confirmed as cholera using bacteriological culture methods. No. 2, which was most probably cholera, was embalmed before autopsy analysis commenced.

**No. 12 occurred in New Brunswick, N.J., not in New York City; the New York City Health Department analyzed the case.

Time in U.S.	Job	Residence	Result*
8.5 yrs	Plasterer	879 Tenth Avenue	Died at home, Sept. 6, 1892.
4 mos	Stableman	318 East Forty-Seventh Street	Died at home, Sept. 10, 1892.
30 yrs	Butcher	768 Eleventh Avenue	Died at home, Sept. 10, 1892.
32 yrs	Housewife	768 Eleventh Avenue	Died at home, Sept. 11, 1892.
life	Minor	411 East Forty-Sixth Street	Died at home, Sept. 11, 1892.
2 yrs	Laborer in tripe factory	411 East Forty-Sixth Street	Recovered. No cultures done.
32 yrs	Butcher	1764 Second Avenue	Recovered. No cultures done.
30 yrs	Housewife	1764 Second Avenue	Died at home, Sept. 13, 1892.
3 days	Sailor/ fireman	*Nevada*	Died as ship was docked at the Hudson River piers at West Twenty-First Street, Sept. 18, 1892.
7 yrs	Coachman	14 First Street	Died at Reception Hosp., Sept. 23, 1892.
10 yrs	Potato dealer	255 West Twenty-Ninth Street	Died at home, Sept. 29, 1892.
	Boatman	New Brunswick, N.J.	Died in N.J., Sept. 18, 1892.

Commerce.[57] Other preparations included bacteriological and chemical analyses of the Croton aqueduct water supply, city-wide inspections of public schools, street cleaning efforts, and the mass printing of hundreds of thousands of handbills in English, Yiddish, Hebrew, Chinese, Italian, Polish, and several other languages on how to avoid contracting cholera.[58]

Despite these efforts the municipal authorities, too, subscribed to the familiar equation: Immigrants equal cholera. The reliability of this formula increased when Health Department president Charles Wilson announced on September 14 that four cases of cholera had been discovered in the city. Most alarming to many New Yorkers was the admission that the first cholera death occurred as early as September 6 and the suspicion that some of the victims had close contact with immigrants.[59] The response of the Health Department was to inspect closely the neighborhoods populated by immigrants.

To be sure, the Health Department had to be especially vigilant for the possibility of infection breeding in the tenement districts of New York's East Side, which was widely known for its unsanitary living conditions and populated largely by Russian Jews, Italians, and Chinese newly immigrated from their respective native lands. Similarly, all efforts to track down the origin of these sporadic cases of cholera, reasonably, had as their endpoint a passenger or contaminated cargo from a "cholera-infected" port. But the following description of the Health Department's actual handling of the eleven cases that appeared in New York City between September 6 and September 29, 1892, reveals far more about its daily operations than do the public gestures of creating a new municipal bacteriology laboratory or holding frequent press conferences. Indeed, the tacit acceptance of steerage immigrants as the cholera vector and the resultant class-oriented quarantine effort, rather than the scientific principles of bacteriology, struck the major chord of the Health Department's administration of the crisis.

In charge of the city cholera efforts was the newly promoted sanitary superintendent Cyrus Edson, already known in the Yiddish-speaking New York community for his harsh handling of Jewish immigrants during the typhus epidemic of March 1892. On September 4, Edson ordered the "careful inspection" of 39,587 tenement houses on the Lower East Side because he determined the slums to be the "breeding places of the allies of cholera, as well as cholera itself." He divided the immigrant tenement neighborhoods of the Lower East Side into one-block-square "cholera districts" during the first week of September. Although cholera had not yet entered the city proper at that point, Edson ordered his large staff of physicians, nurses, and policemen to "hunt up all persons with intestinal diseases" in the immigrant districts.[60] Edson's cholera campaign during the first week of September extended to the closing down of kosher Jewish butchers on the Lower East Side for minor infractions of the sanitary code and the extensive search of "the haunts, drives, cellars, corners and closet abodes" where Russian Jewish and Italian immigrants were observed to "swarm." As a result, hundreds of immigrant tenement dwellers were evicted from their homes during these raids. No provisions for boarding these frightened, displaced immigrants were made by the city and many were forced into the streets.[61] One Yiddish journalist, writing in the Hebrew Trade Union's weekly *Arbeiter Zeitung,* noted with irony the disparity between the frantic actions of the Health Department during a cholera scare and their lax efforts regarding less spectacular public health problems, such as slum housing or tuberculosis, the rest of the year:

> The capitalist society has become clairvoyant. It knows its disasters. It knows their causes. But so far it has not mustered the might to prevent these causes. . . . The filth which grows in the dwellings of the poor and downtrodden develops and grows into the deadly bacillus just as a parent raises a child. The uncleanliness of these "little animals" [germs] cause communicable diseases such as typhus, cholera, and consumption. Today's capitalistic society wants to get rid of these bacilli but without changing the living conditions of the poor. These ends cannot be achieved without such changes; they [contagion, poor sanitation and living conditions] have grown up together.[62]

Most important to the city's cholera containment effort was the prompt response team of physicians, sanitary inspectors, and policemen arriving at any home where a suspicious case of diarrhea was reported. Once a case was reported, a black-wagoned, horse-driven ambulance rushed to the scene. If a Health Department ambulance parked outside a tenement did not create enough of a panic, surely the less than social visit paid by these rubber-suited officials did. Victims of cholera, if still alive, were placed in a large canvas bag with a drawstring around the neck for immediate removal to the Willard Parker Hospital. Amid the screams of their frightened relatives, the dead — a far more common result of cholera that fall — were wrapped in sheets saturated with a bichloride disinfectant and removed for autopsy and analysis at the city's newly installed bacteriological and pathological laboratory.

The homes noted to contain cholera, or some other suspiciously similar diarrheal disease, were disinfected, quarantined, and blockaded by the sanitary police. The names of the afflicted, and their newly quarantined families, were published by midafternoon when the evening dailies reached the newsstands.[63] Subsequent dispatches on the case histories of the unfortunates who actually developed cholera, their families, and rumors that those quarantined were attempting to escape appeared in the daily newspapers alongside lists of cholera victims in New York Harbor and at Quarantine on Hoffman and Swinburne Islands.

Perhaps the best means of detecting the distinctly different handling of

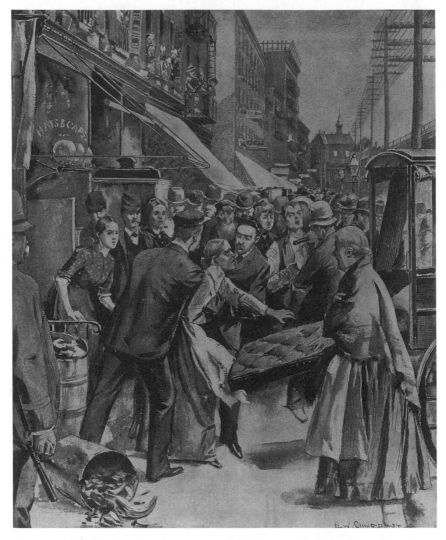

Figure 5.8. The cholera invasion — removing a suspected victim from a house on Second Avenue to the hospital. *Frank Leslie's Illustrated Weekly* 75 (1892).

immigrant cases and those of native-born Americans by municipal health authorities is to review the case histories of some of the unfortunate New Yorkers who developed cholera that fall of 1892. The Health Department spent considerable time during the first week of September denying that a man who died of diarrhea in the city was a victim of cholera. That man was a thirty-five-year-old Irish American plasterer named Charles McAvoy. He had lived in the city for over a decade. He was taken ill with mild diarrhea on the evening of September 5 and his symptoms rapidly progressed to a worsening and violent diarrhea, tremors, muscle cramping, and dehydration. McAvoy lost a wretched battle against the microbe and was dead before the sun set on September 6.[64] Newly graduated Dr. Robert Deshon, who was called in on the case, had never seen a case of cholera. On the evening of September 5, he consulted a senior colleague, Dr. Henry Robinson, who confirmed the young doctor's diagnosis of Asiatic cholera although no specimens were taken for bacteriological culture. Together, the physicians reported their empiric diagnosis to the Health Department, and McAvoy's body was removed to the Willard Parker Hospital that evening for an autopsy and bacteriological analysis to be performed the following morning, September 7, by Drs. Hermann Biggs and Edward Dunham.

There were few pathologists in the United States more qualified to verify or dispute a death due to cholera than Biggs or Dunham. Hermann Michael Biggs, canonized in the history of medicine as one of the pioneers of preventive medicine, was a well-trained, widely published pathologist and bacteriologist anxious to apply the principles of germ theory to the prevention of epidemic diseases. By 1892, Biggs was not only the New York City Health Department bacteriologist and director of the city's bacteriological laboratories, he was also professor of clinical medicine and therapeutics at his alma mater, Bellevue Hospital Medical College.[65]

Edward K. Dunham, while not as prominent as Biggs, was also extremely well qualified in the culture diagnosis of cholera. A graduate of Columbia University and Harvard Medical School, Dunham spent a year (1887) studying in Robert Koch's laboratory in Berlin, where he discovered and described the "cholera-red" or indole reaction, a method that greatly facilitated the biochemical identification of cholera bacilli. The following year Dunham returned to the United States, where he made great professional progress as a bacteriologist with the Massachusetts board of health and subsequently became professor of histology and bacteriology at the Bellevue Medical College of New York in 1891. Biggs was so impressed with the abilities of his younger colleague that he introduced Dunham to the honorable Hugh Grant, mayor of New York, as "one of the world's experts on cholera." Similarly, Sanitary Inspector Cyrus Edson declared in a letter to the U.S. Senate Committee on Immigration that Dunham's abilities were exceptional.[66]

Consequently, when Biggs and Dunham's official autopsy report of September 8, 1892, announced that "the anatomical lesions and microscopical appearances of the intestinal contents found in the body of Charles McAvoy . . . are those commonly found in so-called cholera nostras or sporadic cholera, and are not at all suggestive of cholera asiatica," the case was relegated by most observers to the status of a mere false alarm. Both health board president Charles Wilson and Sanitary Superintendent Cyrus Edson insisted that McAvoy could not possibly have Asiatic cholera. The two health officials characterized Dr. Deshon, the physician who made the diagnosis, as "incorrect and inexperienced."[67]

It was not until a week later that McAvoy's case was announced as "true Asiatic cholera" when his case history was anonymously inserted in the September 14 announcement with eight other cholera deaths. The delay in announcing McAvoy's true cause of death remains curious. Despite their confident statements that cholera cultures were reliable, simple to perform, and capable of giving an answer within thirty-six to forty-eight hours, Biggs and Dunham explained the several-day delay of their postmortem diagnosis by stating that they wanted to be absolutely certain.[68] Yet even with the confirmation of bacteriological evidence of cholera in McAvoy by Dr. T. Mitchell Prudden on September 10, the announcement was further delayed another four days. The New York Herald specifically asked the board of health, on its editorial page, why they were so unwilling to announce a case of cholera in the city instead of hiding behind the alibi of the necessity for "extra vigorous investigation."[69] One unidentified sanitary inspector for the Health Department cast his own aspersions on this delay of announcement:

> If Dr. Biggs can't cultivate bacilli in 48 hours, all I have to say is that I can. I was in the Loomis Laboratory for three years and I did it there in that time. Dr. Biggs has had three days and there is no result yet.[70]

Whether the delay was due to actual difficulties in performing cultures on scant intestinal materials, as later explained by Biggs and Dunham, or was an act of concealment on the part of the board of health in order to avoid the panic a cholera epidemic might produce, remains difficult to ascertain. One reporter for the New York Herald suggested another reason for the delay in announcement: There was great reluctance among the health officials to diagnose a case of cholera in an American citizen who had absolutely no evidence of being "caressed by immigrants."[71]

Another cholera victim announced in the press on September 15 was Peter Callahan, a thirty-year-old Irish stableman who worked on Cherry Street along the East River (near the Jewish Quarter on the Lower East Side). After Callahan's sudden death from diarrhea and dehydration on September 10, his body was quickly removed by a local undertaker for embalmment in contradiction to the New York City sanitary code regulations for contagious disease-related deaths. The premature chemical embalmment of Callahan's remains precluded any substantive autopsy or bacteriological examination. A strikingly different standard for confirming the cause of death was applied to Callahan's case than to McAvoy's. Callahan was a recently arrived immigrant from Ireland and frequently took his meals at some of the eating and drinking establishments on the Lower East Side where he worked. In Callahan's case, the immigrant linkage was enough to compensate for the lack of bacteriological evidence, as the Health Department officials immediately declared this unexamined case to be "true" Asiatic cholera.[72]

But the cholera case that most stimulated the attention of the Health Department and the imagination of those New Yorkers avidly reading about the crisis was the death of a twenty-month-old child named Minnie Levinger. Minnie, the only child of a Hungarian Jewish couple, developed symptoms of cholera on the morning of September 11 and, largely because of the relative ease with which a two-year-old child can develop dehydration, was dead in the arms of her mother by midafternoon.[73]

Although nine people died of cholera that September in New York City, without any clear pattern of distribution or transmission, it was the epidemiological history of the Levinger family that was most widely discussed in the press. Young Minnie, it was discovered, had close contact with four Hungarian Jewish immigrant girls who had just arrived in the United States on August 29 via Antwerp, where cholera was not reported to exist, and were boarding in the same tenement house as the Levingers. An elaborate hypothesis was proposed by Cyrus Edson that linked the child's death to the immigrant girls. The four immigrant girls were immediately quarantined for observation at the Willard Parker Hospital. They were released three weeks later after failing to develop any symptoms of cholera. Minnie's father, Adolph, himself an immigrant only a few years earlier, also developed diarrhea during this same period but his stools were never examined using bacteriological culture methods. Nevertheless, Adolph was classified by the health officials as a cholera patient who had the good fortune to recover.

Some of the yellow journalists reported rumors that the egress of cholera into the city was caused by butchers and grocers who were bringing food and provisions by tugboat to the various passengers quarantined in the harbor. This rumor gained significant power when it was revealed that Adolph Levinger was employed as an unskilled worker in a tripe and meat packing company on East Forty-fifth Street. Edson ordered his inspectors to search carefully all East Side butchers and food handlers for evidence of cholera.[74] Nothing untoward was found.

Ultimately, the immigrant searches and roundups were time-consuming blind alleys. As to an immigrant linkage, all but one cholera victim, Peter Callahan, had lived in the United States for more than a year; most had minimal, if any, contact with the path of cholera and lived in different parts of Manhattan. Hermann Biggs subsequently reported that no evidence was amassed, either epidemiological or bacteriological, which supported the theory that cholera was introduced into New York City or was spread by immigrants and food handlers.[75] How cholera entered the city remains a mystery. Not a few observers suggested that the microbe was imported into the city by health officials and newspaper reporters who had close contact with the "cholera fleet" and who may not have adequately washed before returning to Manhattan.

Despite public statements from Biggs that exonerated immigrants as the cholera vector, the Health Department's expensive manhunt for a scapegoat continued throughout the month of September. Cyrus Edson, on the other hand, angrily denounced Biggs' suggestions that public health efforts concentrate on more productive activities, insisting that "the germs must have come from Europe, some way, possibly in the bags of immigrants who escaped the disease or whose sickness in the city was concealed."[76] Similarly, the mayor of New York City, Hugh Grant, dismissed Biggs' contention that for an epidemic to be spread by immigrants there ought to be a number of cases of cholera among immigrants. Ignoring the fact that the few cases of cholera in New York City occurred among citizens of long standing without a clear epidemic pattern of distribution or spread, Grant announced that "the greatest source of danger to the City" was immigrants and he subsequently blamed New York City's public health problems on them.[77]

By September's close, however, it became clear that cholera in the city had been conquered.[78] Accordingly, searches for "index cases" and elaborate analyses of the possible entry and spread of cholera by immigrants became of less concern to New Yorkers. Perhaps, more characteristically, the hue and cry over cleaning up the Lower East Side and ameliorating its public health problems also lost its momentum and the preexisting conditions of squalor and filth there prevailed.

"Lessons of the Cholera"

On September 16, the last ships to have active cholera on board were placed under quarantine.[79] Both ships originated from Hamburg: a tanker named the *Heligoland* with two cholera deaths during its voyage, and the steamer *Bohemia* which, among several hundred Russian Jewish steerage immigrants, carried fifty-two active cases of cholera and the memories of ten cholera deaths.[80] The placement of these and other ships under Jenkins' quarantine, however, failed to prevent the further spread of cholera and measles among the steerage passengers.

The continued spread of contagious disease among the quarantined passengers was greatly scrutinized by the Special Physicians' Advisory Committee on Quarantine to the New York State Chamber of Commerce, which consisted of Drs. Stephen Smith, Abraham Jacobi, Allan McLane Hamilton, Edward G. Janeway, Hermann Biggs, Richard H. Derby, and T. Mitchell Prudden. In a particularly graphic section of their final report, the committee documented the toilet and sanitary facilities Jenkins had provided for the quarantined immigrants in his charge:

> Their faces and hands were soiled, their clothing dirty, the air in the place was foul, the floor was filthy. There are two water closets near the stern of the boat, accessible from the cabin; one on each side, each with three seats and pans. Adults and children used them promiscuously, the sick and the comparatively well, those with or without diarrhea. The closets, seats, covers and floors were offensive from soiling with filth and feces. The latter was widely distributed. On one set there was a large mass of diarrheal discharge. The pans were also foul. The doctor [Jenkins] assured us that these places were washed and disinfected twice a day, but that we had just come in a time when there might be an accumulation.[81]

Such gross inattention to sanitary issues and the isolation of cholera victims with healthy suspects, the committee report argued, were tantamount to a death sentence for all those quarantined.[82] Perhaps the committee's strongest charge was that the Jenkins quarantine was based more upon class issues than those of bacteriology and modern sanitary and isolation procedures: "It was a system of simple human storage under decidedly unfavorable conditions . . . with what seemed to be a feeling on the part of those in charge that those people all might justly be treated very much like cattle because the natural condition of many of them was that of desperate uncleanliness, and because many of them were accustomed to being herded like brutes."[83]

The combination of new cases of cholera appearing among the immigrants quarantined both on Hoffman Island and aboard the *Bohemia,* a limited physician force, no space to board these passengers, and harsh criticism of his work from just about everyone concerned with or following the epidemic left Jenkins with few options other than finally yielding all control to the U.S. Marine Hospital Service. Surgeon General Wyman arranged to transfer bacteriologist Joseph J. Kinyoun to take over disinfection and quarantine matters in the harbor. In a similar move, Secretary of the Treasury Foster ordered former Supervising Marine Hospital Service surgeon general and a harsh critic of Wyman, Dr. John B. Hamilton, to administer the national quarantine station (Camp Low at Sandy Hook, New Jersey) with the assistance of the larger Marine Hospital Service medical staff based at Ellis Island.[84] By early October, the epidemic in the harbor was declared over and the emergency public health effort was quickly dismantled.

The final tally of cholera cases during the 1892 New York City epidemic was minimal compared with the previous cholera epidemics in New York City during the nineteenth century or to the one going on throughout Europe

Ships	Port of Departure	Date of Arrival in New York	Date of Release from Quarantine	Transferred to SWINBURNE ISLAND				Deaths						
				With Asiatic Cholera	With "Light Cholera" (Diarrhea)	Cholera Suspects	TOTAL	At Sea, Cholera †	Swinburne Island ** — Cholera	Swinburne Island ** — Other Causes	Other Places in Port — Cholera	Other Places in Port — Other Causes	TOTAL DEATHS	Cremated at Swinburne
Moravia*	Hamburg	Aug. 31	All Steerage 9/23	–	–	–	–	22	–	–	1	2	25	3
Normannia*	Hamburg	Sept. 3	Cabin: 9/14 Steerage 9/19	12	6	18	36	5	6	–	6	1	18	13
Rugia*	Hamburg	Sept. 3	Cabin: 9/19 Steerage: 10/8	23	–	19	42	4	8	–	4	–	16	16
Wyoming*	Liverpool	Sept. 7	Cabin: 9/23 Steerage: 9/27	1	–	4	5	–	1	1	2	2	6	6
Scandia*	Hamburg	Sept. 9	Cabin: 9/21 Steerage: 9/29	11	2	13	26	32	1	2	7	2	44	12
Heligoland (tanker)	Hamburg	Sept. 14	Unloaded, went to sea	–	–	–	–	2	–	–	–	–	2	–
Bohemia*	Hamburg	Sept. 15	Cabin: 10/1 Steerage: 10/8	17	–	2	19	11	4	1	4	1	21	10
Totals	–	–	–	64	8	56	128	76	20	4	24	8	132	60

that same year. Forty-four immigrants, mostly East European Jews, died of cholera at the quarantine station; if one includes the seventy-six deaths that occurred on the boats en route to New York Harbor, the total increases to 120 deaths. Another nine deaths from cholera occurred in the city itself (Table 5.1).[85] And while every public official, from the U.S. surgeon general to the health officer of the Port of New York, declared that the handling of the epidemic was an unqualified success, aided largely by "the value of bacteriological examinations in combating disease,"[86] the preceding account suggests that the management of the operation depended far more upon issues of class and national origin than on the "value" of bacteriology.

The modern principles of bacteriology were only sporadically applied to the administration of the 1892 quarantine. To be sure, steam and chemical disinfection of all immigrants and rapid isolation of the ill contributed to the process of disease containment. Yet issues of cursory medical inspections of all passengers from infected ports, ineffective sanitation on the quarantine islands and ships, inadequate medical care for the afflicted, and the commingling of healthy suspects with cholera victims undoubtedly plagued Jenkins' quarantine. Such deficits were most likely responsible for the additional cases of cholera that appeared. For the overwhelming majority of New Yorkers who successfully protected themselves from the immigrant threat, matters worked out fairly well. The quarantined steerage passengers, on the other hand, were forced into a living nightmare or, in the case of the forty-four victims who died at Swinburne Island, worse.

It is difficult to factor in other policies or public health initiatives that may have contributed to the containment of cholera among immigrants in the harbor and its minimal spread into the city itself. Certainly President Harrison's twenty-day quarantine order was a helpful measure in that it significantly reduced the flow of immigrants into the United States and helped lighten Jenkins' overwhelming workload of medical inspection. Moreover, the unusually cool temperatures New York City experienced that fall hindered the spread of cholera,[87] as did the advance notice, by means of telegraphic communication, of the Hamburg epidemic and those ships most

Figure 5.9. Synopsis of sickness and deaths on board the Cholera Fleet, from the time of departure of the infected ships from European ports until the last case of Asiatic cholera was disposed of in lower quarantine, New York Bay. From *Ann. Rep. Comm. Quar.* (1892). *Notes:* *Had immigrants (steerage) on board; 5,300 immigrants were bathed and disinfected on Hoffman Island. †Cholera cases at sea were not confirmed by culture methods. **Other causes include measles, complications following childbirth, marasmus, etc. The *Scandia* and *Bohemia* had a measles epidemic among its children passengers in the steerage. Mothers accompanied their children to the contagious disease hospital on Swinburne Island.

likely to carry cholera. The rapid isolation of the cholera victims in the city by the Health Department and the quarantine of those victims' homes may have been an important factor in limiting the spread of cholera within the city. Finally, the state-of-the-art Croton aqueduct water filtration and supply system that provided fresh, clean, and cholera-free water for New Yorkers as opposed to the flawed system in Hamburg undoubtedly contributed a great deal to the protection of New York City's public health during this crisis.[88]

Of broader interest to the medical historian is the observation that even as late as 1892, many of the same pitfalls described in cholera epidemics that occurred during the early and mid-nineteenth century, ranging from political turf battles to the squandering of scarce resources, dominated the public health efforts while the new science of bacteriology took a back seat.[89] Administrative problems created by the separation of public health powers among municipal, state, and federal government, and the results of the New York state legislature's failure to fund properly or to rebuild the New York quarantine station despite urging by the medical community, became especially obvious during the epidemic. Given a quarantine facility deemed insufficient, arguments over who should control the epidemic's management, and a contentious health officer who had no specific training or experience in the fields of bacteriology and maritime public health and who received his job through patronage politics, chaos might have prevailed. Jenkins may have not been the ideal candidate for this important job, but it seems doubtful that anyone could have satisfied all of its requirements.

In many ways, the cholera epidemic of the fall was an amplification of the typhus fever epidemic that preceded it that winter. Like the later rounds of a game of poker, the stakes—and consequences—associated with the cholera epidemic became much higher. On an administrative level, of course, the typhus fever epidemic was far less complex than the cholera scare. All of the cases of typhus were discovered—after the fact of their eruption—within the confines of New York City and the epidemic's control was clearly vested with the New York City Health Department. In the case of the cholera epidemic, advance notice from Hamburg in the late summer strongly suggested that cholera was traveling the same route as the East European immigrant. This route included inspections divided among federal immigration and public health officials as well as New York State and New York City agents. Such a splintered approach to regulating immigration traffic and public health threats seemed almost destined to inspire the contentious politics that resulted that fall.

On a social level, cholera was one of the most feared epidemic diseases in nineteenth-century America. Although most cholera epidemics of this period did not cross the Atlantic Ocean, their paths of destruction and death were widely reported in American newspapers. These epidemics were not confined to New York Harbor or even New York City; a large number of North American locales, from Texas to Canada, were also visited by these early-nineteenth-century cholera epidemics. Moreover, each American brush with cholera during the nineteenth century was literally imported from foreign sources. Unlike more "domestic" contagious diseases, such as tuberculosis, diphtheria, and even typhus fever, the threat of cholera was capable of eliciting some of the strongest reactions from both the public health authorities and the lay public.

In terms of a scapegoat, the two epidemics were similar in that the principal target was the East European Jewish immigrant. Their differences were largely a matter of scale. The New York City Health Department's efforts to contain typhus among the East European Jewish immigrants who traveled on the *Massilia* or who had contact with them included many harsh public health measures, but these efforts were largely limited to those East European Jews living in or arriving in New York City. Both the rapid control of the epidemic and the people who were most severely affected—newly arrived *grine kuzines* on the Lower East Side—made the issue a local concern. Although Senator William Chandler attempted to make the typhus epidemic in New York City into a clarion call for immigration restriction legislation, the brief rise and fall of the episode did not sustain such an effort. Similarly, Dr. William Jenkins' temporary moratorium on Jewish immigration that Feburary and March at the New York quarantine station was unsustainable in the weeks following the close of the typhus epidemic. What increased the stakes of the cholera epidemic was the widespread perception that it was a national threat intimately tied to immigration traffic. The result of this perception was the Harrison quarantine order, which attempted to prevent the entry of cholera by means of immigration suspension for a period of five months. Ultimately, however, even the perceived threat of cholera's return was not enough to change U.S. immigration law permanently.

But the gravest problems with the New York quarantine efforts—on the local, state, and federal levels—were a too ready acceptance of Russian Jews as the source of cholera, inadequate medical care for those detained, and the elaboration of policies based upon considerations of class and scapegoating more than on deterministic principles of bacteriology. Ironically, as early as October 1892, German public health officials exonerated Russian Jews as the cholera vector, declaring they were "free even from suspicion of disease."[90] Many American public health experts agreed with this clean bill of health. Indeed, the cultural and religious practices of Orthodox Jews, the ethnic group most closely associated with the 1892 epidemic, include a rigorous code of personal hygiene. Dictates requiring ritual hand washing before meals and after defecation, dietary cleanliness, and prohibitions against drinking uncovered water and sharing cups may have played a factor in their "disease-free" status. Out of distrust of previous German assurances that Hamburg was cholera-free and a clear acceptance by the Harrison administration that the immigrants were the principal source of the cholera, the twenty-day quarantine order remained in place until February 1893. The result of this temporary quarantine was the reduction of immigration at major U.S. ports over five months to a mere trickle. In the rush to protect New York City and beyond from a cholera epidemic, the federal, state, and municipal officials developed a plan that intertwined prejudice, or fear, of the large numbers of emigrating Russian Jews, federally mandated moratoria restricting steerage immigration, preferential treatment to cabin-class passengers, and the harsh treatment of undesirable immigrants. Such was the state of the art of quarantine at America's largest port in 1892.

PART III

LEGISLATING QUARANTINE

Attempting to Restrict Immigration as a Cholera Preventive

No one believes that we can prescribe and enforce upon foreign governments and the steamship officers such measures as will keep the cholera from coming here. It will sail into our ports and overtax all the resources of our quarantine and health authorities, and will alarm and distress our whole people, even if it does not widely break into our borders and ravage our homes. If we allow immigration we are largely at the mercy of foreigners. If we suspend it our lives are in our own hands. In suspension alone is there any certainty of safety.

— *Senator William Eaton Chandler, 1893*

CHAPTER 6

Maintaining the Quarantine

Epidemics, historian Charles Rosenberg reminds us, typically end with "a whimper rather than a bang. Susceptible individuals flee, die, or recover, and the incidence of disease gradually declines. It is a flat and ambiguous yet inevitable sequence for a last act."[1] Not surprisingly, daily life in New York City during the winter of 1892–93 soon returned to its normal rhythms and pursuits.

In the daily newspapers and popular periodicals during the months immediately following the cholera epidemic, coverage of public health issues was soon relegated to the back pages of an issue, if it appeared at all. By late October, most American eyes were turned toward the presidential election, which ended on November 8 in Grover Cleveland's favor: Cleveland garnered 5,554,414 votes; Benjamin Harrison attracted 5,190,802.

Soon after the November elections, many Americans focused on abruptly turbulent Fall River, Massachusetts, where dozens of schoolchildren are reputed to have created one of the best-known pieces of Gilded Age doggerel:

> Lizzie Borden took an ax,
> And gave her mother forty whacks;
> When she saw what she had done
> She gave her father forty-one.[2]

On December 1, Lizzie Borden was indicted by the Bristol County, Massachusetts grand jury for the murder of her father and mother.

Yet this is not to say that all consideration of cholera in New York and other American cities died with the last case reported in late September. Surgeon General Walter Wyman and his staff organized an international surveillance of sanitary conditions around the globe connected by means of telegraphic communication. Many prominent cholera experts feared that once the winter chill had lifted, a new epidemic would appear—perhaps in Russia, perhaps in the Middle East—and, again, threaten to spread.[3] In Chicago, physicians and public health workers, anticipating the daily arrival of thousands of visitors to the Columbian Exposition of 1893, began laying plans to stand guard against the possible incursion of a "foreign case of cholera."[4]

Physicians, public health workers, journalists, legislators, and business-men met frequently in Washington, D.C., during the winter of 1892–93 to offer their opinions on how best to prevent a future epidemic at the nation's ports, borders, and immigration centers. Senator William Chandler forced the issue on January 6, 1893, by submitting a bill that distinctly made immigration restriction a public health policy.

Chandler's immigration restriction-cholera bill essentially called for a quarantine in its strictest medieval reincarnation: the absolute noninter-course with disease-ridden countries such as Russia, Italy, and other undesir-able European nations by means of suspending all immigration. The widely publicized association of East European Jewish immigrants with the New York City epidemics made this group the most conspicuous symbol of the nation's ailing public health that winter.

On the other side of the debate were those groups and individuals who remained in favor of open immigration and did not see the past threat of an epidemic as grounds for halting it. Many Gilded Age Americans still strongly believed in the nation's role as the welcoming land of the oppressed or, as Walt Whitman put it, a "teeming nation of nations."[5] Even among those who feared the new immigrants were many who, given the strong American tra-dition of welcoming newcomers, balked at the idea of suspending immigra-tion altogether. Other pro-immigration advocates pragmatically noted that the vast stretches of undeveloped America would remain so without readily available immigrant labor. Assimilated, naturalized immigrant Americans and their offspring were also vociferous proponents of open immigration; more important, naturalized Americans voted, and they demanded advo-cacy from their elected officials. These Americans consequently tended to favor solutions that strengthened and nationalized the medical inspection process but did not severely restrict immigration.

Epidemics and their quarantines are often used by contemporary ob-servers, artists, writers, moralists, philosophers, and historians as a form of communal retrospection—parables that ask how that particular community and its individual members reacted to the challenges of the crisis. In order to ascertain better how American society managed the dual problems of anti-immigrant sentiment and the threat of contagious disease during the winter of 1892–93, it is useful to discuss the development of the National Quar-antine Act of 1893 using the following questions: What were the different viewpoints and proffered solutions? How did racist or anti-immigrant views become embedded in the resultant policy? What role did the science of bac-teriology play in these deliberations? What were the results of the legislation that ultimately passed?

Really a misnomer, the National Quarantine Act that was ultimately

passed did not call for quarantine per se in the form of immigration restriction as a cholera preventive; instead, it specified national regulations of
medical inspection and disinfection for ships and immigrants to be administered by the federal Marine Hospital Service. These regulations established
acceptable protocols for medical inspections and ship sanitation and required more specific medical documentation of the shipping lines before
ships departed for America. In the event of a pending epidemic, the act
authorized the president to halt immigration temporarily.

Like the epidemics that prompted and inspired the new federal "quarantine policy," however, this debate was framed by both by scientific concepts
of health and disease and the many social and cultural barriers that existed
between native-born Americans of the 1890s and their newly arrived immigrant counterparts. How did these native-born Americans view the social
problems associated with immigration of that era? More specifically, how
did Gilded Age Americans view the ethnic composition of their country and
where did East European Jews fit into that society (if at all)?

The reprise of a debate that occurred over a century ago illustrates how
difficult it is to measure the real but elusive factors of nativism and prejudice. The legal solution reached at the end of the nineteenth century was one
that attempted to divorce public health regulations from national immigration policy and the compromises required were not easily reached. Yet by
interpreting the opinions of the president of the United States, legislators,
physicians, public health workers, businessmen, Jewish community leaders,
and others active in the national quarantine debate of 1893, one gets a sense
of how complicated the intermingling of immigration and health issues can
be. Political ramifications, legal theory, medical knowledge, and economic
predictions would all be hammered into shape by the proponent or opponent of immigration restriction to form a product that would fit his argument's needs.

President Benjamin Harrison's Quarantine Policy

Despite Benjamin Harrison's complaints that as the president of the United
States he had no real authority to adapt his emergency quarantine policy to
a broader and continued restriction of immigration, the federal government
was doing precisely that in the aftermath of the 1892 cholera epidemic. Harrison's secretary of the treasury, Charles Foster, who oversaw the administration of both the U.S. Marine Hospital Service and the Immigration Bureau,
extolled the virtues of the federal quarantine policy at the annual banquet of
the Chamber of Commerce of the State of New York. On the rainy evening
of November 15, Foster announced to the well-heeled audience dining on

Table 6.1 *Russian Jewish Immigration to New York City, January 1, 1891–December 31, 1892*

Month	Jewish Immigrants	
	1891	1892
January	2,179	3,276
February	2,185	3,057
March	3,150	2,397
April	2,714	1,468
May	1,225	1,629
June	8,667	4,028
July	8,253	5,673
August	9,109	4,842
September	9,422	1,729
October	5,255	416
November	3,792	121
December	4,310	198
Total	60,261	28,834

Source: S. Joseph, *Jewish Immigration,* 163. Unfortunately, Joseph does not offer a month-by-month analysis beyond December 1892.

terrapin à la Baltimore, canvas-back duck, and filet de boeuf at Delmonico's that the country's success in fending off cholera that fall was a direct result of the "restriction of immigration." Presiding over the banquet hall gleaming with the sparkle of Delmonico's fine silver and china, snowy-white table linens, and a bed of chrysanthemums, Foster pointed out that he thought the twenty-day quarantine policy should remain in place in order to "ward off the threatened and imminent danger" of another epidemic.[6]

Indeed, the Harrison twenty-day quarantine order proved to be an effective means of restricting immigration from Europe for a period of five months. It may be recalled that 1891 and 1892 (before the epidemics) were peak years for East European Jewish immigration, in terms of both actual numbers and the percentage of total immigration to the United States, during the nineteenth century. The number of Russian Jews entering the Port of New York between June and September 1892 — before the presidential circular was issued — averaged about 3,800 per month; between October and December 1892, that monthly average fell to about 267 Russian Jewish immigrants (Tables 6.1, 6.2). An even better measure of how effective a means of immigration restriction the Harrison order was would be to compare 1891 monthly immigration statistics for East European Jews with those of late 1892; the average number of East European Jewish immigrants arriving at

Ellis Island each month during 1891 was about 5,500. East European Jewish immigration was essentially restricted under Harrison's order, out of proportion to the general rates of immigration, by more than 90 to 95 percent.[7]

Such striking results were not lost upon the American press. As the *New York Sun* editorialized in early March 1893: "We have had a very great Jewish immigration last year until it was stopped by the enforcement of the quarantine laws in September and by the President's proclamation. . . . It is not likely that there will be any great addition to our Jewish population this year."[8] The *New York Times* Russian correspondent Harold Frederic more clearly reported the deadly consequences of halting Jewish immigration:

> To attempt to deal in any satisfactory way with the whole question of Jewish persecution in Russia is like setting out to write an Encyclopedia Britannica. The subject is so vast that its bulk fairly frightens one. . . . The most industrious gleaning cannot hope to gather the thousandth part of the past twelve months' tragic

Table 6.2 *General and Jewish Immigration from Eastern Europe to the United States, 1871–1900*

Year	General Immigrants	Jewish Immigrants	Percent Jewish
1871–80	2,810,000	15,000	0.5
1881–84	2,580,340	74,310	2.9
1885	395,350	19,610	4.9
1886	334,200	29,660	8.8
1887	490,110	27,470	5.6
1888	547,000	31,360	5.7
1889	444,430	24,000	5.4
1890	455,300	34,300	7.5
1891	560,320	69,140	12.3
1892	579,660	60,325	10.4
1893	440,000	33,000	7.5
1894	285,630	22,110	7.7
1895	258,540	32,080	12.4
1896	343,270	28,120	8.2
1897	330,830	20,685	6.3
1898	229,300	27,410	11.9
1899	311,715	37,415	12.0
1900	448,570	60,765	13.5

Sources: Based on data from the U.S. Bureau of the Census, Historical Statistics of the United States to 1957 (Washington, D.C.: U.S. Government Printing Office, 1976); S. Joseph, *Jewish Immigration;* S. Kuznets, "Immigration of Russian Jews to the United States."

facts. The scope of the figures staggers the imagination. More families, for example, have been affected by this new and savage enforcement of Ignatieff's May laws and the added ukases than were called to mourn the loss or wounding of relatives on either side during the great American civil war.[9]

Although the threat of cholera had officially ended by early October 1892, steamships continued to stack up at the New York quarantine station and at other U.S. ports of entry through February 1893. Considering the Harrison twenty-day quarantine rule a major inconvenience to commerce, the steamship companies complained vociferously to the Treasury Department about the loss of revenues from diminished transatlantic traffic.[10] Immigration was a boon to this industry, particularly when one considers the volume of steerage passengers. In 1891, for example, over 110,000 people traveled steerage from Liverpool to New York; an additional 82,000 steerage passengers sailed from Hamburg to New York, 68,000 from Bremen, approximately 25,000 each from Rotterdam and Havre, 23,000 from Glasgow, another 20,000 from the less well-known northern European ports, and almost 50,000 from Mediterranean ports also sailed to American seaports that year.[11] Despite the adverse impact of the quarantine regulations on maritime commerce, Secretary of the Treasury Charles Foster announced in mid-November 1892 that the twenty-day rule would remain in effect "indefinitely." The order applied only to steerage immigrants seeking to settle in the United States; it did not affect American citizens or cabin-class passengers who were traveling from the same ports. As Assistant Secretary of the Treasury O. P. Spaulding explained the policy: "This [steerage immigrants] is where the danger [of cholera] lies, and it will not do to take any chances."[12] The measure resulted in the further abridgment of many of the shipping lines' transatlantic schedules and encouraged them to transport only cabin-class passengers in order to avoid the prohibitive costs of quarantine. Those lines that brought the least amount of revenue and had the most likely chance of being associated with an epidemic disease—such as the fleet of steerage steamers that previously carried East European Jews out of Odessa, Hamburg, Rotterdam, and other major European seaports—were the first to be eliminated.[13]

One of the most eloquent opponents of the call to combine quarantine and immigration policies that fall was Gustav Schwab, the New York agent for the North German Lloyd steamship line and the child of German immigrant parents:

The order as now interpreted is nothing more than a return to the Know-Nothingism of years ago, a return to the methods of the Dark Ages. It is nothing more nor less than an attempt to keep immigrants out of the country and that is the most absolute nonsense. To keep out improper persons who come—criminals, the maimed, the blind, and the halt — is quite proper, of course, and that can be done well under the existing law; but this attempt of the government to keep out immigrants on the pretense of keeping out cholera is the most absolute rot. There is very little cholera now in Europe. According to the Treasury Department, however, American citizens and tourists are cholera proof and it is only aliens who come here intending to make their home in this country who are likely to bring the disease here. The absurdity of such a proposition should be plain to anyone possessed of ordinary common intelligence.[14]

Schwab and his fellow steamship agents proposed a responsible plan in early December 1892 that outlined the means for improving the medical inspection and documentation process of steerage immigrants on *both* sides of the Atlantic, promises to hire more physicians to deliver better medical care during the voyages, a system of heavy fines for the less scrupulous shippers who violated the new regulations, improved sanitary conditions aboard the ships' much-reviled steerage compartments, increased disinfection of ships and baggage, and provisions to send those deemed too ill for entry to the United States back to their port of origin.[15] Schwab and the other shipping agents justified their support of this costly plan on "self-interest alone . . . for the occurrence of a single case of cholera on a steamship line is sufficient, in the present state of the public mind, to ruin the business of that line for an indefinite period of time."[16]

Appearing in the daily press that fall were a number of other critics of the Harrison quarantine policy; political opposites Charles A. Dana of the *New York Sun* and E. L. Godkin of the *New York Evening Post* and *The Nation* noted the unheralded precedent of primarily stopping the immigration of one ethnic group (Russian Jews) on the pretext of preventing another cholera epidemic *after* the threat of disease was announced to be over.[17] Godkin, who had experienced the ordeal of quarantine himself during the 1892 cholera epidemic and who was a vociferous critic of its management, accused the Harrison administration of "lawlessly" taking into their own hands a delicate issue that had been wrestled over in Congress for twenty years without resolution. Godkin also accused the president of using issues of public health to create immigration policy:

> The fact is simply this, that the public health has no necessary connection or relation to these goings on. The [Treasury] Department has simply undertaken to stop immigration without any authority of law. Whether immigration ought to be curtailed, and how, are grave questions, to be settled after due investigation by the law-making power. We hope that somebody whose rights are infringed on by these high-handed proceedings will have spirit enough to bring suit for damages against the infringers.[18]

Even the once pro-quarantine and frequently immigration restrictionist editorial board of the *New York Times* called the continuance of the Harrison order an "opera bouffe" and openly asked the government, "Why are they detained?" Answering its own rhetorical question, the *Times* concluded that with the cholera epidemic over there must be political motives behind the continued enforcement of the presidential quarantine order.[19] The newspaper pundits and the shipping men were not alone in asserting the need to separate issues of public health protection from that of immigration restriction. Instituting a rigorous international system of health regulations and inspection procedures at both the ports of disembarkation *and* entry was seen by many businessmen, chambers of commerce, physicians, and public health workers as the best approach to the primary prevention of another cholera epidemic.

Nevertheless, the Harrison administration little heeded these protests and continued to enforce the quarantine order for months after the risk of a cholera epidemic was over. That political rather than public health motivations were behind the continued order on the part of President Harrison becomes evident when his published views and presidential actions on immigration issues are reviewed. In May 1892, for example, Harrison signed the Chinese Exclusion Act, which extended the 1882 act, a law that imposed harsh immigration quotas on Asians and severe regulations on those allowed to settle in the United States.[20] Long an immigration restrictionist, Harrison made his views concerning the huge wave of "Russian Hebrew" immigration more than clear. For example, during his third annual address to Congress on December 9, 1891, the president warned that "the sudden transfer of such a multitude under conditions that strip them [Russian Hebrews] of their small accumulations and . . . depress their energies and courage is neither good for them nor for us."[21] Harrison's unsuccessful 1892 reelection platform also contained strong calls for the immigration restriction of Russian Hebrews.[22]

Even after the 1892 presidential election, when Harrison was relegated to lame duck status by Democrat Grover Cleveland, Harrison insisted that his quarantine order be continued. In his final State of the Union address before Congress on December 6, 1892, Harrison reiterated his views on the need for immigration restriction, specifically tying it to the threat of infectious disease:

> We are particularly subject in our great ports to the spread of infectious diseases by reason of the fact that unrestricted immigration brings to us out of European cities, in the overcrowded steerages of great steamships, a large number of persons whose surroundings make them the easy victim of the plague. This consideration, as well as those affecting the political, moral, and industrial interests of our country, leads me to renew the suggestion that admission to our country and to the

high privileges of citizenship should be more restricted and careful. We have, I think, a right and owe a duty to our own people, not only to keep out the vicious, the ignorant, the civil disturber, the pauper, and the contract laborer, but to check the too great flow of immigration now coming by further limitations.[23]

Many of the president's key cabinet members, such as Secretary of State James Blaine, offered similar unsympathetic or nativistic public comments about the "rising tide of Hebrew immigration."[24] Indeed, Blaine's comments, as well as the pro-immigration restriction views of President Harrison, so aroused and upset the Jewish American community that a series of meetings was held in Washington during 1891–92 between administration appointees and such prominent members of the American Jewish community as Oscar Straus, Simon Wolf, and Jacob H. Schiff. The purpose of these meetings was to counteract what the Jewish American community perceived to be a White House insensitive to the plight of East European Jews.

Complaints about the Harrison policy from a number of groups demanding a separate consideration of immigration and quarantine policy became louder as November progressed to December and the Congressional Committee on Immigration prepared to meet. Clearly, some accord would ultimately have to be reached over how to handle the parallel problems of preventing the entry of dangerous infectious diseases into the United States, via immigrant traffic, and a clarification of the federal government's tolerance toward the "foreign hordes" seeking a better life in the United States. President Benjamin Harrison was probably more successful in temporarily halting immigration than any other U.S. president, before or since, using the grounds of the risk of infectious disease, but the constitutional authority to address such issues on a permanent basis was provided by a congressional act approved by both houses of Congress.[25]

Public Perceptions, Anti-Semitism, and Quarantine

Quarantine as a social policy has the power to isolate more than those labeled "diseased." The stigmatization that results from labeling a particular social group as a potential source of contagion clearly extends to far many more than those who are actually ill. Healthy members of the stigmatized social group also risk being perceived as contagious and dangerous. To some extent, the entire American Jewish community worried about the repercussions of the 1892 epidemics. As Charles Dickens observed in his 1857 novel, *Little Dorrit,* "It is at least as difficult to stay a moral infection as a physical one."[26] And while the stigma of epidemic disease was a transitory one for many American Jews during the winter of 1892–93, it should not be interpreted as harmless.

Throughout the public health crises of 1892 in New York City, there was an irrefutable commingling of public health measures with a less than kindly attitude toward East European Jewish immigrants. Moreover, the stigma of disease was quickly cast over all East European Jews seeking entry to the United States — even after cholera was deemed to be quiescent by public health authorities — with the continued enforcement of the Harrison quarantine circular. The threat of a bill that would completely suspend immigration as a cholera preventive, as proposed by Senator William Eaton Chandler, did little to alter many Americans' perceptions of the East European Jew as a vector of disease.

Jewish historian Ismar Elbogen described 1892 as a year that East European Jewish immigrants became the "principal object of attack" by immigration restrictionists.[27] In response to this attack, the American Jewish community braced itself for the potential repercussions from scientific pronouncements that East European Jews were breeders of infection and a public health threat to the United States.[28]

It should be noted that anti-Semitism and its effects were only too real for American Jews during the 1890s without the added inherent risks of an association with epidemic disease. Despite more optimistic opinions once offered by historian Oscar Handlin, that the Gilded Age was one of "philo-Semitism" and that the Jewish stereotypes of the era involved "no hostility, no negative judgment," one need only randomly sample daily newspapers, popular magazines, plays, and novels of the Gilded Age to detect a real, if not all-pervasive, belief in the inherent undesirability and dangers of allowing too many Jews to settle in the United States.[29] Indeed, as more recent historical scholarship of anti-Semitism during the Gilded Age has revealed, the 1890s was a period when anti-Semitic feelings expressed for decades by native-born Americans "crystallized, intensified, and evolved into more urgent apprehensions."[30]

During much of the Gilded Age, misguided perceptions of Jews were often phrased in terms of a social conspiracy imported along with their suspicious rituals, religion, and language. Given that the East European Jews were the most "foreign" of the Jews settling in America and one of the largest groups to arrive at the eastern seaboard during this period, they received a large share of the American public's disdain and ridicule.

Yet anti-Semitism was not restricted to the many *grine kuzines* stepping off the steerage boats during those years. Perhaps the most common anti-Semitic shibboleth during the late nineteenth century, in counterdistinction to charges that the new Jewish immigrants were all "likely to become public charges," was the complaint about the "uncanny ability" Jews had with money. At a banal level, we find cartoon depictions of Russian Jews involved in some petty business deal where they got "the best" of a Gentile customer, or a hook-nosed Jewish merchant indoctrinating his young son in the crafty business dealings of "the Jew." These complaints were elevated to an art form of anti-Semitism, however, when international economic slumps and depressions of the 1890s were explained as clandestine attempts by German Jewish financiers such as the Rothschilds to control the world's gold supply.[31]

Depictions of Jews in popular literature of the era were also frequently negative. For example, in Henry Adams' popular 1880 novel, *Democracy,* one of the minor characters was a German Jewish businessman Adams named, in sophomoric imitation of Charles Dickens, Hartebeest Schneidekoupon, the surname being the German word for "coupon cutter." As the years went on and Adams watched his patrician influence become irrelevant to political discourse, he fortified his hatred against the "alien" Jews threatening to take over his beloved America.[32]

Less subtle was Ignatius Donnelly's best-selling 1891 utopian novel, *Caesar's Column,* which blamed almost all of the United States' financial and social woes on "the Jewish Race."[33] Similarly, a short story featured in the popular monthly *Cosmopolitan* during 1893 entitled "Omega: The Last Days of the World" detailed the activities of an American Jew who stays firmly rooted to his desk and telephone, making speculative business deals while the world is threatened by total destruction.[34] Even William Jennings Bryan's well-honed and often-quoted "Cross of Gold" speech, which he gave repeatedly in the late 1890s, may be interpreted as an indictment of Jewish domination over the world's gold supply in the language of the more infamous event of Christ's crucifixion.[35] Nativist fears and attitudes were not lost on American Jews during the late nineteenth century. Cultural representations of the Jew as the parsimonious and flesh-extracting moneylender Shylock were common, as were descriptions of newly arriving East European Jews as "riffraff," or "offensive creatures," and so-called humorous portrayals of Jews by penny-novelists, dialect comedians, and cartoonists detailing the capitalistic adventures of huge-nosed, bearded Jews named "Ikey," "Jakie," or "Abie."

If not directly anti-Semitic, many native-born Americans certainly felt uncomfortable about the rising East European Jewish population and, in true late-nineteenth-century American manner, had few qualms about publicly expressing their distrust of the hordes of "hebes and kikes" arriving daily at U.S. ports.[36] Some historians have distinguished this kind of anti-Semitism as a rhetorical or social form of bigotry—one whose bark is far worse than its bite. Yet the constant erosion of a group's social character that such bigotry engenders has the potential to devolve into harsher forms of bigotry.

The widespread stereotyping of Jews as penurious, crafty, and evil foreigners may have even contributed to an atmosphere where subsequent, more dangerous espousals of anti-Semitism were accepted because "millions of well-intentioned Americans . . . had already accepted its ingredients in a form that was not anti-Semitic."[37]

Certainly the differential quarantine policies elaborated in New York City during 1892, where thousands of East European Jews were subjected to stricter regulations and improper health care than the native-born Americans stricken with typhus or cholera, are excellent examples of what can happen in a public health context as a result of such dehumanization and minimization. It may be recalled that, during the typhus epidemic of 1892 the focus of management was on the isolation of the *Massilia* Jews from the city proper rather than on their care at Riverside Hospital on North Brother Island. The ends — avoidance of disease for the native-born residents of New York — justified the means in too many American minds. In a similar vein, leaving East European Jewish and other undesirable immigrants potentially to die of cholera on Hoffman Island was far more acceptable to most Americans in 1892 than that same fate would have been for the socialites stranded in the cabin class of the *Normannia*.

Even the lengthy extension of Harrison's twenty-day quarantine order might have been seen as less imperative to Gilded Age Americans if it had been targeted at native-born American, cabin-class transatlantic passengers, instead of the so-called undesirable steerage immigrants. To be sure, no long-lasting restrictive or punitive policies against American Jews emerged from the rhetorical anti-Semitism of the 1890s.[38] But if you were a Russian Jew living in the United States during the Harrison quarantine, surrounded by subtle (and not-so-subtle) swipes at your heritage and physiognomy, reified by socially justified public health policies that potentially put you at risk, the ready association of East European Jews with contagious disease was a most threatening experience.

New York's German Jewish community in 1892, on the other hand, was a more assimilated and wealthier group of Americans than their newly arrived East European counterparts. Many were well-established, respected members of their communities, although most did not have to go back more than a generation or two to recall their own immigrant roots. Nevertheless, they were filled with ambivalence between protecting their own standing in American society, like many an established immigrant group before or since, and the traditional Jewish commandment of *tzadukah* (the Jewish doctrine of charitable acts, particularly for needy co-religionists). Their response to the quarantine–immigration restriction debate, then, was divided between an understandable desire to avoid stigmatization of their race and enormous charitable relief and sophisticated lobbying efforts to defeat the proposed immigration suspension bill.

At the most squeamish end of this spectrum was the American German Jewish press, which frequently expressed concern in its Friday evening editorial pages about the threat of an American perception of Jews as "the cause" of epidemic disease. In New York City, Abram S. Isaacs, the scholarly editor of the weekly *Jewish Messenger*, recorded the feelings his elite German Jewish readers had about casting the recent epidemics as an all-too-familiar reprise of anti-Semitic persecution:

> Against whom would the first stone have been flung? Why the Jews, of course. That is the lesson of history. The faint, ungenerous murmurings of the press would have grown bolder and more unrestrained. The Jew has always been a favorite scapegoat. By his stripes we are healed, is the popular cry in all ages.[39]

Similar qualms were expressed by Isaac Meyer Wise, the editor of the Cincinnati-based German Jewish weekly, the *American Israelite:*

> Why does not our government make proper quarantine regulations, or see that the quarantine laws we have are properly administered? Small pox, cholera, yellow fever, and other contagious and infectious diseases are brought into this country constantly, but there is no cry that all foreigners must be excluded. But the Jew is a prominent target, he always has been, and always will be, I am afraid—till the millennium comes.[40]

In Detroit, city alderman J. Christopher Jacob proposed a resolution at a city council meeting blocking the entry of Russian Jews into the city since they "brought cholera to this country and should be kept out." Responding "trenchantly" to the "impulsive" alderman, Rabbi Louis Grossman of the Reform German Jewish Congregation Beth-El of Detroit informed Jacob that his resolution was both prejudiced and spurious.[41]

Perhaps no member of the American German Jewish community attacked the Chandler suspension bill more vigorously than the publisher and writer Philip Cowen, who noted on the pages of his weekly newspaper, *The American Hebrew:*

> [Senator Chandler's] project of killing two birds with one stone, of solving, by means of one act of legislation two such problems as Quarantine against possible Cholera and the Restriction of Immigration, is unstatesmanlike, and the result of his labors is the inadequacy of his provision for quarantine and the un-American, inhumane, and economically improvident nature of his provision in regard to immigration. . . . We, the people of the United States, can offer a potent pressure in even the most hardened of politicians, and even the most bigoted of demagogues.[42]

At the same time American German Jews tried to distance themselves from the accusations of being carriers of cholera, however, members of that community organized on behalf of their scapegoated co-religionists. For example, the prominent German Jewish philanthropists and former presidential advisors Jacob Schiff, Simon Wolf, and Oscar S. Straus, backed by an anti-restriction petition from the Council of the American Hebrew Congregations, made eloquent pleas to President Harrison, Secretary of the Treasury Charles Foster, and Senator Chandler not to restrict immigration or to blame the epidemics on Jewish immigrants.[43]

The German Jewish charitable organizations, such as the United Hebrew Charities, the International Order of B'nai B'rith, the Alliance Israélite Universelle, and the Baron de Hirsch Fund, provided excellent service and generous funding for all aspects of care related to the Russian Jewish immigrants during the epidemics of 1892.[44] By early 1893, the Jewish immigration charities began to complain loudly about the "temporary" suspension of immigration. Calling the Harrison quarantine order a policy of "popular prejudice," Myer S. Isaacs, the president of the Baron de Hirsch Fund, was forced to close several branch offices of the immigrant aid agency in different American cities that fall because the "arrival of immigration from Russia has been comparatively few."[45]

Ironically, few of the Jewish charitable organizations devoted to facilitating Russian Jewish immigration worried aloud about problems that might result from the massive numbers of Russian Jews arriving in America during the early 1890s. For example, the B'nai B'rith periodical, *The Menorah*, published an article on the problems of immigration in late 1892 that could almost have been written by an immigration restrictionist instead of the Reform rabbi, William Sparger, who actually penned the piece:

> If these Russian refugees, like their less numerous forerunners, will build up among us that demi-Asiatic *Hassidism* into which oppression and persecution together with a lack of modern culture have forced them, to any considerable extent, they will become a cancer on the body of American Judaism, which will fast consume the blood of our social organism. As long as these people were few in number, they were harmless to the large body of American Jews. But let them come in by the thousands and many thousands, and persist in their obsolete practices and in their exclusiveness, and our good reputation must suffer, through a Judaism which is transplanted from Russian soil and which is as different from American Judaism as is the Russian moujik to the American farmer.[46]

In January 1893, former minister to Turkey and presidential envoy Oscar S. Straus, in his role as American agent for the Baron de Hirsch Fund, wrote to Baron Maurice de Hirsch explaining the singular benefit of the Harrison quarantine order; many tens of thousands of impoverished East European Jews had arrived in America during the fiscal year of July 1891 to June 1892, and the Jewish charitable organizations were rapidly depleting their financial resources. The temporary suspension, Straus observed, would, at least, serve as a respite.[47]

Naturally, the Russian Jewish American community, particularly those who lived in New York City, was far more sensitive to the charges that Jews were importing cholera and other infections into the United States. Unlike their better assimilated German Jewish brethren, who were cushioned somewhat by years of Americanization and financial success, the Yiddish-speaking *grine kuzines* and their predecessors in the Lower East Side of New York were less able to hide behind the veneer of social acceptability. These people, after all, were the embodiment of the disease-carrying East European immigrants so frequently reviled on the front pages of the newspapers and discussed so avidly in Congress. American Jews of East European descent were especially fearful of massive restrictions on immigration, in the name of quarantine, because they would prevent the relatives they left behind in Russia from escaping the Czar's tyranny. Moreover, they feared that any backlash, in terms of new local health regulations, would be most severely felt by the Jewish immigrants living in New York and other urban ghettos along the eastern seaboard and across the nation.

The lone East European Jewish "representative" interviewed in the native-born American press on the immigration–quarantine issue was the much maligned "Chief Rabbi of the Congregations of Israel in New York," Jacob Joseph. A competent rabbi and sermonist from the "Jerusalem of Lithuania," Vilna, Jacob was hired as a compromise candidate by a cooperative of Lower East Side synagogues to oversee Jewish life in New York in 1888. Unfortunately, the job required far more skill in political leadership than scholarship. The Yiddish-speaking, Old World, bearded rabbi was hopelessly miscast in the role of spokesman for the Jewish community of New York. As Abraham Cahan recalled: "Reb Jacob Joseph was like a plant torn out of the soil and transplanted into a hothouse."[48] By 1892, a number of paralytic strokes had rendered Rabbi Joseph even less active in American Jewish affairs. Nevertheless, the rabbi consented to make a statement from his sickbed for the *New York World* on the problems of restricting the immigration of East European Jews as a cholera preventive:

> We love everybody and are thankful to all. We are ever ready to show our gratitude. I cannot intermarry with the Christians because that is against one of our laws. Some of the Hebrews who come here have considerable money, while others are not so well off. But no matter what their condition when they land, you can

depend on it that they will not beg and they will go to work and earn their own living. I am not able to say whether the health of this nation may be more secure by stopping immigration because I am not a physician, but it seems to me that if good sanitary measures are adopted, nothing more will be needed.[49]

The Yiddish press, of course, made its views quite clear on the immigration–quarantine debate. For example, the socialist Yiddish weekly newspaper, the *Arbeiter Zeitung*, followed the debate closely with a jaundiced and scientifically up-to-date eye on the activities of Congress and the immigration restrictionists. Critical of "the swindlers and the heads of this country" who "blinded the eyes of Americans," the *Arbeiter Zeitung* called the action to close immigration as a public health measure a "big slap in the face for America."[50] The politically conservative *Tageblatt* was more respectful of the American leaders they disagreed with than the *Arbeiter Zeitung* but, nevertheless, insisted that the solution to the problems of importing cholera was not restricting immigration but, instead, improving the sanitary conditions of steerage travel and the areas of the American cities where immigrants ultimately settled.[51]

Ambivalence about the foreigners, fears of overtaxing both the private and public charitable system, and other worries were voiced by members of both the more established German Jewish and newly arrived East European Jewish communities, but these were secondary to a far larger argument. The overwhelming consensus of the American Jewish population in late 1892 was that the extension of Harrison's quarantine order was morally unconscionable given the level of Jewish persecution in Czarist Russia; and that Chandler's plan to suspend immigration as a cholera preventive was a transparent move toward a permanent system of immigration restriction.[52]

CHAPTER 7

The Doctors' Prescription
for Quarantine

Historians of medicine and science like to remind us that the pursuit of scientific knowledge rarely occurs in a vacuum. The much popularized account of the lone investigator toiling away in his laboratory oblivious to the call for meals, let alone national politics and other social matters, is a cherished, but problematic, myth. Instead, a significant body of scholarship has shown how scientific inquiry is often a distinct product of the era from which it emerges, influenced by social, cultural, and historical contexts. The American medical profession's debate on quarantine policy at the close of the nineteenth century reflects this social construction of knowledge.[1] Although it was the elite American medical establishment who were most often questioned for advice regarding quarantine and immigration policy during that winter, medical professionals representing different theoretical and therapeutic philosophies ranging from allopathy and homeopathy to hydropathy and balneotherapy gladly offered their opinions on the quarantine debate.[2] Similar to the debate going on within the halls of Congress and across the nation at private citizens' dinner tables, the medical discourse was forced through a prism of anti-immigrant sentiment, differing political ideologies, and, at times, prejudice. Vibrant and colorful in its expression, but often blurred at the edges, the medical profession's debate had less to do with a victory of germ theory and the institution of the laboratory in public health than with a bitter fight over U.S. immigration policy.

The germ theory of disease was certainly discussed and heartily subscribed to by many New York City physicians in 1892–93, but its impact in terms of clinical practice was negligible at best. Moreover, there remained several prominent practitioners, called anti-contagionists, who doubted the veracity of the germ theory, which held that infectious diseases were caused by distinct living organisms (bacteria) that enter a human host, reproduce themselves indefinitely, and cause signs and symptoms that are characteristic of certain types of disease.[3] The entire American medical community did not do an absolute or immediate scientific about-face in the early 1890s.[4] There still remained a wide spectrum of beliefs about the etiology of contagious diseases among experts and the lay public alike. From the distance of a century of events, it is tempting to view the germ theorists overtaking the anti-contagionists much like a giant snowball coming down a large mountain, gaining speed and size with each consecutive revolution; in the reality of daily life as it was experienced in the early 1890s, however, it was more of a snowstorm—difficult to ignore for even the most strident anti-contagionist, but certainly navigable.

Among the guardians against what Abraham Jacobi prematurely derided in 1885 as "bacteriomania"[5] were those who maintained that epidemic diseases were the direct result of filthy conditions and poor sanitary measures. Cleaning up the streets, improving water and sewage systems and the food chain, providing good ventilation, and similar environmental approaches, then, were the issues these sanitarians or anti-contagionists held most dear. Admittedly, by 1892, those who ascribed contagious diseases only to environmental causes were in the minority but they most certainly existed. For example, at a November 23, 1893 meeting of the New York Academy of Medicine's Section on Public Health, Legal Medicine, and Medical and Vital Statistics, chemical engineer Charles Wingate argued with pediatrician Henry D. Chapin that the cause of diphtheria was not the Klebs-Loeffler bacilli, as had been asserted independently by Edwin Klebs in 1883 and by Fredrich Loeffler in 1884, but, instead, the inhalation of foul, damp air and sewer gas. Wingate concluded that prevention tactics ought to focus on sewers rather than children's throats.[6]

Others skeptical of the germ theory, such as the redoubtable Dr. Alfred L. Loomis, elaborated complicated explanations called "contingent contagionism," which incorporated several different explanations for epidemics, including atmospheric contamination by miasmas and rotting organic matter; specific zymotic poisons that found an entry into the human bloodstream and yielded an internal fermentative process—much like the brewing of beer—and a specific disease pattern; spontaneous generation of poisons or organisms that cause disease; and even some aspects of germ theory, under specific geographic or "local" conditions.[7] This doctrine of contingent contagionism was popular among those who were still unwilling to accept the germ theory fully during the late 1880s and early 1890s but who were also hesitant to seem old-fashioned or out of date. Like a large old blanket, this polyglot theory of contingency after contingency could be used to cover and obscure almost any possible explanation of etiology. Contingent contagionism was a pragmatic explanation that resonated greatly during an era in which Harvard philosopher William James defined the two basic classes of human needs as "theoretic and practical."[8]

Although logic suggests that if you do not believe in the concept of transmissible germs, you should not be a proponent of quarantines erected to prevent the entry of germs, this was not necessarily the case in 1892. Even those who did not accept the germ theory and bacteriological concepts of infectious diseases were in favor of restricting immigration as a cholera preventive. For example, there were physicians who at many points during the early 1890s offered skeptical assessments of the germ theory and countered it with the tenets of contingent contagionism, such as Alfred Loomis, Joseph Winters, medical editor and physician George F. Shrady, and, at various times, New York City Health Department Sanitary Supervisor Cyrus Edson. Despite previous complaints that quarantines were often futile in the prevention of epidemic disease, these men used the cholera threat to support a quarantine in the form of immigration suspension during the winter of 1893. All four openly supported Chandler's immigration bill and volunteered their services as prominent medical experts on the matter. Testifying before the Senate Immigration Committee in early December 1892, no one was more clear on the health risks of undesirable immigrants and the need to suspend immigration for "a reasonable period, say a year," than George Shrady, who explained: "The history of every [cholera] epidemic in this country has proven that the disease entered our port on account of defective quarantine, and that it has been carried to us, mainly, by filthy immigrants."[9]

More devout anti-contagionists, on the other hand, openly derided the use of quarantine to prevent cholera epidemics. The well-known anti-contagionist and future reform commissioner of street cleaning for New York City, George E. Waring, was an excellent representative of the anti-contagionist, anti-quarantine viewpoint. Objecting to the "panic of cholera" that appeared to be driving Senator Chandler's immigration suspension crusade, Waring wrote a letter to the editor of the *New York Evening Post* calling for sound sanitary inspections and cleanliness:

> The truth is, it is wiser to render the soil sterile to the seed than to try vainly to keep out the seed by clumsy expedients, which are about as efficacious as if a tortoise were set to catch a butterfly. . . . Quarantine has never done more than to delay the introduction of an epidemic from foreign sources. It has never prevented it. It may well be questioned whether the brutality of quarantine methods has not led to much more suffering and death among its victims than to lives saved by a temporary suspension of the disease against which it is directed.[10]

Equally diverse was the spectrum of opinion regarding the need for immigration suspension among those who subscribed to the germ theory of disease. Again, as we find with the other social groups involved in the debate, the participants' perceptions of and beliefs about the value of immigration played a significant role in the conclusions reached by different germ theorists. For example, the consensus of most American bacteriologists and public health experts in late 1892 was that careful sanitary inspection of the food and water chain was sufficient to prevent the return of cholera, and that a return to the ineffective doctrine of nonintercourse and exclusion was unneccessary.[11] Some of the strongest advocates of this solution, such as T. Mitchell Prudden and William H. Welch, were also publicly in favor of open immigration or, at least, of separating the public health issue from the immigration debate.[12]

Far more sanguine in his criticism of an immigration suspension bill explained as a cholera preventive was Dr. Henry Walcott, chairman of the Massachusetts board of health. Walcott argued for viewing public health as but one factor in an effort to meet the challenges of modern society. Reforms in the public health laws, he argued, must consider all aspects of science and even statecraft in order to create laws that best protect the nation from disease "with the least disturbance or injury to the rights of others."[13] More emphatically, in an editorial for the *Boston Medical and Surgical Journal,* Walcott insisted that the issue of immigration restriction was entirely different from that of quarantine regulation: "This is a question of national economics, not a question of medicine, until it has been shown that these emigrants are diseased."[14]

The multitalented physician, sanitarian, librarian, and public health expert John Shaw Billings of the U.S. Army described this problem of conflation even more succinctly in an unsigned editorial for *The Medical News:*

> Many persons are of the opinion that the time has come when it is desirable to check immigration to this country, to prevent paupers and unskilled laborers from coming here, on the ground that we have more than enough of them already; and these persons use the danger of importation of cholera merely as an argument in favor of the action that they advise. Among them are a number of practical politicians who believe that such an action will tend to secure what is known as the labor vote.[15]

Billings insisted that modern sanitary measures were capable of both protecting the health of the nation and preventing "injurious restrictions" to immigrants and maritime commerce.[16]

There were other germ theorists, however, who openly advocated a quarantine in the form of immigration suspension. Dr. Edward O. Shakespeare, the well-known bacteriologist and author of the encyclopedic 950-page *Report on Cholera in Europe and India to the 49th U.S. Congress,*[17] essentially supported a national system of quarantine similar to that proposed by Surgeon General Walter Wyman, but he rarely missed an opportunity to describe the new immigrants with such adjectives as "pestiferous" or "filthy." In the several articles Shakespeare wrote on the quarantine question that year, he concluded by recommending a complete suspension of immigration in the name of public health. As he opined in an editorial he wrote for

Dr. Simon Baruch's New York City-based journal, the *Dietetic and Hygienic Gazette,*

> What, indeed, can more harass and impede the course of maritime commerce, or the movements of men of affairs, than the necessity which frequently arises for the holding of a ship on quarantine because she carries a lot of filthy passengers of the immigrant class, either afflicted with contagious diseases or accompanied by personal effects, the unpacking of which in America is liable to let loose the seeds of a pestilence? The temporary suspension of immigration during times of unusual danger of importing, with this class of travelers also such a disease as Asiatic cholera, would render it possible to safely expedite maritime commerce and the ocean voyages of business men as well as of all others whom experience has taught bring with them practically no dangerous contagions.[18]

In New York City, a like-minded Joseph D. Bryant, the former commissioner of the board of health of New York City, spoke to the press on one day about the abilities of bacteriology and sanitary science to defeat any epidemic, and the need to exclude "the infection-breeding and infection-carrying agents—the immigrants themselves" on another.[19] Across the East River, the medical director of the Brooklyn Naval Yard, Albert L. Gihon, M.D., explained the need to suspend the immigration of Russian Jews because of their inherent susceptibility to the germ of cholera:

> Now if their houses are foul, what do you think of ships? You probably never have seen a Russian Jew when he starts for this country. He is a man who probably has never washed in his life; he is a man who certainly has worn the rags upon him as many years as these rags would hold together. You put that man in a crowded steerage, he becomes seasick (this same thing applies to the women); he vomits, his dejecta are thrown out in that bunk; it becomes saturated with seasickness, and then he becomes choleraic.[20]

In Baltimore, the medical staff at the Johns Hopkins Hospital, including the world-renowned physician and ardent supporter of the germ theory, William Osler, conspired to meet at a time when they knew their colleague and strident opponent of quarantine, Dr. William Henry Welch, would be out of town. The result of their clandestine meeting on September 1, 1892, was a highly publicized memorial petitioning the president of the United States to suspend all immigration to prevent a cholera epidemic.[21]

The diversity of opinion among these well-known and respected physicians was not lost upon those who had to make the final decision: the members of Congress. Savvy Senator John Tyler Morgan (D-Ala.) dismissed the medical debate with a complaint about the all-too-common problem of relying on physicians to answer a political question:

The doctors may disagree and probably will become a little strenuous and prag-
matical about their respective authority and dignity, and the like of that. They are
always quarreling with each other. It is part of the business of the profession, I believe, to underrate, undervalue, and quarrel with each other in their opinions, etc.
Perhaps that is all right, but it is not very convenient, and it is not a very useful
thing in an epidemic; it produces strife and contention. . . . The king of terrors
[cholera] seems to have no power at all unless he has got a doctor for a leader in
some way or other.[22]

One Part Medicine and Two Parts Politics: The New York Academy of Medicine Quarantine Committee

Perhaps the most instructive example of the way in which the American
medical profession's debate was driven more by nativism, politics, and class
than by medical theory and practice was the work of one body of physicians
who were fairly prominent in the national quarantine debate: the Quarantine
Committee of the New York Academy of Medicine. This committee evolved
out of the Advisory Committee to the New York State Chamber of Commerce of 1892. Political skirmishes and nativist beliefs significantly detracted
from the committee's influence on the legislation that ultimately passed into
law. Indeed, the New York Academy of Medicine's prescriptive report on
national quarantine issues was suppressed by those who were opposed to its
content in an attempt to delay its official appearance until after the passage
of the National Quarantine Act of 1893.

It may be recalled that, during the 1892 cholera epidemic, the Special
Advisory Committee to the New York State Chamber of Commerce played
a widely publicized role in examining the New York quarantine station and
identifying its inadequacies. The committee consisted of pediatrician Abraham Jacobi, surgeon Stephen Smith, pathologist Hermann Biggs, psychiatrist Allan McLane Hamilton,[23] T. Mitchell Prudden, Professors A. L. Loomis
and Edward G. Janeway of Bellevue, and Dr. R. H. Derby, a prominent New
York practitioner.[24]

The committee was originally commissioned by the New York State Chamber of Commerce, a strong alliance of New York businessmen, merchants,
and traders. Officially chaired by Alexander Orr, himself an Irish immigrant
and successful produce merchant, and Seth Low, then president of Columbia University and future mayor of Brooklyn and New York, the unofficial
leader of this group was Dr. T. Mitchell Prudden, director of the Physiologi-
cal and Pathological Laboratory of the Alumni Association of the College of
Physicians and Surgeons.[25]

A descendant of one of the founders of the New Haven Colony and educated at Yale University and Columbia's College of Physicians and Surgeons, Prudden was, by 1892, one of the best-known pathologists and bacteriologists in the United States. His opinions on the quarantine debate were actively sought after and highly regarded. Prudden's accomplishments included authoring two popular textbooks of pathology and histology,[26] introducing the methods of Koch and other European bacteriologists to American medical students at the College of Physicians and Surgeons in New York, and enjoying an established international scientific reputation.

Equally important to Prudden's professional activities was his successful career as a best-selling author of books on bacteriology and public health for the lay public. Beginning in the late 1880s, Prudden embarked on an active literary presence in such popular periodicals as *Harper's Weekly, Harper's Monthly, The Century, Popular Science Monthly,* and *The Christian Union.* In 1889, he published his first book for the popular audience, *The Story of the Bacteria,* which ultimately went through several editions and hundreds of printings, followed by similar public health primers such as *Dust and Its Dangers* (1890) and *Drinking Water and Ice Supplies and Their Relations to Health and Disease* (1891). One of the major missions of these slim volumes was the demystification of cholera and other "conquered" epidemic diseases as a source of panic or threat. Always stressing his case in positivistic, assured tones, Prudden explained that cholera could be handled on a "rational and tangible basis" of careful attention to the water supply, disinfection, and proper sanitation.[27] The control of cholera, Prudden insisted, need not be accomplished by harsh immigration restrictions. Instead, he proposed enacting public health laws that protected the nation's food and water chain and regulated the medical inspection of immigrants as the most effective means of preventing the entry of infectious diseases into the United States.

The Chamber of Commerce Quarantine Committee's report under Prudden's leadership was confrontational and bold in its conclusions. So negative were the committee's findings of the New York quarantine station's administration that the report's initial release was temporarily delayed during the fall of 1892. When the document was released in December 1892, it was filled with graphic descriptions of the inadequate facilities at Quarantine, unmonitored water sources and toilet facilities, the improper handling of potentially contagious fecal matter, and strong condemnations of the gross incompetence of Dr. William T. Jenkins. One committee member, Dr. Hermann Biggs, became especially nervous over the report that detailed, one by one, Jenkins' errors and acts of negligence. Biggs initially did not sign the first draft in late October 1892 because he was "a member of the Health Department and, therefore, in a sense a subordinate of a gentleman [Dr. William Jenkins] who is a member of that Board ex officio."[28] Biggs somehow gained

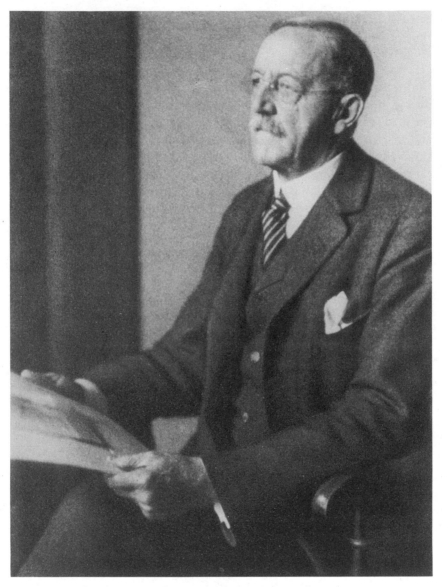

Figure 7.1. T. Mitchell Prudden, M.D. From Lillian Prudden, ed., *Biographical Sketches and Letters of T. Mitchell Prudden, M.D.* (New Haven: Yale University Press, 1927).

enough courage to endorse the final version presented to the Chamber of Commerce in December 1892, which was just as strong in its condemnation of Jenkins.

The opinions of the members of the Chamber of Commerce committee were especially important in the national policy debate of 1893 because all of these physicians had been present as consultants and inspectors of the New York quarantine station during the cholera epidemic of 1892; a few of them, such as Biggs and Prudden, had extensive knowledge of the bacteriological and public health mechanisms of cholera prevention. Further, all of these physicians were prominent members of the New York Academy of Medicine. Founded in 1846 at the suggestion of New York surgeon Valentine Mott, the academy was by 1892 one of the most prestigious and active medical societies in the United States. Consequently, these physicians' views on how to prevent the entry of contagious diseases into a large seaport like New York carried a great deal of weight in the national deliberation of the issues of cholera and quarantine.

At a meeting of the New York Academy of Medicine on January 31, 1893, the Chamber of Commerce committee was asked to report its final findings on the inadequacies of the New York quarantine station. After a supportive response from an audience consisting of many of the "most eminent medical men of this city," Dr. Richard Derby proposed that their commission be extended as a formal committee of the academy. By overwhelming consensus, a committee of twenty-one was appointed to travel as soon as possible to Washington, D.C., to advise Congress on national quarantine legislation; to draft a bill that met both the needs of the medical profession and protected the public health; and to organize a collective medical voice among other medical societies across the nation.[29]

Opposed to the entry of potentially ill immigrants into the United States and anxious to introduce language to that effect in the academy's "quarantine bill" was the senior professor of clinical medicine at Bellevue, Alfred L. Loomis. He also opposed the extension of the quarantine committee's commission because he feared their actions would be too heavily influenced by Prudden's inspection solutions rather than a complete suspension of immigration.

Educated at Union College and the New York College of Physicians and Surgeons in the mid-1850s, Loomis became a fashionable New York practitioner and consultant who specialized in auscultation and diseases of the chest. His textbooks on the topics of physical diagnosis, medicine, and diseases of the chest were extremely popular among New York medical students and went through several editions. One of Loomis's long-held beliefs was the importance of restricting immigration as a public health measure. Despite a

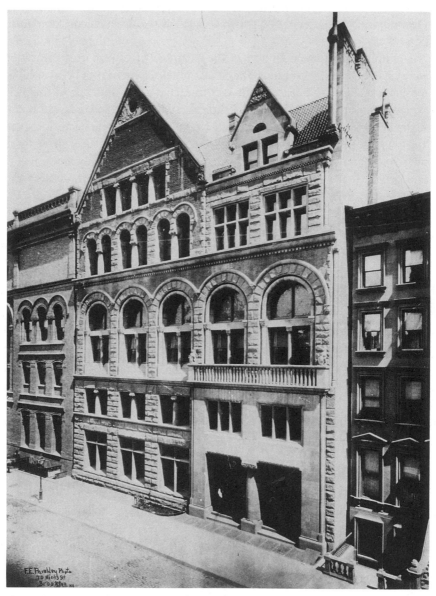

Figure 7.2. New York Academy of Medicine, 17 West 43rd Street, circa 1890. Collection of the New York Academy of Medicine.

long career as first an anti-contagionist and later a contingent contagionist, Loomis held fairly consistent opinions on immigrants as a vector of disease over the span of his professional career. One of Loomis's favorite clinical anecdotes, which he repeated in lectures to his medical students, published papers, and many medical textbooks, was a recounting of his experience as a resident physician at Bellevue Hospital during an especially severe typhus fever epidemic in early 1861:

> Immediately, I commenced investigations in order to ascertain the origin of the fever in these cases. I found that the fever had its origin in the upper story of a rear tenement house in Mulberry Street, in the most filthy portion of the city. The first case was that of a little girl, who had been brought into the house, ten days before she sickened, from a ship which had come from Ireland, and which had cases of typhus fever on board.[30]

By 1877 and extending well into the early 1890s, Loomis lectured medical students at Bellevue Hospital and the Medical Department of University of the City of New York that filth diseases such as typhus fever and cholera invariably came from "certain endemic centres"; by the early 1890s Loomis consistently identified these centers of disease as the "undesirable" nations of Russia, Italy, and Ireland.[31] Loomis extended his nativist viewpoints at the Senate Immigration Committee's hearings in December when he emphatically testified to Senator William Chandler that the only way of preventing a return of the cholera was to suspend immigration, particularly from the more undesirable regions, for at least one year.[32]

A man of forceful personality, Loomis was one of the "grand old men" of New York medical circles who, in his capacity as professor and attending physician at Bellevue, had taught clinical medicine to most of the committee members. Although he is frequently recalled by medical historians as the teacher who once derided Koch's discovery of the tubercle bacillus and tried to persuade his then-student William Henry Welch not to abandon a promising medical career for the fad of bacteriology, Loomis remained a powerful and persuasive medical authority until his death in 1895. He also served as the president of the New York Academy of Medicine from 1889 to 1892.[33]

An excellent example of Loomis's political strength in New York medical circles can be seen in his conduct on the Chamber of Commerce–New York Academy Quarantine Committee. Over the objections of the other members, Loomis insisted that the committee's report insert a final prescription that would "put an end to the perpetual menace of immigration."[34] After a lengthy debate and vote, Loomis's anti-immigrant clause was ultimately removed from subsequent drafts of the document by the other committee members. When the final draft of the report was read at a meeting held on January 31, 1893, the offensive passage was replaced with a less nativist conclusion that there existed a need "to secure legislation as will most effectively protect this city and the country at large from the threatened invasion of cholera." Loomis refused to sign the "altered" version of the report and vowed to fight the committee as fiercely as possible, although his name was later recorded in the press as one of its endorsers. Finally, in a dramatic and angry manner, Loomis announced that he was resigning his appointment on the quarantine committee that evening.

Loomis's subsequent actions were described by T. Mitchell Prudden as an attempt to do everything he could "to block, delay, and otherwise obstruct the work of the Quarantine Committee." In a memorandum to himself over the proceedings, Prudden criticized Loomis for his "blundering," "malicious intermeddling," and an "absolute lack of personal knowledge of quarantine affairs." More to the point, Prudden diagnosed the cause of Loomis's interference as the result of the committee's failure to make recommendations more in line with Loomis's desire for a complete ban on immigration.[35]

Loomis continued to attack the quarantine committee's work in a series of public statements to the New York press corps throughout the early weeks of February 1893. The committee's response to Loomis's campaign was to delay announcing its formal report until after the National Quarantine Act, then being deliberated by Congress, was enacted, in the hopes of avoiding battles among its members and influencing the policies of the newly elected but not yet inaugurated president, Grover Cleveland.[36]

The episode climaxed at a poorly attended academy meeting on the evening of February 16, 1893, the day after the Harris–Rayner National Quarantine Bill was signed into law by President Harrison. At the meeting, Loomis "caused a mild sensation" by complaining that the quarantine committee had gone well beyond its commission as a medical advisory body. Loomis charged that the committee was now threatening to become a political group dedicated to keeping immigration open and meddling in affairs best controlled by the public health authorities. Insisting that these issues were not in the proper domain of the academy and that the passage of the National Quarantine Act obviated the need for further deliberation, Loomis demanded that the committee be disbanded. The academy's president, Dr. D. B. St. John De Roosa, pointed out to Loomis that he had no authority to make such a motion given that he was no longer a member of the quarantine committee. In response, Loomis insisted that the motion was not his, but instead one made on behalf of the absent Dr. Abraham Jacobi.

When news of the meeting got out, there was, obviously, great consternation among the members of the academy's National Quarantine Committee. Perhaps most angry at Loomis was Abraham Jacobi, who had not authorized in any shape or form the disbanding of the committee. The internationally known pediatrician, himself an immigrant from Germany only forty years earlier, announced to the academy that he deeply resented Loomis's using his name in the spurious motion of February 16.

At a much better-attended emergency meeting on February 24, 1893, Jacobi publicly disavowed the action taken by Loomis and chastised the physician for "exceeding his authority."[37] Although the matter was resolved at this meeting by reinstating the committee, the damage caused by the delay tactics had already been done. A national quarantine bill had been passed into law. And while the National Quarantine Committee continued to be a prominent advisory board on issues of public health, maritime quarantine, and similar matters to the federal government for several years, it did not participate in writing the legislation that ultimately remained in effect well into the twentieth century.

CHAPTER 8

The Congress Responds

Senator Chandler
and the Immigration Question Redux

Few American politicians studied the problems, vagaries, and emotions of American immigration policy during the 1890s more intensely than William Eaton Chandler. His position as chairman of the Senate Immigration Committee insured that he would play an active role in the quarantine debate of late 1892 to early 1893.

A review of Senator Chandler's public speeches during the late 1880s and early 1890s reveals that he was deeply concerned with the "overwhelming incursion of Jews from Russia."[1] Refuting the complaints of several Jewish Americans that he was inspired to create new restrictions against Russian Jews by religious bigotry, Chandler insisted that his only motivation was the inherent "undesirability" of Russian Jews as potential residents of the United States. Chandler repeatedly and publicly inflamed Jewish American citizens involved in the relief efforts of Russian Jews with questions hinting at their participation in conspiracies that might lead to national ruin. For example, Chandler predated the interrogatory techniques of the infamous Senator Joseph McCarthy when he attacked the motives of Simon Wolf, the well-known American German Jewish lawyer, philanthropist, and presidential advisor in early 1893:

> The Russian Jews are swarming to this country, and I think they are not desirable immigrants, as I think of the Hungarians and many of the Italians. . . . New York City is vitally interested in this question. The Jewish immigrants are not agriculturists. They do not go West. They stay in the seaboard cities. They swarm into New York City. . . . Public sentiment has not yet been strong enough to make it possible to pass a law making new exclusions. But shall we receive a whole nation of Jews as Jews, who are not desirable citizens; and if we object and argue the question, shall we be vilified by you because we even venture to use the word 'Jews'? And, now frankly tell me, Mr. Wolf, are you or have you at any time been in the employ of the Hirsch Society?[2]

In early January 1893, Chandler took the floor of the U.S. Senate and charged without any proof that an illegal scheme was under way by the steamship companies, Jewish bankers, and U.S. immigration officials to allow more Russian Jewish immigrants into the country against the orders of the Harrison quarantine rule. Chandler suggested that if the huge wave of East European Jewish immigration over the past two years continued, the United States faced epidemic disease, economic ruin, and a destruction of the labor market.[3]

Not surprisingly, Chandler's declarations resonated among the laboring classes in America. Organized labor unions, such as the Knights of Labor, the National Labor Union, and the American Federation of Labor, were steadfastly in favor of immigration restriction legislation in order to protect the interests of the working man in the United States during the last two decades of the nineteenth century. Immigrants, the unions' broken record continuously played, drove down wages, pushed American citizens out of jobs, and would somehow lead to the downfall of the United States of America.[4] The perceived health risks of immigration, as evidenced by the recent near-miss at disaster with cholera in New York, only strengthened these views.

Labor leader and founding member of the National Labor Union, Robert Blissert, reminded the rank and file at their annual meeting in December 1892 that the evils of immigration needed to be arrested immediately in order to protect the health of the nation from "a race of undersized and miserable people growing up among us. There are 100,000 of these people living and working in that section bounded by Broadway, the East River, Houston Street and Division Street."[5] This geographically defined epicenter of disease, incidentally, was New York City's Jewish Lower East Side.

Echoing the same conflation of public health risks and immigration were Henry Abrahams, the secretary of the Central Labor Union; Edward L. Fanning of the Order of United American Mechanics; R. H. Campbell of the International Typographical Union; William Weibe, the former president of the Amalgamated Iron Workers; and John A. Hitt of the Locomotive Engineers Brotherhood. All of these union representatives called for a legislative policy that would close "the gates to that class which constitutes the scum of Europe," East Europeans and Italians.[6]

The comments of Samuel L. Gompers, president of the American Federation of Labor, were representative of the irony that ensued when the established immigrant citizens of the working class and their sons called for the restriction of newer immigrants. At the A.F. of L.'s annual convention in Philadelphia in December 1892, Gompers—who was both a Jew and an immigrant from England—defended labor's immigration restrictionist views and the need to protect both the physical and the economic health of the United States.[7] The American German Jewish weekly newspaper, *The Jewish Messenger,* was quick to criticize the labor leader, who "in his anxiety to remain chief of the Federation has no word to say in favor of his unfortunate brethren driven from Russia to fight tyranny in a class that ought to be most sympathetic." [8]

In the immediate aftermath of the cholera epidemic of 1892, it was not primarily the traditional fears that immigrants would become public charges or bring economic ruin that Chandler and others brooded over. Instead, it was the fear of contagion imported by undesirable immigrants that drove the discourse. Recalling the brief but unsustainable panic engendered by the typhus epidemic on New York's Lower East Side and the more recent incursion of cholera into New York City, Chandler reasoned that if he could convince Congress and the American public that the undesirables he had been warning about threatened aspects of American life even more basic than economic or character concerns — in fact, life itself — headway might be made.

Most remarkable about Chandler's public statements during this period were the comments from anti-immigration constituents that he used to fortify his plans to restrict the entry of Russian Jews and other undesirable immigrants. Before the epidemics, constituents' letters to Chandler in favor of immigration restriction were almost exclusively couched in the language of economic concerns or fears of the foreigners' potential to weaken the nation's political process and the American way of life. Soon after the news of the epidemics and their presumed vector became public, however, the anti-immigrant complaints received and quoted by Chandler were largely supported by the threat of imported disease.

One constituent's letter to Chandler during the typhus fever epidemic represents an excellent and early example of this shift:

> They [Russian Jewish immigrants] make it difficult for the poorer class of our native population to get along in life. They introduce filth disease and jeopardize the health and lives of respectable Americans by introducing forms of sickness not indigenous to the soil by reason of our cleanly habits and a liberal expenditure of money for sanitary inspection and the maintenance of health of American cities. In God We Trust is our motto, but we should remember that God helps those who helps [sic] themselves.
>
> [Signed] An American. [9]

Another immigration restrictionist named J. W. Van Buskirk of Bayonne, New Jersey, warned Chandler about the health risks of immigration several times during the early summer of 1892:

> Russian Jews are, in fact, the dregs of Europe. Thieves, Scoundrels, etc. that are now being landed on our shores. . . . I think the Quarantine [is] not rigid enough by any means and think that it should be enforced . . . to the fullest extent. [10]

Throughout the late fall and early winter of 1892, Chandler substantiated his own anti-immigrant views with the comments of like-minded constituents who wrote to him. For example, Chandler's accusations that the steam-ship lines planned to smuggle Russian Jews into the United States may have originated from an American residing in Hamburg that fall named C. M. Ready who wrote him about the unsanitary and filthy "small lots of Russian and Polander Jews and others in a deplorable condition. . . . All these pau-pers are shipped to New York by the North German Lloyd!"[11]

Chandler also corresponded with many common laborers and working-men such as Phillip Mulligan, a Brooklyn carpenter:

> As a workman I say that the people most injurious to the country looking at it from a patriotic standpoint are the Jewish and the Italians. The Jews will not do hard work. It is plain to everyone who reads the papers that you thoroughly understand the question and are acting in the best interests of the country. Don't let the steamship agents put you off the track: I think your object is to protect the working man and keep out the cholera.[12]

Occasionally, Chandler received more virulent examples of the "average American's" distrust of unrestricted immigration, such as this missive from Sarah Gaylord of Springfield, Illinois:

> In regard to this Emigration bisness [sic] . . . you will have the thanks of thou-sands who are waching [sic] this bisness [sic] Oh, we don't [need] any more over here dirty low lived creatures breeding all kinds of diseases. We have the Negroes and the Indians to take care of that and that is enough for any country. You make the emigrant laws as strict as you will.[13]

By the beginning of December 1892, Chandler galvanized his anti-immigration crusade by devising a plan to suspend all immigration as a means of preventing cholera's return in 1893. Using the power he held as chairman of the Senate Committee on Immigration, Chandler proposed to force a bill through the Senate and House suspending all immigration for a minimum of one year with the hope that a more permanent and complete restriction package might be enacted during that period.[14] In preparation for his legislative attack, Chandler announced to the press that a series of hear-ings would be held in New York City's stately Fifth Avenue Hotel during the first week of December in order to formulate such a bill to introduce in the Senate.

At the hearings of the Immigration Committee, Chandler polled several prominent New York physicians, shipping agents, and immigration offi-cials on the best possible means of preventing cholera the following sum-mer. The transcripts of these hearings reveal mixed, ambivalent, and fre-quently contradictory responses on the issue of restricting immigration as a cholera preventive. For example, while many of those testifying agreed with Chandler that Russian Jews were the vector of cholera and should be refused entry, several of the shipping men and some of the physicians testifying strongly disagreed and instead advocated preventive public health measures such as improving ship sanitation and medical inspection on *both* sides of the Atlantic.[15] Despite the conflicting testimonies, Chandler announced on the steps of the Fifth Avenue Hotel on December 6 that the hearings unequivocally confirmed the need for an absolute suspension of all "undesirable immigration."

Perhaps the loudest salvo discharged by William Chandler against undesirable immigrants was at the onset of the second session of the Fifty-second Congress on January 6, 1893. That morning, Chandler delivered a long-winded diatribe on the "public health evils of immigration" and proposed his bill calling for the "suspension of all immigration for one year" in order to protect the nation against "the danger from cholera in 1893."[16] The "stormy petrel" concluded his speech by announcing to his colleagues: "I am in favor of every possible step which can be devised for the protection of this country from cholera during the coming season."[17] Later that afternoon, Chandler's counterpart in the House of Representatives, Immigration Committee Chairman and Congressman Herman Stump of Baltimore, submitted a similar bill calling for the suspension of immigration as a cholera preventive.

Chandler's quarantine, of course, was based not on the immediate threat of an epidemic, nor on the well-known bacteriological nature of cholera's transmission, incubation, and spread to others. Instead, it was an opportunistic attempt to ban all undesirable immigration under the guise of public health. The motives of Chandler and his restrictionist colleagues were made more evident by the other clauses of the proposed bill, including some of Chandler's personal favorite exclusions such as no entry for those over the age of twelve years who could not read or write their own language; those who lacked $100 in assets (the "head tax"); and the long-standing restriction against the acutely ill, physically infirm, or disabled. The bill also called for the restriction of "substandard" steerage steamships and regulations outlining improved means of medical inspection, voyage documentation, and ship sanitation.[18]

Chandler's desire to close the gates to immigrants was especially obvious to Oscar Solomon Straus, the American Jewish attorney, importer, and former ambassador to Turkey during Grover Cleveland's first term as president. In early December 1892, Straus formulated a Special Committee on Quarantine of the New York Board of Trade and Transportation to address the issue.[19] Representing the interests of the businessmen, shippers, and exporter-importers who relied upon the commerce of New York Harbor, Straus polled leading sanitarians and public health officials, municipal and state leaders, and others across the nation on how best to mount a defense against the entry of infectious diseases.

It is not surprising that the American business community, especially those concerns that had transactions with foreign countries, was interested in the debate over enacting a quarantine law. As medical historian Erwin Ackerknecht discussed in his seminal study of anti-contagionism in the early to mid-nineteenth century, the issue of maritime commerce was intimately tied to the regulations of quarantine. Since the quarantine of a port specifically meant a restriction on free trade, merchants, industrialists, and shippers were destined to become involved in the debate.[20]

The overwhelming majority of the American business community not only favored strong quarantine regulations but wanted the federal government, rather than state or municipal authorities, to administer them. Such a position reflected the businessmen's concerns over the potential for markedly different quarantine regulations between different ports and states if the state authorities held sway; in that case, businessmen in one locale suffered economically if their port was subjected to more stringent regulations than another. Indeed, this happened frequently during the nineteenth century before a clear set of national regulations was established. For example, between 1800 and 1847 the Port of New York had far more exacting rules and regulations pertaining to ships carrying rags or goods from foreign ports than the nearby entrepôts in New Jersey, such as the Elizabeth and Perth Amboy seaports. Consequently, it was not uncommon for a ship rejected or anticipating rejection at the New York port simply to enter the United States via the more lenient New Jersey ports.[21] Given the inevitability—in the eyes of the businessmen—that quarantine regulations would be strengthened, it was considered best for all commercial interests if the rules enacted were consistent, uniform and, above all, protective no matter where goods or people entered the country.

In the final report of the National Board of Trade's Quarantine Committee, endorsed by literally hundreds of businessmen, shippers, merchants, public health experts, and municipal and state government officials and released on January 6, Straus strongly advocated a separate consideration of the issues of immigration and quarantine policy:

> The more perfect we make the system of quarantine under scientific regulations, with ample facilities to enforce them, the less will be the restrictions and the burdens upon commerce. . . . The general question of immigration, and whether it has the same value for our country as in past decades, is foreign to the subject, and care should be taken under the pretense and cover of quarantine laws that the opponents to immigration, as such, be not permitted to effect their purpose contrary to the will of the majority of the people of several states. That classes

of immigrants shall be admitted to this country is one question; what system of quarantine and sanitary inspection of vessels, cargoes and passengers shall be adopted is another question, and it is the opinion of this Committee that the best results will be attained by separating the two subjects in legislation.[22]

Another harsh critic of the Chandler proposal was the commissioner of immigration at the Port of New York, John B. Weber. It may be recalled that Chandler and Weber frequently battled over the issue of immigration. Perhaps partly because of his 1891 trip to Russia's Pale of Settlement, where he witnessed firsthand the persecution of Jews, and partly out of his firm conviction that immigration was beneficial to the United States, Weber beseeched an auditorium filled to capacity at the Cooper Union in New York City on the evening of January 4, 1893, to beware of demagogues stuck in "the rut of prejudice" who proposed the suspension of immigration as a cholera preventive:

> Naturalization of aliens, because of the viciousness of local control, has been permitted to degenerate into a farce, and now the evils and weaknesses of both quarantine and naturalization have been confounded with and saddled upon immigration, and the load is too much for it to carry. It is distinct and separate from the others and should be considered and determined by itself solely upon its own merits and defects. It is admitted that if the bars be put up so high that no one can climb over them, we can dispense with Quarantine regulations and in the course of a few years our courts would have no one to naturalize; so you can get rid of a corn by amputating the foot. . . . I don't believe in cross-eyed politics or cross-eyed policies. I want to strike where I look. I don't believe in squinting at cholera and striking at immigration.[23]

On Capitol Hill, several senators and congressmen joined in the public debate and announced their objection to Chandler's assertion that specific ethnic groups, such as the Russian Jews and Italians, posed the principal threat of cholera and other infectious diseases. For example, in a sophisticated rebuttal to Chandler's contention that it was only the poorer class of immigrants traveling steerage from places such as Russia, Poland, Hungary, and Italy who threatened the health of the United States, Senator Henry Dawes (R-Mass.) argued that germs rarely discriminated along lines of class or wealth: "An immigrant's character does not depend upon the amount of money he has. I suppose that a man may be of excellent character and habits and cleanly and be very poor at the same time."[24] Similarly, Senator Roger Q. Mills (D-Tex.), who had participated in relief efforts for the cholera epidemic of 1849, recalled helping well-dressed patients as well as impoverished ones:

> The germs can come through goods; they come in the clothing of the saloon passengers, as well as in that of those in the steerage of the vessel, for pestilence is

no respecter of persons. Whatever scientists may say to the effect that nobody but those who are clothed in rags and poverty can carry disease, it is a fact that the wealthiest and best people of the country will be stricken with it as well as the lowliest and the humblest.[25]

In a more combative vein, the chairman of the Senate Committee on Epidemic Diseases, Senator Isham Harris (R-Tenn.), declared his opposition on the pages of the *New York Times:*

> I shall vote against it and take great pleasure in voting against it. The question of immigration is a tremendous one and the question of sanitation is only one of a thousand considerations affecting it. It should not be considered with reference to sanitation alone as the provisions of Senator Chandler's bill seem to show that he so regards it.[26]

Instead of endorsing Chandler's nativistic approach, the majority of the Congress favored a separate consideration of public health and immigration issues by creating a system of national quarantine regulations and setting aside the decision to restrict or halt immigration.

Like many an astute politician, Chandler knew the importance of numbers in the American democratic process. Sensing the almost insurmountable opposition to his quarantine–immigration suspension bill, he quickly retreated to create a separate immigration restriction bill. In this bill, he called for new excludable classes while still advocating the most stringent of medical exclusions possible for the final version of the quarantine bill that resulted that winter.[27]

The Passage of the National Quarantine Act of 1893

The actual enactment of a bill into law in the United States of America's legislative process is rarely an issue of one side against another; instead of clear shades of black and white, it is far better described as a muddy grey. The laws enacted are frequently results of differing opinions, needs, and perceptions of the issues at hand. Given the many voices and interests involved, a process of consultation, calculation, and compromise was necessary in order to draft a suitable quarantine bill that would be passed by both houses of Congress.

The version of the 1893 quarantine bill that was ultimately passed into law was co-written by Senator Isham Harris (R-Tenn.) and Congressman Isador Rayner (D-Md.). What an odd pair these two legislators must have made walking together along the halls of the Capitol. Harris, a tall, courtly, yet forceful Civil War secessionist, and the short, balding Raynor, the son of Bavarian Jewish immigrants, studiously polled their colleagues to fashion a bill that would both protect national public health interests against the entry of epidemic disease and pass through a Congress hesitant to enact the harsher immigration restriction legislation proposed by Chandler. The congressional poll taken by Harris and Rayner indicated that those representing the majority of the American electorate were not yet ready to support a complete suspension of immigration regardless of the shouting, activism, or bigotry of the restrictionists. More broadly, an opinion poll on the "Immigration Question" taken by Joseph Pulitzer's *New York World* in December 1892 revealed that while the overwhelming majority of Americans felt free to discredit the ethnic group of their choice, most hesitated to slam the door to newcomers.[28]

The Harris–Rayner compromise bill mirrored the suggestions of the businessmen, physicians, sanitarians, and others to separate the issues of immigration and quarantine completely and, instead, focus on the public health needs of the country's seaports and borders. The bill began by calling for the creation of a national system of quarantine regulations, specific procedures for the medical inspection of immigrants and cargos, and other nationalized standards of public health to be administered by the burgeoning U.S. Marine Hospital Service but with the cooperation and consent of state or local health authorities. This concession was, perhaps, most difficult for Senator Isham Harris, who had long been an advocate for the re-creation of a National Board of Health. During the 1880s and early 1890s, Harris proposed in session after session of Congress a bill to create a new and politically independent national board of health. And each time, as one historian of the National Board of Health noted, "the bill went to committee and stayed there."[29]

As part of the public health reforms of the 1870s, in response to the threat of cholera and yellow fever epidemics, sanitarians and politicians concerned with the nation's public health turned to the problem of enforcing national standards of quarantine and medical inspection without infringing on the sensitive doctrine of state rights, which traditionally reserved public health as a function of state or local government. With the passage of the National Board of Health Act of July 1, 1879, an eleven-member committee, including the prominent public health reformers Stephen Smith, James Cabell, and John Shaw Billings, was organized to oversee such issues. Their work was frequently thwarted by a distinct lack of adequate financial and political resources. Largely due to aggressive political maneuvering by then Supervising Surgeon General John Hamilton, the vacuum of public health power was quickly filled by the Marine Hospital Service during the 1880s. The National Board of Health continued to exist, mostly as a paper committee without any real administrative powers, until the passage of the final version of the National Quarantine Act in February 1893. An article in the law extinguished the National Health Board's commission in deference to the expanding Marine Hospital Service.[30] Understandably there were ill feelings between the victorious members of the Marine Health Service and the disenfranchised National Board of Health members (and their supporters) over issues of control of the nation's public health.

Also at issue were the political maneuverings of the current supervising surgeon general of the Marine Hospital Service, Walter S. Wyman, to increase his agency's federal powers and responsibilities. Wyman, as discussed earlier, attempted to arrange a clandestine "economic" quarantine of the Port of New York before President Harrison's executive order was issued; the supervising surgeon general was also a key advisor to Harrison in elaborating and perpetuating the twenty-day quarantine rule that essentially halted immigration for five months. As late as December 28, 1892, Wyman publicized his nativistic beliefs when he reminded the nation about the undesirable "character" and the inherent health threat of the "new immigrants" from Eastern and Central Europe:

> The order for expulsion of Jews from Russia, heretofore enforced in certain limited districts, is now being enforced all over the empire. This means that a large number of immigrants from badly infected districts will try to reach the United States, and no one can view these matters without serious concern. . . . It is not so much the number of immigrants as their character that is exciting the public.[31]

The officially stated policy of the U.S. Marine Hospital Service that winter, however, was to design and implement a means of controlling every quarantine station across the nation through one federal agency and to apply better methods of disease prevention, including chemical disinfection of all ships and immigrants, adequate isolation facilities, and the application of the science of bacteriology to the inspection of immigrants.[32] Other sanitary objectives included more stringent methods of documenting a ship's health, at both departure and arrival; supervised medical care during the voyage; and a stronger federal presence in the nation's major seaports. Providing an excellent example of his intellectual malleability, Wyman reined in his bigotry against Russian Jews in support of managing a far more powerful public health agency than the one he currently controlled. By mid-January 1893, rather than supporting Chandler's plan of immigration restriction, Wyman was a vocal supporter of the Harris–Rayner bill.[33]

Another attempt at compromise, aimed at those who represented states with strong quarantine stations already in operation (e.g., New York City, Baltimore, Boston, and New Orleans), was a modification of the law's language so as to ensure federal control but not to trample on the individual state's or municipality's right to be involved in local public health matters.

Despite its plan to establish a national system of quarantine under the aegis of the Marine Hospital Service, the bill did not negate the individual state's right to maintain its own quarantine station. It was suggested that, in the event of national emergency, "state officers might surrender local stations to the Secretary of Treasury, who was authorized to receive and pay for them if he considered them necessary to the United States."[34] This was a subtle if indirect means of insinuating a precedent for federal superiority in the event of an epidemic.

The final and most important compromise of the Harris–Rayner bill, however, was in deference to the immigration restrictionists led by Chandler. Simply put, if their more expansive suspension of immigration was not to be enacted, the restrictionists wanted some legal stipulations that would prevent another public health power struggle such as that which characterized the recent incursion of cholera at New York City. At the insistence of Chandler, the Harris–Rayner bill included an article that gave the president power in the case of an emergency, such as an impending epidemic of cholera, yellow fever, or any other "loathsome," contagious epidemic disease, to suspend all immigration on a temporary basis.[35] Adroitly, Harris was able to appease his pro-immigration colleagues without incurring the wrath of Chandler by removing the words "immigrant" or "immigration suspension" from the bill in favor of a clause that prohibited "in whole or in part, the introduction of persons and property from such countries or places as [the president] shall designate and for such a period of time as he may deem necessary." Although, as immigration historian John Higham reminds us, this executive power has never been invoked by a president, its appearance into law should, at the least, be interpreted as a minor victory for Chandler and the immigration restrictionists in their attempt to conflate federal immigration and public health policy.[36]

After three readings of the bill and lengthy arguments on its exact language, the National Quarantine Act was passed and referred to the House of Representatives for approval on January 10, 1893. A defeated Chandler closed the discussion with a promise to resubmit his bill to suspend undesirable immigration at the next opportune moment.[37]

Down the long corridors and through the stately arches of the Capitol building, in the House of Representatives, there was formidable opposition to the Harris–Rayner quarantine bill but it had little to do with either the subjects of immigration or national quarantine. Instead, it was based on issues of state rights to control public health matters and, more significantly, the power-hungry Tiger of Tammany Hall.[38] In many respects, the attempt by Tammany-associated legislators to overturn the national quarantine bill in order to protect a local franchise (the New York quarantine station) suggests Arthur M. Schlesinger Sr.'s elegant thesis on what he called the "state rights fetish": "Economic interest or some local advantage has usually determined the attitude of states and parties toward questions of constitutional construction."[39]

During most of the nineteenth century, along the Atlantic seaboard, control over quarantine matters rested largely within municipal and state governments. The New York quarantine station, which figured largely in the epidemics of 1892, was then under the control of Tammany Hall. As a pivotal player in the daily commerce of the busy New York Port, the control of the station was a lucrative patronage plum to be bestowed only on a "friend of Tammany." When he heard about the proposed legislation in mid-January 1893, Tammany Boss Richard Croker instructed his former aide and now a U.S. congressman, Bourke Cockran, to look into the matter.[40]

Born in County Sligo, Ireland, in 1854, Cockran immigrated to New York City in 1871. The burly, statuesque Celt, who possessed a "commanding figure," a "leonine head, deep-set eyes, a thoughtful forehead" and a "deep and resonant voice,"[41] quickly rose to prominence in the Democratic Party and Tammany Hall during the 1880s before being elected to the U.S. Congress in 1886. In the quarantine matter, Croker ordered Cockran to create an amendment to the proposed bill that would erode all attempts by the national government to control the quarantine system in general and the New York station in particular.[42] Cockran was not working alone, however. Under similar orders from Boss Croker, Dr. William Jenkins of the New York quarantine station sent telegrams to several Democratic congressmen, urging them to support Cockran in order to protect Tammany dominance over the quarantine station.[43]

On the morning of January 21, Cockran began his oration to the House, in a thick but elegant Irish brogue, with a defense of immigration and an attack upon the propensity to confuse it with issues of public health: "For one hundred years the immigration into this country has continued without any of the dangers or evil consequences," he stated. The main problem with the bill, as Cockran explained it, was the expansion of the federal government into what had traditionally been a state or municipal domain. Cockran parlayed his eloquence on the sanctity of state rights into an actual amendment that essentially rendered the national quarantine bill impotent. Specifically, Cockran's amendment read as follows:

Provided, that nothing in this act contained shall be construed to authorize any Federal officer to relax, modify, or suspend any rules, precautions, or regulations which may have been or which may hereafter be adopted by State or municipal authorities for the exclusion of contagious or infectious diseases from any port of the United States where quarantine regulations have been established by State or municipal authority until such vessel shall have complied with such regulations.[44]

Cockran's intentions were readily apparent to his congressional peers. Upon acceptance of the amendment by the house speaker, cries of "Oh No!" were recorded on the pages of the *Congressional Record*.[45] Almost immediately, a largely anti-Tammany press waged a national campaign against this obvious tactic of legislative emasculation and chastised the self-interest of Tammany Hall. As the editorial page of the *New York Tribune* angrily declared:

[Cholera] can be kept out of the United States only by incessant vigilance and skill and fidelity at every point. The country realizes its danger and the peculiar loss and misery which an invasion of the pestilence [cholera] in the year of the World's Fair would produce. But because Tammany controls the administration of quarantine at this one port through its control of an incompetent and discredited Health Officer [William T. Jenkins], and cannot endure the thought of relaxing its grip upon a single morsel of patronage and plunder, it strains every nerve to keep the whole land in peril. Thus far it has succeeded.[46]

Cockran, facing national scorn for the creation of the iron-clad Tammany amendment, had little choice but to back down and take a more politically prudent tack. Denying that Boss Croker or Dr. William Jenkins had anything to do with his introduction of the amendment but acknowledging that its presence would result in the failure to pass any quarantine legislation that session, the Tammany congressman withdrew the clause on January 31:

Mr. Rayner and I endeavored to see Senator Harris to-day and to tell him that we were not only willing to support his original bill without any amendment, but we were willing to do all in our power to pass it through the House. . . . I am a strict party man, and I think, reasonably stalwart in my partisanship, but I do not believe that the means adopted for the preservation of the public health is a legitimate subject of party contention.[47]

The Rayner–Harris version of the national quarantine bill passed the House on February 8, 1893, and was sent to the White House for presidential signature the following day. The bill remained on President Harrison's desk until February 15, 1893, when the "Little General" signed it into law. Shortly after that trying activity, President Harrison left Washington, D.C., for a duck-hunting trip in Canada. As the *New York Tribune* opined, while worrying about the recrudescence of cholera in southern Europe (e.g., Italy and France) and the expected return of warmer weather, "this reform has not been accomplished any too soon."[48]

A Postmortem Examination

With the passage of the National Quarantine Act of 1893, the "quarantine year" of 1892–93 drew to an ambiguous close. At first seen as a novel call to arms by those in favor of immigration restriction, the epidemics ultimately inspired a conscious legislative effort to separate the issues of public health from those of immigration. Running through these events, however, were the common threads of political maneuvering and negative perceptions of undesirable immigrants. More an entr'acte than a finale, the events of the year represent the insidious intertwining of the fear of imported disease, social scapegoating, and immigration policy that continues to make episodic appearances in American society to the present day.

Beginning with the National Health Board acts of the late 1870s and extending well into the first decades of the twentieth century, the U.S. federal government gradually increased and strengthened its role in protecting the public health. Given that the domain of public health was traditionally assigned to state or local administration during this era, this was a difficult and contentious move. Although there were a number of different proposals to create a national health administration during the late nineteenth century, immense care was taken to avoid entering into political battle with state and local health officials who had no intention of giving up their control. The centralization of public health responsibilities (which led to the creation of the U.S. Public Health Service out of the U.S. Marine Hospital Service in 1902) and subsequent federal involvement in the domain of public health required a slow, painful, and complicated process of "cooperative federalism."[49] The political machinations of Tammany Hall during the epidemics in New York City of 1892 and the deliberations over the National Quarantine Act of 1893 indicate how difficult this centralization process could be. Indeed, the U.S. Public Health Service could not boast a truly national system of quarantine until March 1921, when the last remaining local quarantine station was handed over to federal control. Not surprisingly, given the powerful forces of patronage and lucre, the last holdout was the quarantine station of New York Harbor.[50]

More broadly, the National Quarantine Act represents the changing focus of public health matters in American society in the late nineteenth century. As historian Alan Marcus has noted, "The emergence of the bacteriological view, coupled with the socio-technological transformation of America, converted disease prevention from a local to a national problem and Americans adopted a coordinated disease prevention system in hope of securing its resolution."[51] Rapid urbanization, industrialization, and immigration during the late nineteenth century raised many disruptive challenges for American society. The National Quarantine Act of 1893 was one response to one set of these challenges, a small part of what historian Robert Wiebe called the "search for order" that characterized the era. A major goal of this regulatory law, and others like it, was the application of scientific, centralized administration to public health issues.[52] The National Quarantine Act of 1893 might be best seen, then, as a vital brick among many along the road the federal government continued to build during the twentieth century in its assumption of public health responsibilities. Among the beneficiaries of this process were the public health experts who expanded the scope of their power and authority in monitoring health concerns of Americans.

The National Quarantine Act of 1893 is a document reflective of its time in other respects as well. In it, Americans attempted to grapple with some of the complex and confusing social issues—both new and perennial—surrounding public health and immigration. In 1893, negative perceptions of the "immigrant menace" were superseded by a national consensus that suspending immigration as a form of quarantine was an inappropriate means of protecting the public health and one that violated traditional national principles of the United States as a welcoming nation for the world's oppressed people.

Most of the regulations that resulted were not based on the traditional, more restrictive definition of quarantine as total nonintercourse and lengthy isolation. Instead, the act mirrored the fine-tuning process then being elaborated by public health workers and physicians to prevent the entry of "foreign" epidemics by means of medical inspection, rigid sanitary regulations, and the isolation of those found to be ill with a contagious disease based on bacteriological concepts of disease incubation and transmission. And while bacteriological methods were less reliable in reality than many proponents claimed during the winter of 1892–93, the perception held by most Americans was that medical science was more than adequate to prevent the entry of epidemics. The conquest of cholera in New York City—an epidemic whose previous visits to the United States were devasating—actually strengthened the popular perception that scientific knowledge could protect the country's borders from the incursion of epidemic diseases. As the late nineteenth and early twentieth centuries progressed, in concert with both the rapid rise in reliability of bacteriological and disinfectant measures and a worldwide decrease in the incidence of the classic epidemic diseases such as cholera, typhus fever, and plague, American faith in the value of a national public health system only increased.[53]

Inserted into the act was the controversial but never-employed presidential power to halt immigration unilaterally if the threat of an imported contagion appeared imminent. Both as a concession to the immigration restrictionists and a tacit acceptance by the U.S. Congress that immigration might equal contagious disease, this clause reflects the ambivalence many Americans felt about the benefits and costs of open immigration. This ambivalence was not lost on East European Jews and other immigrants who were living in the United States at the time. Indeed, it may have contributed to the animosity and fear that accompanied subsequent confrontations between immigrants and the public health authorities. The fact that the presidential powers clause was based upon the Harrison quarantine order that successfully halted immigration for five months made it even more offensive to immigrant observers.

As a rationale for restricting immigration, however, the 1892 cholera epidemic, not unlike the typhus fever epidemic, was successful only in inspiring a vociferous but short-lived nativist response. In many ways, perhaps, the failure to suspend immigration permanently as a cholera preventive was a function of the biological metaphor chosen. In order to legislate a long-standing "quarantine" against immigrants to protect the public health, a long-standing public health threat was required. The brief rise and fall of a widely feared epidemic disease such as cholera or typhus may have engendered fearful (and frequently bigoted) responses and policies among many Americans, but they were simply not sustainable long enough to effect permanent immigration restriction as a public health reform.

Instead, one might argue that immigration restrictionists required a stronger and more permanent metaphor of disease to characterize the health risks of immigration. Immigration restrictionists during the early twentieth century found this metaphor in the authoritative language of eugenics and inherited deleterious traits. Diseased newcomers, the eugenists would assert, not only threatened the present with their propensity toward contagion and poverty; they also threatened the future of American society as they passed on their defective genes and protoplasm, in multiplicity, generation after generation, long after the admission of the "neurasthenic" Jew or "criminally minded" Italian at Ellis Island.[54]

It would be less than accurate to conclude that the National Quarantine Act of 1893 represents the progressive improvement in federal administration of immigration or that scientific methods of immigrant inspection triumphed. Prejudice, abuses of power, and political avarice framed and informed the management of the epidemics and their aftermath, frequently to the immigrant's disadvantage. More seriously, immigration was temporarily halted by the Harrison quarantine order long after the threat of cholera abated. It remains difficult to estimate exactly how many more Russian Jews lost their lives or were unnecessarily persecuted because they were not permitted to flee from Czarist Russia to the United States during the winter of 1892–93; conservative estimates suggest at least 25,000 to 50,000 lives were significantly and negatively affected by the measure.

"The Microbe as Social Leveller"

Our own troubles, together with the troubles of others, have dampened our joy at being in America at last. We have seen and heard so many sad things on Ellis Island that we are quite worn out. Our whole family huddles in one spot, standing shoulder to shoulder, staring at the large noisy [New York] City which is still a good distance away. . . . If you've never traveled on sea, if you've never sailed for ten days and ten nights, if you've never been imprisoned on Ellis Island, if you've never seen with your own eyes nor heard with your own ears all the troubles and tribulations, all the sorrows and miseries of the immigrants, if you've never floundered in a flood of tears, and if you've never yearned impatiently for your friends and relatives to deliver you from bondage — if you've never experienced any of these things, you cannot understand how one feels — how we felt — when our feet were finally on American soil.

— Sholom Aleichem

The French social and cultural historian of medicine François Delaporte once declared: "Disease does not exist. . . . What does exist . . . [are] practices."[1] In discussions with other historians about the social construction of disease, I frequently lapse into my persona as physician and rejoin that disease is socially constructed until you happen to contract one. There is, after all, a critical synergy between the social and biological elements of the experience of illness. The microbes causing the 1892 epidemics played an integral role in the drama that resulted. Cholera and typhus fever attacked with a rapidity and vengeance. The former infection yielded a massive attack of diarrhea and dehydration; the latter, a several-week bout with excruciating pain and fever-induced delirium. They were disgusting and painful diseases to be avoided at all costs. At the same time, however, these contagious diseases were strongly associated with the urban poor and foreign-born.

As a result of this association, cultural and social responses to immigrant-imported epidemics framed the events of the quarantine year of 1892–93.

Ultimately, there is an aggressive and dangerous nature to quarantine that, as the Yiddish writer Sholom Aleichem suggests, can only be truly understood by those who find themselves in one. The narratives of the unfortunate human beings who experienced quarantine in 1892 provide some insight to those of us who are fortunate enough to live among the healthy. We need to pay close attention to these experiences and others like them. The East European Jewish immigrants of 1892 are certainly not the only, nor the last, social group to be scapegoated by disease, but their individual stories help us consider larger processes of stigmatization and social responses to disease in American society. The rather unique circumstantiality of these events — a pariah group, dreaded and contagious diseases, and the political maelstrom of an era marked by economic strife and anti-immigrant sentiment — make them especially compelling.

In terms of morbidity and mortality rates alone, one might conclude that the 1892 epidemics were successfully managed by the public health authorities. Compared to previous epidemics in New York City during the late nineteenth century, these attacked far fewer New Yorkers and caused far fewer deaths; they were also rapidly contained and extinguished. But, as one epidemiologist has observed, "Vital statistics succeed most in divorcing one from his or her personhood."[2] As the preceding narratives of the quarantined suggest, public health success is a relative term. A person's definition of successful containment of an epidemic changes markedly depending on which social group that person identifies with, and whether that person or his or her loved ones are targeted as "contagious" to others.

On February 11, 1893, the health officer of the Port of New York, William Jenkins, and members of the New York City Health Department were honored at a testimonial dinner and reception for over four hundred in recognition of their "brilliant service" during the epidemics of 1892.[3] Less than seventy-five city blocks from this feast at Jaeger's Hall on Madison Avenue and Fifty-ninth Street, tailor Isaac Mermer ate bread and herring with his five children, Sara (age 18), Celia (age 17), Abram (age 13), Pincus (age 11), and Clara (age 8), on the Lower East Side. Mermer, it may be recalled, lost his wife, Fayer, to typhus fever during the epidemic. He nearly lost his own life and those of his children, who overcame both typhus and quarantine on North Brother Island. The Mermers undoubtedly would have reached a strikingly different conclusion about the quarantine process in New York City from those who gathered to celebrate the work of Jenkins, Edson, and their staffs.

Historian Alan Kraut has identified several themes surrounding the interactions of disease and immigrants in the United States over the past two centuries. The most pervasive theme is the fear of foreigners, particularly when they are associated with deadly disease. Second is the role that medical or scientific advances play in explaining or arbitrating conflations of immigration and public health policies. A third focus of these interactions is the immigrant responses to being scapegoated as vectors of disease. These responses have often been ignored by contemporary observers and historians largely because of barriers of language and culture. Finally, there exist a large number of complex social responses by institutions and individuals to the threat of "diseased" immigrants.[4] All these themes may be seen in the 1892 epidemics and the aggressive use of quarantine to contain infectious disease among the East European Jewish immigrants.

During the Gilded Age, many Americans were alarmed by the rising tide of immigrants making their way to the United States. For many reasons—cultural and language differences, class distinctions, economics, and bigotry—"dirty Hebes," "lazy WOPS," and other undesirable immigrants became a symbol for all that was ailing a rapidly changing nation.[5] There was a wide spectrum of responses, ranging from simple avoidance to racial slurs, physical violence, and calls for immigration restriction. A majority, though, had ambivalent feelings about immigrants. In times of social and economic stress these ambivalent Americans were often pushed in the direction of immigration restriction. Labeling immigrants as "contagious"—in the face of an epidemic—temporarily fortified anti-immigrant rhetoric into specific and insensitive plans of action.

In 1892, the newly arrived East European Jewish immigrants were a convenient scapegoat for that era's unsavory blend of cataclysmic thought about an America overridden with foreigners.[6] There was, of course, a long tradition of subtle, and not-so-subtle, anti-Semitism in nineteenth-century America. Perceptions of the Jew as an enemy of Christianity and an evil usurer certainly contributed to the scapegoating process. Native-born American interpretations of the impoverished, "dirty," Yiddish-speaking immigrants helped erect a social quarantine around them long before the arrival of the typhus-ridden *Massilia* or the "cholera fleet" from Hamburg.

History teaches us that society has no shortage of means available to dehumanize and minimize so-called undesirable groups of people. The grave risks of this minimization process are magnified when combined with the threat of contagious disease. It is at this moment that rhetorical scapegoating may be transformed into a mentality of quarantine. Not only does the infectious disease become the "enemy" but, so, too, do the human beings (and their contacts) who have encountered the microbe in question. A common symptom of the quarantine mentality is to do everything possible to prevent the spread of an epidemic, often at the neglect of the human or medical needs of those labeled contagious.

The containment of the 1892 epidemics was characterized by the Health Department's rapid removal and isolation of the ill, closing off gates and ports of entry into New York City, and any other available means of stemming the tide of disease and death. The tenet of *salus populi suprema lex esto* (literally, Let the safety of the people be the highest Law, or as the health officials interpreted it, the health of the public outweighs that of the individual suspected of being ill) was the immediate concern of those charged with epidemic containment.

The health officials controlling the 1892 epidemics boasted state-of-the-art scientific management. The bacteriological hyperbole was vital to the development of institutions such as the Health Department of New York City and the federal Marine Hospital Service as well as the advancement of individuals who made their careers in these institutions. Rapid containment of contagious diseases, innovative public health programs, and a healthy dose of public relations were essential to the rise of the public health enterprise in the United States during the late nineteenth century. On closer examination, we find that the 1892 quarantines were dictated more by issues of social status than by the strict principles of germ theory. These influences were most seriously felt by the immigrants placed in quarantine, their families, and, to a lesser extent, the American Jewish community of New York City. One need only recall the markedly different experiences of the typhus-exposed *Massilia* passengers who were dragged out of their tenements by the sanitary police compared to the lenient *cordon sanitaire* provided for the native-born American Devlin family in Harlem, or the care of the cabin-class passengers of the *Normannia* and their immigrant counterparts in the steerage during the cholera epidemic, to substantiate such a statement.

The treatment of the quarantined was often a secondary concern during most phases of an epidemic, and this was certainly true of the public health efforts of 1892 in New York City. I define treatment for contagious diseases, especially during the late nineteenth century, more broadly than a specific medicinal or definitive vaccine therapy. Instead, I would argue that all aspects of an isolated patient's experience comprise his or her treatment, including nourishment and fluids, nursing care, medical care, and the provision of bathing, and clean, healthful living conditions. The quarantine officers of the 1892 epidemics were charged not only with the rapid removal of the ill but also with the treatment and care of those afflicted with typhus and cholera.[7] Their failure to provide even minimal levels of sanitary precautions, to furnish proper food and water, or to budget for additional physicians and nurses in a timely manner most likely contributed to additional cases of typhus and cholera and to an environment hardly conducive to health for the other isolated immigrants.

A far worse condemnation of the quarantines administered in New York City over a century ago is provided by the physical state of the isolation islands themselves. During the 1880s and 1890s, special advisory committees sponsored by the New York Academy of Medicine and other prominent medical or community organizations inspected the New York quarantine station on an annual basis. These reports consistently revealed inadequate sanitary facilities and overcrowding. By the criteria of 1892 medical and public health standards, little was done to provide for even the most basic needs of the quarantined. The lack of significant funding for municipal, state, and federal public health needs remained a glaring problem in late-nineteenth-century and early-twentieth-century America.

One must also consider the social status of the typical patient placed in an American public contagious disease hospital during the late nineteenth century. Inmates were almost exclusively drawn from the ranks of the socially disenfranchised, immigrants, African Americans, and the poor. When the reports of the sanitary inadequacies at the New York quarantine station were made public in late 1892, a pervasive attitude among many middle-class and wealthy New Yorkers was that the immigrants should be more appreciative of what *was* provided for them, and not complain. The immigrants who were exiled to the quarantine islands—North Brother, Hoffman, and Swinburne—were unlikely to agree. They recalled the horror of quarantine at first hand; those who survived the experience described it as similar to "the ordeals endured by cattle about to be slaughtered."[8]

Even in times of relative public health calm during the late nineteenth and early twentieth centuries, the milieu of cultural insensitivity and acrimony widened the distance between local health authorities and the immigrant communities of New York. Russian Jews, Catholic Italians, Chinese, and other newcomers had every expectation that a visit from a Health Department official in 1892 would result in a restriction of their rights to practice religious and cultural customs and, often, far worse. The Health Department's selective enforcement of the sanitary code's regulations on burial of those who died of typhus fever in 1892 is an excellent example. The intense guilt an Orthodox East European Jew experienced at the mere thought of a loved one's remains not being handled according to the strict requirements of the Torah reminds us of the importance of understanding a particular group's cultural and religious beliefs in the mounting of any public health effort. The reality was that the public health authorities of 1892 ignored the advice of numerous established American Jews concerning several cultural issues, including Jewish burial practices and observing the kosher food regu-

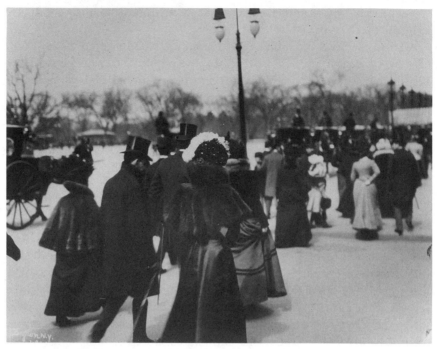

Figure E.1. New Yorkers enjoying the 1892 Easter Parade, Fifth Avenue at Fifty-ninth Street. Byron Collection, Museum of the City of New York.

lations for the detained in order to prevent starvation. This arrogant exercise of power did little to improve relations between immigrants and the health authorities.

More oppressive and counterproductive were the harsh means the public health authorities and the Police Department often used to enforce the sanitary code. Public health surveillance and sanitary law enforcement are, of course, vital functions of a municipal or state Health Department; too frequently, however, during the last decades of the nineteenth century, these functions degenerated into the vindictive destruction of businesses, such as overturning pushcarts, the eviction of the urban poor, and, at times, physical brutality. Partly haunted by pogroms and similar experiences in the Russian Pale but also motivated by the health authorities', at times, cruel enforcement practices, immigrants typically fled or hid from the public health doctors. Sanitary Inspector Cyrus Edson might have castigated the immigrants for this "devious" behavior, but to an immigrant on the Lower East Side fearful of being bashed about the head with a billy club and dragged off to an island of death, fleeing made a great deal of sense. In the event of an epidemic, such a contentious relationship, mediated by cultural indifference, frequent violations of religious or cultural codes, abusive force, and fear, potentially contributed to the spread — rather than the containment — of disease.[9]

An encouraging footnote to these events was the passage of the National Quarantine Act of 1893. Relying on traditional American ideals about the value of immigration and the powerful authority of the nascent science of bacteriology, the U.S. Congress's legislative response was to divorce — as much as was politically acceptable — the federal government's role in preventing the entry of contagious disease from its role in elaborating immigration policies. The National Quarantine Act remains only a footnote because the law really did not settle all the problems its advocates initially intended in the aftermath of the epidemics associated with immigrants. Inadequate financial resources and political battles frequently eroded the authority of the federal government in similar, subsequent public health crises.

As early as 1900, only seven years after the passage of the quarantine act, a devastating epidemic of bubonic plague erupted in the Chinatown district of San Francisco. Under the leadership of Supervising Surgeon General Walter Wyman and his assigned representative, Assistant Surgeon Joseph J.

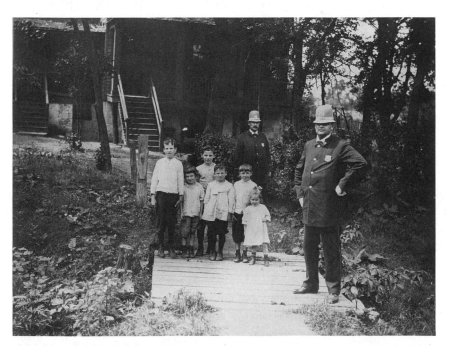

Figure E.2. Children in quarantine under police guard, Hoffman Island. Courtesy United States History, Local History, and Genealogy Division, the New York Public Library, Astor, Lenox, and Tilden Foundations.

Kinyoun, a harsh and racially insensitive quarantine effort was mounted against Asian immigrants.[10] In 1924, Mexican Americans and Chicano immigrants were improperly quarantined for pneumonic plague in Los Angeles.[11] Sadly, the insinuation of ethnic stereotyping and anti-immigrant sentiment into quarantine and similar public health policies has yet to extinguish itself. Issues of class, prejudice, and negative social perceptions continue to color the interface of public health issues and immigration. Nevertheless, the intention of the National Quarantine Act of 1893, despite the political machinations surrounding its passage, was a wise and valuable one: The elaboration of policies of isolation and quarantine to protect the public health should be a function separate from that of the control or restriction of immigration. Political and economic interests and negative stereotyping of immigrants have too frequently perverted this process in American society.

Historian Mirko Grmek has coined a term, *pathocenosis,* to describe the equilibrium of health in a relatively closed and ecologically stable population. When this equilibrium is disrupted by human migration, famine, climate, and other social or physical upheavals, "new" and deadly epidemics may flourish.[12] As the twentieth century has progressed, the "classic" epidemic diseases such as cholera, yellow fever, smallpox, and typhus have steadily declined in the United States. Their episodic visitations have been controlled with modern disinfection techniques, international sanitary surveillance methods, increased access to communications technology, medical inspection, and, if necessary, the isolation of the contagious. But epidemic diseases — both the old and the new — do not yet appear to be conquered, despite hopeful predictions of only a generation or two ago. A number of factors, ranging from newly emerging human migration patterns to the discovery of drug-resistant strains of bacteria and viruses, threaten to disrupt the pathocenosis we have come to take for granted during much of the second half of the twentieth century.

Like epidemics, anti-immigrant sentiment and scapegoating have appeared episodically throughout American history. One might argue that there are recognizable risk factors for both. Writing these words in an era where immigrants are again a symbol of American anger and are again subject to American scapegoating, I am reminded of John Higham's wise synthesis of American immigration history: "History may move in cycles but never in circles. . . . With every revolution some new direction opens, and some permanent accretion is carried into the next phase. Each upthrust of nativism left a mark on American thought and society."[13] Each time an epidemic erupts, as with each new wave of nativism, a different play with different scenes and actors evolves. And yet we find past dramas of epidemics and nativism culturally embedded in our contemporary responses to these dilemmas.

In an article entitled "The Microbe as Social Leveller" published in the *North American Review* in late 1895, New York City's newly appointed commissioner of health, Cyrus Edson, compared the germ theory of disease to the political philosophy of socialism. Recalling the 1892 typhus fever and cholera epidemics, Edson warned:

> It is not only in material things that the prosperity of each is dependent on that of his fellows. Disease binds the human race as with an unbreakable chain. More than this, the development of the world has enlarged this chain until now all nations are embraced in its band.[14]

By 1895, Edson's writings reflected an almost evangelical conversion to germ theory. But he was also quick to remind his readers that immigrants, such as "the poor, ignorant, down-trodden peasant of such a country as Russia," were a serious and constant threat to the public health of the United States.[15] Although the socialist metaphor was uncharacteristic of its author, the all-too-easy segue from a discussion of epidemic disease to the identification of a foreign scapegoat was common to many Americans of the Gilded Age.

Today, a little more than a century after Edson's article appeared in print, we find a return to the perception of immigrants as vectors of disease in the popular media. Today's potential scapegoats include Latino, Asian, African, Cuban, and Haitian immigrants.[16] Concurrent with an era of newly emerging public health problems and epidemic diseases, it is almost predictable that at some point anti-immigrant rhetoric may again include a conflation of nativism, disease, and the quarantine mentality. For example, journalist Peter Brimelow of *The National Review* recently published a polemic against immigration that, with historical perspective, reflects little more than a new strain of an old infection: "Quite possibly, disease incubated in the teeming human petri dishes that Third World cities now comprise may be the chance factor that finally crystallizes immigration as a political issue in the United States."[17]

"Chance" is *not* the descriptor I would choose to characterize future collisions of public health crises and immigrant scapegoating. The presence of serious public health risk factors, including rising rates of tuberculosis among foreign-born Americans, newly emerging and poorly understood infectious diseases, shrinking economic resources to maintain adequate disease control, and the restriction of public health and medical care for legal and illegal immigrants all point to potential episodes where the appearance of epidemic disease may, again, become associated with a scapegoated alien group.[18] How we attempt to handle these potential crises will be as much a measure of our society's perceptions of health, disease, and individual human rights as it is a measure of our medical, scientific, and technological expertise.

At present, the isolation or quarantine of people with specific contagious diseases is neither an antiquated practice nor a theoretical discussion. It remains an occasional reality of public health control. Some, but not many, contagious diseases, such as influenza, may be casually transmitted simply by breathing in a closed space, such as a hospital room, where an ill person is. As a pediatrician, I routinely isolate babies admitted to a children's hospital with respiratory syncytial virus (RSV) in order to prevent the spread of disease to others. The recent management of the drug-resistant tuberculosis epidemic in New York City, where recalcitrant patients were admitted to an isolation facility on Roosevelt Island in the East River,[19] and the handling of HIV/AIDS patients in Cuba[20] are widely publicized applications of quarantine. More dramatically, with the outbreak of an infectious disease we do not yet fully understand, Ebola virus, we find a return to quarantine in its oldest and strictest sense: During the summer of 1995, the gates of Kikwit, Zaire, were closed and the virus eventually burned itself out.[21] What appears to be different today from the quarantines of 1892, at first glance, is a decided attempt by public health workers to pay close attention to both individual rights and societal obligations in the containment of modern-day epidemic disease.[22]

The unresolved tension between protecting the public health and protecting the individual needs of the contagious person suggests a literary device commonly employed by Sholom Aleichem and many other Yiddish writers of the late nineteenth century—a mode of discussion I like to call the doctrine of *an der anter hant* ("on the other hand").[23] An oft-repeated anecdote should illustrate. A brilliant young Talmud student named Yankel left his shtetl to search for a wise, one-armed rabbi. After years of futile search, he returned to his shtetl. A perplexed friend asked, "Reb Yankel, why in the Great One's name did you waste so much time and effort looking for this one-armed rabbi?" Yankel replied: "So I could find, maybe, a teacher who would not answer my questions 'On the one hand, it is such-and-such . . . but on the other hand, it could be this-and-that . . .' "

In the consideration of human life, however, there can be no "other hand." The microbe as an agent of illness and death is the ultimate social leveler. It binds us and, when transmitted through a filter of fear, has the potential to divide. But when the quarantine of the contagious is mandated because the disease in question either is easily transmitted or is too poorly understood to take any "chances," there is an absolute moral imperative to avoid stigmatization and to provide humane, safe, and compassionate medical care for those stricken by or suspected of having a contagious disease. Adequate housing facilities, attention to individual rights, economic and recreational needs, cultural and religious differences, and the emotional difficulties patients may experience in isolation are elements as essential to a quarantine as the hue and cry of the roundup of victims. Most important, these measures must be applied equally and fairly to all who are ill with a particular contagious disease rather than relying on policies of scapegoating. These human considerations, unfortunately, can only reduce but never cure the many problems caused by the experience of quarantine. They remain vital considerations, nevertheless. The burden of illness is wearing enough for those stricken with contagious disease without the added social layers of separation.

Notes

Abbreviations

The following abbreviations are used in the notes to designate primary and secondary source materials.

Amer. J. Med.	*American Journal of Medicine*
Amer. J. Med. Sci.	*American Journal of Medical Science*
Amer. J. Pub. Health	*American Journal of Public Health*
Amer. Med. Surg. Bull.	*American Medical and Surgical Bulletin*
Ann. Intern. Med.	*Annals of Internal Medicine*
Ann. Med. Hist.	*Annals of Medical History*
Ann. Rep. Comm. Quar.	*Annual Report of the Commissioners of Quarantine of the State of New York* (Albany: J. B. Lyons, 1892)
Ann. Rep. N.Y.C. Health Dept.	*Annual Report of the Health Department of the City of New York* (New York: Martin Brown, 1892)
Arch. Pediatr. Adolesc. Med.	*Archives of Pediatrics and Adolescent Medicine*
Boston Med. & Surg. J.	*Boston Medical and Surgical Journal*
Brit. Med. J.	*British Medical Journal*
Brooklyn Med. J.	*Brooklyn Medical Journal*
Bull. Hist. Med.	*Bulletin of the History of Medicine*
Bull. N.Y. Acad. Med.	*Bulletin of the New York Academy of Medicine*
Comp. Stud. Soc. Hist.	*Comparative Studies in Society and History*
Int. J. Derm.	*International Journal of Dermatology*
JAMA	*Journal of the American Medical Association*
J. Amer. Culture	*Journal of American Culture*
J. Ethnic Studies	*Journal of Ethnic Studies*
J. Hist. Med. Allied Sci.	*Journal of the History of Medicine and Allied Sciences*
J. Inf. Dis.	*Journal of Infectious Diseases*
Maryland Med. J.	*Maryland Medical Journal*
Med. Exam.	*Medical Examiner*
Med. Hist.	*Medical History*
Med. Rec.	*Medical Record*
Milbank Q.	*The Milbank Quarterly*
N. Amer. Rev.	*North American Review*
New Engl. J. Med.	*New England Journal of Medicine*

N.Y. Med. J.	*New York Medical Journal*
Pub. Amer. Jew. Hist. Soc.	*Publications of the American Jewish Historical Society*
Trans. N.Y. Acad. Med.	*Transactions of the New York Academy of Medicine*
Trans. Stud. Coll. Physicians of Phila.	*Transactions and Studies of the College of Physicians (Philadelphia)*
Weekly Abst. San. Rep.	*Weekly Abstract of Sanitary Reports Issued by the Supervising Surgeon General of the Marine Hospital Service 1892,* vols. 6–7
Western J. Med.	*Western Journal of Medicine*
WHO Chronicle	*World Health Organization Chronicle*
Yale J. Bio. Med.	*Yale Journal of Biology and Medicine*

Preface and Acknowledgments

1. The social construction of disease, or "framing diseases," has been discussed by a number of medical historians. See, for example, Charles E. Rosenberg and Janet Golden, eds., *Framing Disease: Studies in Cultural History* (New Brunswick, N.J.: Rutgers University Press, 1992); Charles E. Rosenberg, *Explaining Epidemics and Other Studies in the History of Medicine* (New York: Cambridge University Press, 1992); Peter Wright and Andrew Treacher, eds., *The Problem of Medical Knowledge: Examining the Social Construction of Medicine* (Edinburgh: Edinburgh University Press, 1982); François Delaporte, *Disease and Civilization: The Cholera in Paris, 1832,* trans. Arthur Goldhammer (Cambridge, Mass.: MIT Press, 1986).

2. See, for example, Arthur Kleinman, *The Illness Narratives: Suffering, Healing, and the Human Condition* (New York: Basic Books, 1988); Howard Brody, *Stories of Sickness* (New Haven, Conn.: Yale University Press, 1987).

3. *Ann. Rep. N.Y.C. Health Dept.* 128–41.

4. *Landsmanshaftn* is the Yiddish word for a cooperative social group formed in the New World by East European immigrants who came from the same village or region in Europe. These social groups developed into support groups for subsequent newcomers, offering advice and help in adjusting to life in America. They continued to flourish for several decades, long after immigration to the United States from Eastern Europe was all but closed. See Michael R. Weisser, *A Brotherhood of Memory: Jewish* Landsmanshaftn *in the New World* (New York: Basic Books, 1985); Radomer Aid Society of Metropolitan Detroit, *Annual Report* (Detroit: Radomer Aid Society, 1995–1996); *Constitution of the Radomer Aid Society,* 1933 (trans. Marc and Esther Fox, 1995, in author's possession).

Introduction: The Concept of Quarantine

The epigraph is quoted from Stan Stesser, "Letter from Japan: Hidden Death. Why Some Japanese with AIDS Feel They Have No Other Choice," *The New Yorker,* November 14, 1994, 62–90 (quote from p. 87).

1. See, for example, *New York Times*, June 7, 1993, A1, A17; June 25, 1993, A18; November 21, 1993, A1, A20; September 24, 1994, A1; September 27, 1994, A5; September 29, 1994, A1.

2. Charles E. Rosenberg, "What Is an Epidemic? AIDS in Historical Perspective," in *Explaining Epidemics and Other Studies in the History of Medicine* (New York: Cambridge University Press, 1992), 279.

3. Charles E. Rosenberg, *The Cholera Years: The United States in 1832, 1849, and 1866* (Chicago: University of Chicago Press, 1987), 4, 241.

4. Asa Briggs, "Cholera and Society in the Nineteenth Century," *Past and Present* 19 (1961): 76–96 (quote from p. 76).

5. For example, see Charles F. Mullet, "A Century of English Quarantine, 1709–1825," *Bull. Hist. Med.* 23 (1949): 527–45; John C. McDonald, "The History of Quarantine in Britain during the 19th Century," *Bull. Hist. Med.* 25 (1951): 22–44; Anne Hardy, "Cholera, Quarantine and the English Preventive System, 1850–1895," *Med. Hist.* 37 (1993): 250–69; George Rosen, *A History of Public Health* (New York: MD Publications, 1958); Margaret Humphreys, *Yellow Fever and the South* (New Brunswick, N.J.: Rutgers University Press, 1992); John H. Ellis, *Yellow Fever and Public Health in the New South* (Lexington: University Press of Kentucky, 1992); John Duffy, *The Sanitarians: A History of American Public Health* (Urbana: University of Illinois Press, 1992); Oleg P. Schepin and Waldemar V. Yermakov, eds., *International Quarantine* (Madison, Conn.: International Universities Press, 1991), 125–58; Guenter Risse, "Epidemics and History: Ecological Perspectives and Social Responses," in Elizabeth Fee and Daniel Fox, eds., *AIDS: The Burdens of History* (Berkeley: University of California Press, 1988), 33–66; John H. Powell, *Bring Out Your Dead: The Great Plague of Yellow Fever in Philadelphia in 1973* (Philadelphia: University of Pennsylvania Press, 1949); Charles-Edward A. Winslow, *The Conquest of Epidemic Disease: A Chapter in the History of Ideas* (New York: Hafner, 1967). For more literary versions of the drama of epidemic disease and quarantine, see Giovanni Boccaccio, *The Decameron*, trans. John Payne (New York: Modern Library, 1931); Daniel Defoe, *A Journal of the Plague Year* (New York: Modern Library, 1948); Albert Camus, *The Plague*, trans. Stuart Gilbert (New York: Modern Library, 1948); Henrik Ibsen, *An Enemy of the People*, trans. James McFarlane (Oxford: Oxford University Press, 1988); Sinclair Lewis, *Arrowsmith* (New York: Harcourt Brace, 1925); Lawrence Dworet and Robert Ray Pool, *Outbreak* (Warner Brothers Pictures, Hollywood, Calif., 1995); Richard Murphy, *Panic in the Streets*, adaptation by Daniel Fuchs; from a story by Edna and Edward Anhalt (Twentieth Century Fox Pictures, Hollywood, Calif., 1950). For recent journalistic accounts of contemporary epidemic diseases, see Laurie Garrett, *The Coming Plague: Newly Emerging Diseases in a World Out of Balance* (New York: Farrar, Straus, and Giroux, 1994); Richard Preston, *The Hot Zone* (New York: Random House, 1994); Randy Shilts, *And the Band Played On: Politics, People, and the AIDS Epidemic* (New York: St. Martin's, 1987).

6. There are many doctrines for avoiding contagion in the Five Books of Moses. For a useful description, see Fielding H. Garrison, *A History of Medicine*, 4th ed. (Philadelphia: W. B. Saunders, 1929), 67–70; Winslow, *Conquest of Epidemic Dis-*

ease, 79-82; Elinor Lieber, "Skin Diseases: Contagion and Sin in the Old Testament," *Int. J. Derm.* 33 (1994): 593-95. See, for example, Leviticus 13:45-46: "And the leper in whom the plague is, his clothes shall be rent, and the hair of his head shall go loose, and he shall cover his upper lip, and shall cry 'Unclean, Unclean.' All the days wherein the plague is in him he shall be unclean; he shall dwell alone; without the camp shall his dwelling be." From a translation of the Old Testament, J. H. Hertz, ed., *Pentateuch and Haftorahs: Hebrew Text and English Translation and Commentary,* 2nd ed. (London: Soncino, 1971), 465.

7. Hippocrates, *Nature of Man* (chap. 9), in G. E. R. Lloyd, ed., *Hippocratic Writings* (London: Penguin, 1978), 266; Thucydides, *The Peloponnesian Wars* (New York: Penguin, 1978); an elegant historical analysis of the concept of infection as understood by the ancient Greeks is offered by Owsei Temkin, "An Historical Analysis of the Concept of Infection," in Owsei Temkin, *The Double Face of Janus and Other Essays in the History of Medicine* (Baltimore: Johns Hopkins University Press, 1977), 456-71; see also Mary Douglas, *Purity and Danger: An Analysis of the Concepts of Pollution and Taboo* (London: Routledge, 1994, reprint edition); Mirko Grmek, *Diseases in the Ancient Greek World* (Baltimore: Johns Hopkins University Press, 1989).

8. Winslow, *Conquest of Epidemic Disease,* 74.

9. William W. Ford, "A Brief History of Quarantine," *Johns Hopkins Hospital Bulletin* 25 (1914): 80-86; Vivian Nutton, "The Seeds of Disease: An Explanation of Contagion and Infection from the Greeks to the Renaissance," *Medical History* 27 (1983): 1-34; William H. McNeill, *Plagues and Peoples* (Garden City, N.Y.: Doubleday/Anchor, 1976), 124-35. For a discussion of migrations and epidemic disease in the context of imperialism and colonization, see Philip D. Curtin, *Death by Migration: Europe's Encounter with the Tropical World in the Nineteenth Century* (New York: Cambridge University Press, 1989); Ronald L. Numbers, ed., *Medicine in the New World, New Spain, New France, and New England* (Knoxville: University of Tennessee Press, 1987); John Duffy, *Epidemics in Colonial America* (Baton Rouge: Louisiana State University Press, 1953).

10. Hippocrates, *Nature of Man,* chap. 12, lines 40-49; Rosen, *History of Public Health,* 62-65; John Gerlitt, "The Development of Quarantine," *CIBA Symposia* 2 (1940): 566-80; Carlo Cipolla, *Cristofano and the Plague: A Study in the History of Public Health in the Age of Galileo* (Berkeley: University of California Press, 1973), 71-100; idem, *Public Health and the Medical Profession in the Renaissance* (Cambridge: Cambridge University Press, 1976), 28-29; Fielding H. Garrison, *An Introduction to the History of Medicine,* 3rd ed. (Philadelphia: W. B. Saunders, 1924), 181; McNeill, *Plagues and Peoples,* 170-98; Ann G. Carmichael, *Plague and the Poor in Renaissance Florence* (Cambridge: Cambridge University Press, 1986). Some ports enacted thirty-day periods of isolation for plague during the fourteenth century, but these were ultimately extended to forty days by the close of the century. Current medical thinking estimates the incubation period for bubonic plague to be two to ten days and pneumonic plague to be one to two days.

11. Gunther E. Rothenberg, "The Austrian Sanitary Cordon and the Control of the Bubonic Plague: 1710-1871," *J. Hist. Med. Allied Sci.* 28 (1973): 15-23.

12. Schepin and Yermakov, eds., *International Quarantine*, 9–27; Rothenberg, "Austrian Sanitary Cordon and the Control of Plague"; N. Howard-Jones, "The Scientific Background of the International Sanitary Conferences, 1851–1938," *WHO Chronicle* 28 (1974): 229–47, 369–84, 414–26, 455–70, 495–508. Claude Quetel discusses the geographical spread of syphilis from the fifteenth to the twentieth centuries in *History of Syphilis* (Baltimore: Johns Hopkins University Press, 1990).

13. David F. Musto, "Quarantine and the Problem of AIDS," *Milbank Q.* 64, suppl. 1 (1986): 97–117.

14. John Higham, *Strangers in the Land: Patterns of American Nativism, 1860–1925* (New York: Atheneum, 1963), 99–101; Alan M. Kraut, *Silent Travelers: Germs, Genes, and the "Immigrant Menace"* (New York: Basic Books, 1994; Baltimore: Johns Hopkins University Press, 1995).

15. See, for example, Henry Steele Commager, *The American Mind: An Interpretation of American Thought and Character since the 1880s* (New Haven, Conn.: Yale University Press, 1950). Commager referred to the 1890s as "the watershed of American History"; Richard Hofstadter, *The Age of Reform: From Bryan to FDR* (New York: Alfred A. Knopf, 1955); Robert H. Wiebe, *The Search for Order, 1877–1920* (New York: Hill and Wang, 1967); Alan Trachtenberg, *The Incorporation of America: Culture and Society in the Gilded Age* (New York: Hill and Wang, 1982).

16. Irving Howe, *World of Our Fathers: The Journey of the East European Jews to America and the Life They Found and Made* (New York: Harcourt Brace Jovanovich, 1976), 51–61. For contemporary documentation of this fear, see, for example, Henry George, *Social Problems* (Chicago: Belford, Clarke, 1884), 40–46, 161–62; and Josiah Strong, *Our Country*, ed. Jurgen Herbst (Cambridge, Mass.: Belknap Press of Harvard University Press, 1963), 41–58; U.S. Congress, *Reports of the U.S. Immigration Commission: Emigration Conditions in Europe* (Washington, D.C.: U.S. Government Printing Office, 1911), 12–18.

17. Roy Lubove, *The Progressive and the Slums: Tenement House Reform in New York City, 1890–1917* (Pittsburgh: University of Pittsburgh Press, 1962), 51–55; Keith Fitzgerald, *The Face of the Nation: Immigration, the State, and National Identity* (Stanford: Stanford University Press, 1996), 102–26.

18. Gerald Sorin, *A Time for Building: The Third Migration, 1880–1920* (Baltimore: Johns Hopkins University Press, 1992), 57; John R. Commons, *Races and Immigrants in America* (New York: Macmillan, 1920), 63–106.

19. The manuscript copy of Emma Lazarus's poem, "The New Colossus," is in the collections of the American Jewish Historical Society, Waltham, Mass.

20. William James, "What Makes a Life Significant?" in Ralph B. Perry, ed., *William James's Essays on Faith and Morality* (New York: Meridian-New American Library, 1962), 285–310 (quote from p. 288); see also Trachtenberg, *Incorporation of America*, 140.

21. Harvey Cushing, *The Life of Sir William Osler* (London: Oxford University Press, 1940), 1:215–16.

22. Abraham Jacobi, "Inaugural Address delivered before the New York Academy of Medicine, February 5, 1885," in A. Jacobi, *Miscellaneous Addresses and Writings*

(New York: Critic and Guide, 1909), 7:170; see Terra Ziporyn, *Disease in the Popular American Press: The Case of Diphtheria, Typhoid Fever, and Syphilis, 1870–1920* (New York: Greenwood, 1988).

23. Quarantine Act of April 29, 1878 (20 Stat., 37) cited in *Weekly Abst. San. Rep.*, 7:531–32.

24. John Duffy, *A History of Public Health in New York City, 1625–1866* (New York: Russell Sage Foundation, 1968), 330–55; idem, *A History of Public Health in New York City, 1866–1966* (New York: Russell Sage Foundation, 1974), 200–207; Alvah H. Doty, "The Health of the Port of New York," *Medical News*, April 22, 1905, (offprint), New York Academy of Medicine Rare Book and Manuscript Collection, New York.

25. For the history of the New York City Health Department, see Duffy, *History of Public Health in New York City, 1625–1866, 1866–1966,* 2 vols.; David Blancher, "Workshops of the Bacteriological Revolution: A History of the Laboratories of the New York City Department of Health, 1892–1912" (Ph.D. diss., CUNY, 1979); C. F. Bolduan, "Over a Century of Health Administration in New York City," *Department of Health of the City of New York Monograph Series,* no. 13, March 1916; Gert H. Brieger, "Sanitary Reform in New York City: Stephen Smith and the Passage of the Metropolitan Health Bill," *Bull. Hist. Med.* 40 (1966): 407–29; David Rosner, ed., *Hives of Sickness: Public Health and Epidemics in New York City* (New Brunswick, N.J.: Rutgers University Press, 1995).

26. Jacob Riis, *The Making of an American* (New York: Macmillan, 1902), 200–233. Riis was a police reporter for the *New York Tribune* (1877–88) and the *New York Sun* (1888–99). He covered the New York City Police, Health, and Fire Departments as well as the Coroner's Office and the Excise Bureau. The Police Department was located on Mulberry Street, in the heart of the city's immigrant community. There, Riis came in contact with many of the immigrants and impoverished New Yorkers he was to document in his well-known book, *How the Other Half Lives: Studies among the Tenements of New York* (New York: Charles Scribner's Sons, 1890).

27. I am grateful to Professor Allan Brandt for pointing out this political relationship. See also E. Fee and E. M. Hammonds, "Science, Politics and the Art of Persuasion: Promoting the New Scientific Medicine in New York City," in Rosner, ed., *Hives of Sickness,* 155–96.

28. William J. Hartman, "Politics and Patronage: The New York Custom House, 1852–1902" (Ph.D. diss., Columbia University, 1952), 297–318; Stephen Skowronek, *Building a New American State: The Expansion of National Administrative Capacities, 1877–1920* (Cambridge: Cambridge University Press, 1982), 52–60.

29. Adapted from "Report of the Health Officer," *Ann. Rep. Comm. Quar.,* 5. The major ports of entry for immigrants coming to the United States during the year 1892 were New York (509,467); Baltimore (48,525); Boston (34,332); and Philadelphia (32,465). While there were other points of entry, such as the West Coast ports and the Canadian and Mexican borders, the above-noted locations constituted well over 95 percent of all immigration to the United States in 1892.

30. John Higham, *Send These To Me: Immigrants in Urban America* (Baltimore: Johns Hopkins University Press, 1984), 3–28, 29–70; George J. Borjas, *Friends or*

Strangers: The Impact of Immigrants on the U.S. Economy (New York: Basic Books, 1990).

31. Herman J. Schulteis, *Report on European Immigration to the United States of America and the Causes Which Incite the Same; with Recommendations for the Further Restriction of Undesirable Immigration and the Establishment of a National Quarantine, Submitted January 19, 1892* (Washington, D.C.: U.S. Government Printing Office, 1892), 25. Joseph Barondess was a magnetic Russian Jewish labor union activist in New York's Lower East Side during the late nineteenth century. I am grateful to Dr. Jeremiah Barondess of the New York Academy of Medicine for sharing memories of his grandfather.

32. Rosenberg, *Explaining Epidemics*, 286; Kraut, *Silent Travelers;* Naomi Rogers, *Dirt and Disease: Polio before FDR* (New Brunswick, N.J.: Rutgers University Press, 1992); Higham, *Strangers in the Land*, 99–102; Richard Evans, *Death in Hamburg: Society and Politics in the Cholera Years, 1830–1910* (New York: Oxford University Press, 1987).

Chapter 1. The Russian Jews of the SS Massilia

The epigraph is quoted from Mary Antin, *The Promised Land* (Boston: Houghton Mifflin, 1912), 174–77; idem, *From Plotzk to Boston* (New York: Markus Weiner, 1985), 37, 42–43. For contemporary literary interpretations of the trauma of quarantine, which frequently separated families and children on both sides of the Atlantic Ocean, see Sholom Aleichem, "Off to the Golden Land," *Jewish Immigration Bulletin* (February 1917): 7–10. This short story tells the poignant tale of a little girl left behind at a German quarantine station while her parents continued on their journey to America. See also idem, *Mottel Peyse Dem Khazns* (*The adventures of Mottel the cantor's son*), trans. Ilya Schor (New York: Henry Schuman, 1953), which depicts the experiences of two Russian Jews isolated at the quarantine hospital on Ellis Island in 1915. Not coincidentally, these immigration stories coincide with Sholom Aleichem's own immigration from Russia to America in 1915.

1. "Typhus Fever in New York," editorial, *Boston Med. & Surg. J.* 126 (1892): 199–200; *New York World*, February 12, 1892, 1:4.

2. Charles Murchison, *A Treatise on the Continued Fevers of Great Britain* (London: Longmans, Green, 1884); Thomas McCrae, "Typhus Fever," in William Osler, ed., *Modern Medicine: Its Theory and Practice* (Philadelphia: Lea Brothers, 1907), 2: 231–44; Hans Zinsser, *Rats, Lice and History* (Boston: Little, Brown, 1935); S. B. Wolbach, J. L. Todd, and F. W. Palfrey, *The Etiology and Pathology of Typhus* (Cambridge, Mass.: Harvard University Press, 1922).

3. Murchison, *Treatise on the Continued Fevers of Great Britain*, 120–24 (quote from pp. 121–22).

4. George Rosen, "Tenements and Typhus in New York City, 1840–1875," *Amer. J. Pub. Health* 62 (1972): 590–93; A. L. Gelston and T. C. Jones, "Typhus Fever: Report

of an Epidemic in New York City in 1847," *J. Inf. Dis.* 136 (1977): 813–21; W. Osler, *The Principles and Practice of Medicine* (New York: Appleton, 1892), 39–43.

5. The daily newspapers frequently made such assumptions. For example, the *New York Times* equated immigration with typhus on its editorial page (February 13, 1892); *New York Press,* February 18, 1892, 1; February 21, 1892, 1; *New York World,* February 15, 1892, 1.

6. Charles F. Roberts, "Report on Typhus Fever in New York in 1892," *Ann. Rep. N.Y.C. Health Dept.,* 30–31, 122–43. The mortality and morbidity statistics for the typhus epidemic, as recorded in this annual report, are somewhat confusing as they include another forty subsequent, sporadic cases of typhus that occurred in the summer and fall months of 1892 as well. These were unlikely to be related to the *Massilia* episode. At some points in the annual report, the number of cases is incorrectly tabulated. Consequently, I have limited this study to those two hundred cases that occurred between February 1 and April 1, 1892.

7. Harold Frederic, *The New Exodus: A Study of Israel in Russia* (New York: G. P. Putnam's Sons, 1892), 20.

8. The most common social interactions between Jews and Russians in the marketplaces and public spaces of the Pale of Settlement are well documented in *Tracing An-sky: Jewish Collections from the State Ethnographic Museum in St. Petersburg* (Amsterdam: Museum Catalogue, Joods Historisch Museum, 1992).

9. Herman J. Schulteis, *Report on European Immigration* (Washington, D.C.: U.S. Government Printing Office, 1893), 42.

10. For contemporary accounts of the various persecutions of Jews in Russia, refer to M. G. Landsburg, ed., *History of the Persecution of the Jews in Russia* (Boston: privately printed, 1892, Collections of the New York Public Library); J. B. Weber and W. Kempster, *Report of the Commission on Immigration Upon the Causes Which Incite Immigration to the United States. The Situation of the Jews in Russia,* U.S. Immigration Commission, 1891–92 (Washington, D.C.: U.S. Government Printing Office, 1891); Baron de Hirsch Fund Papers, *Annual Reports, 1891–1893,* American Jewish Historical Society, Waltham, Mass.; Frederic, *The New Exodus,* 1–35, 257–58; "The Jews of Russia Within the Pale of Settlement," *American Jews' Annual for 1891–1892,* 86–92; E. S. Mashbir, "The Real Cause of the Persecution of the Jews in Russia," *The Menorah* 11 (1891): 333–41; 12 (1892): 97–105; Peter Wiernik, "The Jew in Russia," in Charles S. Bernheimer, ed., *The Russian Jew in the United States* (Philadelphia: J. C. Winston, 1905), 18–32; Herman Rosenthal, "The Pale of Settlement," in *The Jewish Encyclopedia* (New York: Funk and Wagnalls, 1907), 9:468–71; for secondary accounts, see Irving Howe, *World of Our Fathers,* 2nd ed. (New York: Schocken, 1989); Mark Zborowski and Elizabeth Herzog, *Life Is With People* (New York: Schocken, 1962); Maurice Samuel, *The World of Sholom Aleichem* (New York: Alfred A. Knopf, 1943); S. M. Dubnow, *History of the Jews in Russia and Poland,* vol. 2, *From the Death of Alexander I until the Death of Alexander II (1825–1894)* (Philadelphia: Jewish Publication Society, 1918); Arcadius Kahan, *Essays in Jewish Social and Economic History* (Chicago: University of Chicago Press, 1986); I. Michael Aronson, *Troubled Waters:*

The Origins of the 1881 Anti-Jewish Pogroms in Russia (Pittsburgh: University of Pittsburgh Press, 1990).

11. Pierre Botkine, "A Voice for Russia," *The Century Magazine* 23 (1893): 611–15.

12. Abraham Cahan, "The Russian Jew in America," *Atlantic Monthly* 82 (1898): 128–39 (quote from pp. 131–32).

13. *Shtetl* is the Yiddish word for the tiny villages where East European Jews lived in the Pale of Settlement. See Leo Rosten, "Shtetl," in *The Joys of Yiddish* (New York: Pocket Books, 1970), 373–76. Recent scholarship suggests that there were some attempts by local governments to quell some of the anti-Jewish pogroms during 1881; see Aaronson, *Troubled Waters*, 125–44.

14. John B. Weber and Walter Kempster, "Letter from the Secretary of Treasury Transmitting a Report of the Committee of Immigration upon the Causes which Incite Immigration to the United States" (Washington, D.C.: U.S. Government Printing Office, 1892); *New York Times*, February 25, 1892, 9:1; Landsburg, ed., *History of the Persecution of the Jews in Russia*.

15. "The Emigration Situation in Russia," *Reports of the Immigration Commission: Emigration Conditions in Europe*, U.S. Senate, 61st Cong., 3rd sess., doc. 748, vol. 12 (Washington, D.C.: U.S. Government Printing Office, 1911), 279–80.

16. Howe, *World of Our Fathers*, 7.

17. Herman Rosenthal, "Odessa," in *The Jewish Encyclopedia* (New York: Funk and Wagnalls, 1907), 9:377–85; Ronald Sanders, *Shores of Refuge: A Hundred Years of Jewish Emigration* (New York: Schocken, 1988), 6–10; Steven J. Zipperstein, *The Jews of Odessa: A Cultural History, 1794–1881* (Stanford, Calif.: Stanford University Press, 1985).

18. *Congressional Record* (Senate), February 15, 1892, vol. 23, pt. 2 (52nd Cong., 1st sess.), 1132 (speech of Senator W. E. Chandler); *New York Sun*, February 12, 1892, 1:4; *New York Herald*, February 12, 1892, 5:4.

19. *Arbeiter Zeitung* (N.Y.), February 19, 1892, 1:2.

20. Schulteis, *Report on European Immigration*, 44.

21. *Arbeiter Zeitung* (N.Y.), February 19, 1892, 1:2.

22. *Permanent Plan of the Organization of the Central Committee of the Baron de Hirsch Fund* (New York: Press of Stettiner, Lambert, 1891); *Annual Reports of the Baron de Hirsch Fund for 1891–1893*, Collections of the American Jewish Historical Society, Waltham, Mass.; Maurice de Hirsch, "Refuge for the Russian Jews," *The Forum* 11 (1891): 627–33; M. S. Isaacs, "The Baron de Hirsch Fund," *The Menorah* 11 (1891): 265–70; Samuel J. Lee, *Moses of the New World: The Work of Baron de Hirsch* (New York: Thomas Yoseloff, 1970); Samuel Joseph, *History of the Baron de Hirsch Fund: The Americanization of the Jewish Immigrant* (Philadelphia: Jewish Publication Society, 1935).

23. Schulteis, *Report on European Immigration*, 12.

24. *New York Sun*, February 17, 1892, 4:4.

25. *Congressional Record*, February 15, 1892, vol. 23, pt. 2, 1132.

26. Herman Schulteis actually disguised himself as a "pauper immigrant" at sev-

eral European ports in 1891 (including Hamburg, Marseilles, Liverpool, and Naples) in order to assess their medical inspection processes. He documented minimal sanitary surveillance and inadequate medical inspections at these ports. Schulteis, *Report on European Immigration,* 6; *New York Times,* February 2, 1892, 9:5.

27. E. W. Smith, *Passenger Ships of the World, Past and Present* (Boston: G. H. Dean, 1963), 163; *Record of American and Foreign Shipping, 1893* (New York: American Shipmaster's Association, 1893), 674; S. G. E. Lythe, "Gourlay's of Dundee: The Rise and Fall of a Scottish Shipbuilding Firm" (Dundee: Abertey Historical Society, Publication no. 10, 1964); Records of the Gourlay Yard, City of Dundee District Council Archives, Scotland. For an excellent description of the types, speeds, and specifications of steamships carrying immigrants and cabin-class passengers in the 1890s, see Philip Taylor, *The Distant Magnet: European Emigration to the U.S.A.* (London: Eyre and Spottiswoode, 1971), 145–66.

28. "Rigging Plan with Midship Sections Line Plan of the *S.S. Massilia,*" Records of the Gourlay Brothers Shipyard, Dundee, Scotland, City of Dundee, Scotland District Council Archives, University of Dundee; *Arbeiter Zeitung* (N.Y.), February 19, 1892, 1:2; *New York Times,* February 13, 1892, 1:5; Deborah Dwork, "Health Conditions of Immigrant Jews on the Lower East Side of New York, 1880–1914," *Med. Hist.* 25 (1981): 1–40. Howe presents a general description of "the ordeal of steerage" in *World of Our Fathers,* 39.

29. *New York Times,* February 13, 1892, 1:5.

30. *Baltimore News-American,* September 2, 1892, 6; Howard Markel, "Cholera, Quarantines and Immigration Restriction: The View from Johns Hopkins, 1892," *Bull. Hist. Med.* 67 (1993): 691–95. For descriptions of the medical inspection process at Ellis Island and the New York quarantine station, see Alfred C. Reed, "Immigration and the Public Health," *Popular Science Monthly* 83 (1913): 320–38; idem, "Going through Ellis Island," *Popular Science Monthly* 82 (1913): 5–18; L. E. Coper, "The Medical Examination of Arriving Aliens," in *Medical Problems of Immigration* (Easton, Pa.: American Academy of Medicine Press, 1913), 31–42; Alvah H. Doty, "The Means by Which the Importation of Infectious Diseases through Immigration May Be Prevented or Diminished," in *Medical Problems of Immigration,* 43–49; Alan M. Kraut, *Silent Travelers: Germs, Genes and the "Immigrant Menace"* (New York: Basic Books, 1993; Baltimore: Johns Hopkins University Press, 1995), 50–77.

31. *New York Times,* February 14, 1892, 2:1; *Ann. Rep. Comm. Quar.,* 7–8, 30–31, 66–69. Jenkins' career as health officer of the Port of New York is discussed in subsequent chapters. Ironically, some pundits blamed Jenkins for the typhus epidemic even though he was not yet in charge of the quarantine station when the *Massilia* landed. See, for example, *New York Commercial Advertiser,* February 12, 1892, 4:1.

32. *Weekly Abst. San. Rep.* 7:201–2; John B. Weber and Walter Kempster, *Report of the Commission on Immigration on the Causes which Incite Immigration to the United States,* abstract, American Jewish Historical Archives, Waltham, Mass. In fact, each U.S. consul in Russia endorsed the papers of more than 25,000 émigrés to America that year.

33. See, for example, *Annual Reports of the Supervising Surgeon General of the Marine Hospital Service, 1890 to 1900*.

34. *New York Times,* February 2, 1892, 9:5.

35. Letter from U.S. Commissioner of Immigration J. B. Weber to Assistant Secretary of the Treasury A. B. Nettleton, February 19, 1892, William E. Chandler Papers, vol. 85 (1892), items 5900–5903, Library of Congress, Washington, D.C.

36. Testimony of John B. Weber before the U.S. Senate Immigration Committee, March 5, 1892, 13–25; John B. Weber, *Autobiography of John B. Weber* (Buffalo, N.Y.: J. W. Clement, 1924), 98–128; Regulations, *Annual Report of the U.S. Immigration Bureau for 1892* (Washington, D.C.: U.S. Government Printing Office, 1893), 1–35.

37. The twenty-three *Massilia* passengers who were considered likely to become public charges were sent back to Russia at the expense of the Febre line. For similar "likely to become a public charge" cases, see "Immigration Investigation," 415–16; *New York Herald,* February 12, 1892, 5:4. For accounts of the "likely to become a public charge" exclusionary statutes, see Patricia R. Evans, "'Likely to Become a Public Charge': Immigration in the Backwater of Administrative Law, 1882–1933" (Ph.D. diss., George Washington University, 1987); E. P. Hutchinson, *Legislative History of American Immigration Policy, 1798–1965* (Philadelphia: University of Pennsylvania Press, 1981), 85–158.

38. For a discussion of the historical symbolism of the Statue of Liberty, see John Higham, "The Transformation of the Statue of Liberty," in *Send These to Me: Immigrants in Urban America,* rev. ed. (Baltimore: Johns Hopkins University Press, 1990), 71–80; for an example of the immigrant response to the Statue of Liberty, see Edward Steiner, *From Alien to Citizen: The Story of My Life in America* (New York: Fleming H. Revell, 1914).

39. *New York Herald,* February 16, 1892, 3:1.

40. Jacob Riis, manuscript of *How the Other Half Lives,* 142–43, Jacob Riis Papers, box 3, New York Public Library Manuscript Collection.

41. Abraham Cahan, *Yekl and the Imported Bridegroom and Other Stories of the New York Ghetto* (New York: Dover, 1970), 13–14.

42. Moses Rischin, *The Promised City: New York's Jews, 1870–1914* (Cambridge, Mass.: Harvard University Press, 1962), 79–81; R. Sanders, *The Downtown Jews: Portrait of an Immigrant Generation* (New York: Harper and Row, 1969); Howe, *World of Our Fathers,* 148–49; Abraham Cahan, *The Rise of David Levinsky* (New York: Harper Brothers, 1917); Ira Rosenwaike, *Population History of New York City* (Syracuse, N.Y.: Syracuse University Press, 1972), 82–85.

43. Lincoln Steffens, *The Autobiography of Lincoln Steffens* (New York: Harcourt, Brace, 1931), 244.

44. Hutchins Hapgood, *The Spirit of the Ghetto: Studies of the Jewish Quarter of New York* (New York: Funk and Wagnalls, 1902).

45. William Dean Howells, *Impressions and Experiences* (New York: Harper and Brothers, 1896), 136–38.

46. Henry James, *The American Scene,* ed. Leon Edel (Bloomington: Indiana University Press, 1968), 131.

47. Arnold Bennett, *Your United States: Impressions of a First Visit* (New York: Harper and Brothers, 1912), 187.

48. *Report of the Sanitary Aid Society of New York, 1890* (New York: New York Public Library), 8. See also the society's annual reports for 1884–91. The society did much to document the horrid living conditions in the Tenth Ward of the Lower East Side and published their findings in the newspapers as well as issuing complaints to the New York City board of health. See letters of the Sanitary Aid Society to New York City Mayors Hugh Grant and Thomas Gilroy, Mayor's Papers, boxes 88-GHJ-22 and 89-GTF-9, 1889–93, Municipal Archives of the City of New York.

49. *Grine kuzine,* literally "the green cousin" or "greenhorn," is the Yiddish pejorative for a newly arrived immigrant, just off the boat and completely alien to the American scene.

50. *The Jewish Messenger,* September 4, 1891, 4:4.

51. For a discourse on the effects the "combined forces of smells and odors" had on the French in the eighteenth and nineteenth centuries, see Alain Corbin, *The Foul and the Fragrant: Odor and the French Social Imagination* (Cambridge, Mass.: Harvard University Press, 1986); no social history of the "American experience" with such olfactory forces presently exists.

52. Susan L. Braunstein and Jenna W. Joselit, eds., *Getting Comfortable in New York: The American Jewish Home, 1880–1950* (New York: The Jewish Museum, 1990); Howe, *World of Our Fathers,* 148–68; Roy Lubove, *The Progressives and the Slums* (Pittsburgh: University of Pittsburgh Press, 1962); Bernheimer, ed., *The Russian Jew in the United States,* 41–51, 281–303; Richard Plunz, *A History of Housing in New York City: Dwelling Type and Social Change in the American Metropolis* (New York: Columbia University Press, 1990), 35–47.

53. Letter from Dr. M. J. Burstein to the Baron de Hirsch Fund, May 18, 1890, Baron de Hirsch Papers, box 37A, General Correspondence Regarding Immigration, American Jewish Historical Archives, Waltham, Mass.

54. Jacob A. Riis, manuscript of *Children of the Poor,* 1892, 71, New York Public Library Manuscript Collection, New York; *Annual Report of the New York City Department of Street Cleaning, 1892* (New York: M. B. Brown, 1893). For a discussion of these issues, see Jenna W. Joselit, *Our Gang: Jewish Crime and the New York Jewish Community, 1900–1940* (Bloomington: Indiana University Press, 1983), 23–53.

55. See, for example, Richard Wheatley, "The Jews in New York," *The Century Magazine* 43 (1892): 323–42, 512–32; I. B. Ben David, "Goldwin Smith and the Jews," *N. Amer. Rev.* 153 (1891): 257–71; "Prejudice Against the Jews. Its Nature, Its Causes and Remedies. A Consensus of Opinion of Non-Jews," *American Hebrew,* April 21, 1893, 805–17; Leonard A. Greenberg, "Some American Anti-Semitic Publications of the Late 19th Century," *Pub. Amer. Jew. Hist. Soc.* 37 (1947): 421–25.

56. *New York Sun,* March 21, 1892, 5; John Shaw Billings, *Vital Statistics of the Jews in the United States,* U.S. Census Bulletin no. 19 (Washington, D.C.: U.S. Government Printing Office, 1890); idem, "Vital Statistics of the Jews," *N. Amer. Rev.* 152 (1891): 70–84. For other medical descriptions of health on the Lower East Side, see Maurice Fishberg, "Health and Sanitation of New York," in Bernheimer, ed., *Russian Jew*

in the United States, 281–303; idem, *Health Problems of the Jewish Poor* (New York: Philip Cowen, 1903); Friedrich L. Hoffman, "Longevity and Mortality of the Jews," *Med. Exam.* 13 (1903): 21–25; see also Jenna W. Joselit, "Perceptions and Realities of Immigrant Health Conditions, 1840–1920," *U.S. Immigration Policy and National Interest,* appendix A to the Staff Report of the Select Committee on Immigration and Refugee Policy (Washington, D.C.: U.S. Government Printing Office, 1981); Dwork, "Health Conditions of Immigrant Jews on the Lower East Side," 1–40.

57. Milton Reizenstein, "General Aspects of the Population: New York," in Bernheimer, ed., *The Russian Jew in the United States,* 44; Cahan, *Yekl,* 24. For a more sociological interpretation of the ghettoization of Jews, in both Europe and the United States, see Louis Wirth, *The Ghetto* (Chicago: University of Chicago Press, 1928).

58. George M. Price, *Russkye Yevrei v Amerike* (St. Petersburg, 1893), was subsequently translated by Leo Shpall as "The Russian Jews in America," *Pub. Amer. Jew. Hist. Soc.* 48 (1958–59): 28–62, 78–133 (quote from pp. 108–9).

59. See letters to New York City Department of Health, Mayor's Papers—H. J. Grant, 1892, Municipal Archives of the City of New York. See also a series on health conditions that appeared in *The Jewish Messenger* in the fall of 1891 (August 28, 5:3; September 4, 4:4; September 11, 4:4; September 18, 5:2). For contemporary commentary on the health hazards of sweatshop life, see "Where Dwell the Victims of the 'Sweater,'" *New York Herald,* August 21, 1892, 8. The point, here, being that chronic, indolent problems such as unsanitary housing were given less prompt attention than, say, an epidemic.

60. Jacob A. Riis, *How the Other Half Lives: Studies among the Tenements of New York* (New York: Charles Scribner's Sons, 1890), 118–19.

61. Charles Rosenberg, *The Care of Strangers: The Rise of America's Hospital System* (New York: Basic Books, 1987), 15; David Rosner, *A Once Charitable Enterprise: Hospitals and Health Care in Brooklyn and New York, 1885–1915* (New York: Cambridge University Press, 1982).

62. George Price describes these experiences in "The Memoir of Doctor George Price," trans. Leo Shpall, *Pub. Amer. Jew. Hist. Soc.* 47 (1957): 101–10 (quote from pp. 105–6); see also *The American Hebrew,* October 4, 1882, 95; October 20, 1882, 114–19. On October 14, 1882, violence erupted among the quarantined Russian Jews. The resultant rioting was marked by police brutality, mob revolt, and law enforcement actions that made "the Jewish barracks [look] more like a military hospital" (Price, "Memoir," 108).

63. "Bourgeoisie and the Cholera" (editorial), *Arbeiter Zeitung* (N.Y.), September 26, 1892, 2:1. For other accusations of anti-Semitism and harassment on the part of the Health Department, see the *New York Jewish Tageblatt,* March 4, 1892, 1:4; March 18, 1892, 1:3; and *Arbeiter Zeitung* (N.Y.), February 19, 1892, 2:2. See also H. D. Stein, "Jewish Social Work in the United States, 1684–1954" (Ph.D. diss., Columbia University School of Social Work, 1958), 84, for a description of the fear these Jews felt for such physicians. Some of the best descriptions of the disparate social and class spheres of immigrants and physicians assigned to their care in the nineteenth

century can be found in two essays by Charles Rosenberg, "Social Class and Medical Care in 19th Century America: The Rise and Fall of the Dispensary" and "Making It in Urban Medicine: A Career in the Age of Scientific Medicine" which, most recently, appear in Rosenberg's *Explaining Epidemics and Other Studies in the History of Medicine* (New York: Cambridge University Press, 1992), 155–77 and 215–42.

64. Steffens, *Autobiography,* 206–7. In a subsequent chapter, entitled "Clubs, Clubbers and the Clubbed" (pp. 208–14), Steffens further documents that impoverished, elderly Russian Jews who espoused socialist beliefs in the streets of the Lower East Side were a favorite target of such brutal measures by New York City policemen.

Chapter 2. The City Responds to the Threat of Typhus

1. Edson's biography is compiled from a variety of sources: *Who's Who in New York City and New York State* (New York: L. R. Hamersly, 1904), 206; *Medical Record* 43 (1893): 465; *New York Times,* June 29, 1893, 9:3; (obituary) December 3, 1903, 1:3; David McCullough, *The Great Bridge* (New York: Simon and Schuster, 1972), 520, 534; Edward Robb Ellis, *The Epic of New York City* (New York: Coward, McCann, 1966), 374–75.

2. For discussions on the diagnosis of contagious diseases, circa 1892, see, for example, William Osler, *The Principles and Practice of Medicine* (New York: Appleton, 1892).

3. J. W. Brannan, "A Plan to Provide Bedside Instruction in Contagious Diseases in New York City," *Trans. N.Y. Acad. Med.* 10, 2nd ser. (1893): 382–94. This plan entailed utilizing the contagious disease hospitals of the New York City Health Department, and was to be supervised by Dr. Cyrus Edson. For secondary accounts of the prominent role germ theory played in American medical thinking during the final decades of the nineteenth century, see P. A. Richmond, "American Attitudes toward the Germ Theory of Disease," *J. Hist. Med.* 9 (1954): 428–54; H. D. Kramer, "The Germ Theory and Early Public Health Reform in the United States," *Bull. Hist. Med.* 22 (1948): 233–47; Charles Rosenberg, *The Care of Strangers: The Rise of America's Hospital System* (New York: Basic Books, 1987), 295–96.

4. Croker was constantly directing Grant on how to run the city of New York. Letters from Croker to Grant during this period include orders ranging from patronage appointments of Tammany "friends" to the direction of municipal funds; Hugh Grant Papers, New-York Historical Society, New York. For other accounts of the Croker–Grant combine, see Gustavus Myers, *The History of Tammany Hall* (New York: Dover, 1971), 268–76; M. R. Werner, *Tammany Hall* (New York: Doubleday, Doran, 1928), 303–481; Oliver Allen, *The Tiger: The Rise and Fall of Tammany Hall* (New York: Addison-Wesley, 1993), 170–205; E. Vale Blake, *History of the Tammany Society* (New York: Souvenir, 1901), 132–51.

5. For accounts of the obvious ploy of Tammany to control the Health Department as they did other arms of New York City government, see *New York Times,* June 25, 1892, 8:1; June 26, 1892, 9:6; *New York Herald,* June 25, 1892, 4:6, 6:4; June 26, 1892, 18:3, 24:1; *New York Tribune,* June 25, 1892, 1:4, 6:2; June 26, 1892, 6:3; and

N.Y. Med. J. 55 (1892): 486; 56 (1892): 49–50. Edson tells his side of the story about his appointment in a journal he co-edited with Dr. Simon Baruch, the *Dietetic and Hygienic Gazette*. Ewing was dismissed, the editorial explains, because he was too busy with his private practice. See editorial, "Audi Alteram Partem," *Dietetic and Hygienic Gazette* 8 (1892): 190. Edson remained a Tammany loyalist during his public health career, rising to commissioner of the board of health in 1893. He left this post in 1895, when William Strong was elected as reform mayor. Edson, like many other Tammany holdovers, was forced to resign at the end of June 1895. See *New York Times*, March 31, 1893, 2:7; June 29, 1895, 9:3.

6. Jacob Riis, *How the Other Half Lives: Studies among the Tenements of New York* (New York: Charles Scribner's Sons, 1992), 93. This quaint description refers to the city's Jewish and Italian Quarters; idem, *The Making of an American* (New York: Macmillan, 1922), 200–33.

7. Cyrus Edson, "The Contagion of Leprosy," *N. Amer. Rev.* 152 (1891): 759–62 (quote from p. 761).

8. Cyrus Edson, "Typhus Fever," *N. Amer. Rev.* 154 (1892): 505–7 (quote from pp. 506–7).

9. Ibid. Edson offered similar opinions of the health risks among "five cent" or "cheap" lodgers of the Lower East Side and similar neighborhoods in a meeting of the Section on Public Health of the New York Academy of Medicine on the evening of January 18, 1893. See minutes of the New York Academy of Medicine Committee on Public Health, Rare Book Collections of the New York Academy of Medicine, New York.

10. Cyrus Edson, "Grapple of the Plague," *New York Herald*, March 13, 1892, 12.

11. Getsl Zelikowitch, "The Cruelty of Typhus or the Terrible Sword of the Doctor," *Yiddishe Tageblatt* (N.Y.), March 18, 1892, 1:3.

12. "Averting a Pestilence," interview with Dr. Cyrus Edson, *New York Times*, August 7, 1892, 1:1. For even more strident views by Edson espousing immigration restriction as a panacea for epidemic disease, see "Immigration Report, Feb. 22, 1893," U.S. Senate (52nd Cong., 2nd sess.) *Reports*, no. 1333 (serial #3073), Y4. IM6: IM6, pp. 11–12.

13. Charles Rosenberg, "Making It in Urban Medicine: A Career in the Age of Scientific Medicine," *Explaining Epidemics and Other Studies in the History of Medicine* (New York: Cambridge University Press, 1992), 229.

14. The New York City Metropolitan Health Bill of 1866 has been extensively described in the historical literature. See, for example, Stephen Smith, *The City That Was* (New York: Frank Allaben, 1911); Gert H. Brieger, "Sanitary Reform in New York City: Stephen Smith and the Passage of the Metropolitan Health Bill," *Bull. Hist. Med.* 40 (1966): 407–29; Charles F. Bolduan, "Over a Century of Health Administration in New York City," Department of Health of the City of New York, Monograph series no. 13, March 1916, 13–17; C. E. Rosenberg, *The Cholera Years: The United States in 1832, 1849 and 1866* (Chicago: University of Chicago Press, 1987), 192–212; Susan W. Peabody, "Historical Study of Legislation Regarding Public Health in the States of New York and Massachusetts," *J. Inf. Dis.*, suppl. no. 4 (1909): 1–158; John B. Blake,

"Historical Study of the Development of the New York City Department of Health," undated manuscript, William H. Welch Medical Library, The Johns Hopkins University, Baltimore, Md.

15. According to the sanitary code of the city of New York, all physicians attending to a patient who either died from or was ill with a contagious disease (e.g., typhus, cholera, scarlet fever, measles, typhoid, smallpox, or diphtheria) were required to report it to the Contagious Disease Division of the Health Department. Innkeepers had a similar obligation. See *Sanitary Code of the Board of Health of the Department of Health of the City of New York, 1892* (New York: M. B. Brown, 1892), secs. 131-133, 47-48. Letters from New Yorkers asking the Health Department to order a neighbor to keep a dog quiet at night, an unkempt liveryman to do a better job in cleaning his stables, or butchers and tanners not to create a stench with their wares make up the vast majority of petitions and complaints to the Health Department during the 1890s which still survive. See Health Department correspondence and records, Mayor Hugh Grant Papers, 1889-92, box 88-GHJ-21, Municipal Archives of New York City.

16. Testimony of Dr. Cyrus Edson, *Immigration Investigation*, U.S. Senate Committee on Immigration; U.S. House of Representatives Committee on Immigration and Naturalization, March 1892 (Washington, D.C.: U.S. Government Printing Office, 1892), 372-73 (quote from p. 373). "The Death Scare of the Epidemic," *Arbeiter Zeitung* (N.Y.), September 2, 1892, 1:2. For Edson's opinion on the value of quarantine, see Cyrus Edson, "Defenses against Epidemic Diseases," *The Forum* 10 (1890): 475-81.

17. *Sanitary Code of the Board of the Health Department*, 5. Edson had ample communication resources, including telephones and the ability to receive and send telegrams. The board of health's annual budget for 1892 included a line for $9,000 in contingency expenses for such needs. See *Proceedings of the Board of Aldermen of the City of New York* 207 (1892): 314-24; for examples of Edson's frequent use of telegraphic communication, see letter books of the U.S. Supervising Surgeon General (Walter Wyman), 1892, and incoming correspondence files of the U.S. Marine Hospital Service for 1892, RG 90, National Archives, Washington, D.C.. For a history of telegraphy in the United States, see Edwin Gabler, *The American Telegrapher: A Social History, 1860-1900* (New Brunswick, N.J.: Rutgers University Press, 1988).

18. *Annual Report of the United Hebrew Charities of New York City for the Year 1892* (New York: Philip Cowen, 1892), 1-20.

19. Irving Howe discusses the activities of contract physicians or "society doctors" hired by Jewish *landsmanshaftn* (a lodge generally consisting of people from the same shtetl or district in Eastern Europe) and other benevolent organizations in *World of Our Fathers: The Journey of the East European Jews to America and the Life They Found and Made* (New York: Harcourt, Brace, Jovanovich, 1976), 188-89. Many immigrants who consulted these society physicians regarded them as inferior and sought out the more expensive, American-trained doctors for the most serious medical conditions. Two benefits of the society doctors, however, aside from expense were the lack of language and cultural barriers between doctor and patient. See Hannah Kliger, ed., *Jewish Hometown Associations and Family Circles in New York:*

The W.P.A. Yiddish Writers' Group Study (Bloomington: Indiana University Press, 1992); A. J. Rongy, "Half a Century of Jewish Medical Activities in New York City," *Medical Leaves* 1 (1937): 151–63; M. A. Lipkind, "Some East Side Physicians at the Close of the Nineteenth Century," *Medical Leaves* 4 (1942): 103–9.

20. *New York World*, February 12, 1892, 1:4; *New York Times*, February 12, 1892, 5:6; *New York Tribune*, February 12, 1892, 1:3; *New York Evening Post*, February 12, 1892, 1:5; *New York Herald*, February 12, 1892, 5:4; *Ann. Rep. N.Y.C. Health Dept.*, 128; J. W. Brannan and T. M. Cheesman, "A Study of Typhus Fever," *Medical Record* 41 (1892): 713–16; "Typhus Fever," *Sanitarian* 28 (1892): 272–75; R. M. Wyckoff, "The Recent Incursion of Typhus Fever in New York," *Maryland Med. J.* 26 (1892): 463–65.

21. The "mulberry rash" of typhus fever is the result of hemorrhagic lesions originating from the etiologic organism's (*Rickettsia prowazekii*) ability to burrow through tiny blood vessels. It typically begins in the axillary folds (armpits) after four to five days of nonspecific fever and pain and rapidly invades the trunk and extremities. The rash consists of three types of lesions: papular rose spots that blanch with pressure; dark red spots that are only slightly changed in color by pressure; and petechial lesions (bruises) that are unaffected by pressure. The diffuse, mottled appearance with red and purple components of this rash is the reason for its quaint name. See Osler, *Principles and Practices of Medicine*, 39–43; T. E. Woodward, "A Historical Account of the Rickettsial Diseases with a Discussion of Unsolved Problems," *J. Inf. Dis.* 127 (1973): 583. Typhus and typhoid fever were frequently confused by physicians in the nineteenth century; see, for example, Dale C. Smith, "Gerhard's Distinction between Typhoid and Typhus and Its Reception in America, 1822–1860," *Bull. Hist. Med.* 54 (1980): 368–85.

22. Osler, *Principles and Practice of Medicine*, 40.

23. Robert Koch, "Erste Kohferenz für Eröterung de Cholerafrage," *Berliner Klinische Wochenschrift* 30 (1884): 20–49 (quote from p. 33). Koch's four postulates of germ-transmitted diseases are: (1) the causative organism must be observed in all cases of the disease in question; (2) the causative organism must be isolated and grown in pure culture; (3) the culture must be capable of reproducing the disease when innoculated into a suitable experimental animal; and (4) the organism must be recovered from the experimental animal. See John Walton, Paul B. Beeson, and Ronald B. Scott, eds., *The Oxford Companion to Medicine* (New York: Oxford University Press, 1986), 1:636.

24. Osler, *Principles and Practice of Medicine*, 42.

25. Riis, *How the Other Half Lives*, 109.

26. *Immigration Investigation*, 380–81.

27. Ibid., 381.

28. Ibid., 381, 375.

29. Kimberly Pellis, "Pasteur's Imperial Missionary: Charles Nicolle (1866–1936) and the Pasteur Institute of Tunis" (Ph.D. diss., Johns Hopkins University, 1995); Victoria Harden, *Rocky Mountain Spotted Fever: History of a Twentieth-Century Disease* (Baltimore: Johns Hopkins University Press, 1990), 69–71; idem, "Epidemic Typhus," in Kenneth F. Kiple, ed., *The Cambridge World History of Human Disease*

(New York: Cambridge University Press, 1993), 1080–84; Erwin H. Ackerknecht, *History and Geography of the Most Important Diseases* (New York: Hafner, 1965), 32–43.

30. *New York Sun,* February 12, 1892, 1:3.

31. *New York World,* February 12, 1892, 1:4.

32. Howe, *World of Our Fathers,* 69; Riis, *How the Other Half Lives,* 115. Alan M. Kraut, "The Butcher, the Baker, the Pushcart Peddler: Jewish Foodways and Entrepreneurial Opportunity in the East European Immigrant Community, 1880–1940," *J. Amer. Culture* 6 (1983): 71–83.

33. *New York Sun,* February 13, 1892, 1:7; *New York Times,* February 14, 1892, 2:1. Steam bathhouses were a particular favorite repast among the East European Jewish community. A number of charitable groups hoping to improve the hygienic conditions of Lower East Side Jews applied this cultural activity to the construction of inexpensive public bathhouses. See, for example, the work of the New York Association for Improving the Conditions of the Poor (AICP) in constructing and administering such a facility on Grand and Broome Streets in the Lower East Side called "The People's Baths." The AICP erected a "building prominent . . . and large enough to attract the attention of passers-by" and a special lamp was erected to attract attention. The AICP also took out advertisements about the bathhouse in daily newspapers, "especially those which meet the eye of the working classes." See New York Association for Improving the Conditions of the Poor, minutes of meetings of the board of managers for the fiscal year 1891–92, 126–27, Community Service Society Collection, Columbia University Manuscript Collection, New York. The work of Simon Baruch, M.D., in establishing public baths in New York City has been described by Patricia Spain Ward, *Simon Baruch, Rebel in the Ranks of Medicine, 1840–1921* (Tuscaloosa: University of Alabama Press, 1994); Irving Howe has called the work of German Jews and native-born Americans to provide bathing facilities for immigrants "a fetish of cleanliness." Interview with Irving Howe, April 23, 1993, transcript in the author's possession.

34. *Second Annual Report of the Good Samaritan Dispensary in the City of New York. 1892,* 14–15; *List of Cases Treated by the Good Samaritan Dispensary in the City of New York,* January 1, 1892–January 1, 1893, 4–10, pamphlet collections of the New York Academy of Medicine, New York; Helen Campbell, *Darkness and Daylight or Lights and Shadows of New York Life* (Hartford, Conn.: Hartford Publishing, 1898), 319–34; Howard Markel, "Henry Koplik, M.D., the Good Samaritan Dispensary of New York City, and the Description of Koplik's Spots," *Arch. Pediatr. Adolesc. Med.* 150 (1996): 535–39.

35. *New York Sun,* February 12, 1892, 1:2.

36. *Arbeiter Zeitung* (N.Y.), February 19, 1892, 1:2.

37. Quote from *New York Times,* February 18, 1892, 8:3. Given the realities of steerage, it seems highly doubtful that the Russian Jewish and Italian passengers aboard the *Massilia* had no contact. In that relatively few of the Italian passengers stayed on in New York City, they were of little concern to the municipal health authorities. My review of the national press during this period, however, uncovered relatively few reported cases of typhus among the Italian passengers. The Trenton typhus scare is

described in *New York Tribune,* February 17, 1892, 1:1; and in a letter from Cyrus Edson to Mayor Hugh J. Grant, February 16, 1892, Mayor's Papers (Hugh Grant Administration), box GHJ-21, Municipal Archives of New York City.

38. *Weekly Abst. San. Rep.* 7:77; *New York Times,* February 14, 1892, 2:1; *New York Herald,* February 27, 1892, 4:2.

39. *New York Tribune,* February 23, 1892, 1:3; *New York Herald,* February 23, 1892, 8:6.

40. *New York Sun,* February 24, 1892, 1:5. For an excellent description of the "Seven Cent Lodging Houses" in New York in the 1890s, see Riis, *How the Other Half Lives* (chap. 8: "The Cheap Lodging Houses"), 82–91; Cyrus Edson, "Remarks on Municipal Lodging Houses," *Minutes of the Committee on Public Health of the New York Academy of Medicine,* January 18, 1893, bound folio manuscript, 59–69, Rare Book and Manuscript Collection of the New York Academy of Medicine, New York.

41. *New York Herald,* February 20, 1892, 3:6; *Ann. Rep. N.Y.C. Health Dept.,* 132–33.

42. *New York Tribune,* February 23, 1892, 1:3; *New York Times,* February 24, 1892, 5:4; *New York Tribune,* February 24, 1892, 1:2; *New York Sun,* February 24, 1892, 1:5; *New York Tribune,* March 1, 1892, 4:4; *New York Herald,* March 1, 1892, 3:6.

43. Christopher Columbus was a popular symbol among the East European Jews, representing all that was both good and bad about America. See, for example, the popular Yiddish music-hall song "Lebn Zol Kolumbus" (Long Live Columbus) by Arnold Perlmutter and Herman Wohl (1918), reprinted in Jerry Silverman, *The Yiddish Song Book* (New York: Stein and Day, 1983), 158–59.

44. H. Winthrop and H. S. Williams, *Toward North Brother Island* (Rensselaerville, N.Y.: The Center for Community Renewal on Man and Science, 1987), 22, 25–39 (quote from p. 26); J. J. Walsh, *History of Medicine in New York: Three Centuries of Progress* (New York: National Americana Society, 1919), 3:730–37. North Brother Island had a long career of service to New York City, evolving from a contagious disease hospital in the 1880s to a five-hundred-bed public tuberculosis sanitarium in the early twentieth century to a dormitory for students during World War II. It became a drug addiction treatment center between 1951 and 1963 with the island's "isolation" as a major factor in the program in terms of permitting good control of the drug-free environment and "facilitating a psychological break with a patient's old environment and way of life." Today it is an abandoned island with dilapidated buildings and "acres of forest and pheasants." Quotes are from Winthop and Williams, p. 26. I am grateful to Professor Barron Lerner of Columbia University, Dr. Katherine C. Parsons of the Manomet Observatory for Conservation Sciences, and Michael J. Feller, chief naturalist of the New York City Department of Parks and Recreation, for arranging my visit to North Brother Island on May 27, 1995.

45. See "Minutes of the Medical Board of the Hospital (Riverside and Willard Parker) of the Health Department of the City of New York," 1894–1905, New York Academy of Medicine, Rare Book and Manuscript Collection, New York.

46. George Soper, "The Work of a Chronic Typhoid Germ Distributor," *JAMA* 48 (1907): 2019–22; William H. Park, "Typhoid Bacilli Carriers," *JAMA* 51 (1908): 981–82; George Soper, "Typhoid Mary," *The Military Surgeon* 45 (1919): 1–15. For a recent

social-historical analysis of Mary Mallon as a carrier of typhoid fever, see Judith W. Leavitt, " 'Typhoid Mary' Strikes Back: Bacteriological Theory and Practice in Early 20th Century Public Health," *ISIS* 83 (1992): 608–29 and idem, *Typhoid Mary: Captive to the Public's Health* (Boston: Beacon, 1996); J. Andrew Mendelsohn, "Critiques and Contentions: 'Typhoid Mary' Strikes Again. The Social and the Scientific in the Making of Public Health," *ISIS* 86 (1995): 268–77.

47. Winthrop and Williams, *Toward North Brother Island*, 26.

48. Minutes of the Medical Board of the Hospitals of the New York City Health Department (see entries for February 3, 1894, and April 10, 1894). For a contemporary account of the inadequate contagious disease facilities in New York during the 1890s, see A. Jacobi, "Report on the Prevention of Contagious Diseases to the Medical Society of the County of New York, Nov. 23, 1891," in A. Jacobi, *Miscellaneous Addresses and Writings* (New York: Critic and Guide, 1909), 8:151–56; C.-E. A. Winslow, *The Life of Hermann M. Biggs* (Philadelphia: Lea and Febiger, 1929), 91–106; David Blancher, "Workshops of the Bacteriological Revolution: A History of the Laboratories of the New York City Department of Health, 1892–1912" (Ph.D. diss., CUNY, 1979).

49. Minutes of the Medical Board of the Hospitals of the New York City Health Department (MS) (see entries for February 3, 1894, and April 10, 1894).

50. Ibid., entries for February 3, 1894; April 10, 1894; June 12, 1894; April 8, 1895; October 13, 1896; December 13, 1902; J. W. Brannan, "A Plan to Provide Bedside Instruction in Contagious Diseases in New York City," *Trans. N.Y. Acad. Med.* 10, 2nd ser. (1893): 382–294. Brannan was the president of the Riverside Hospital medical board.

51. *New York Times*, February 16, 1892, 1:5.

52. Winthrop and Williams, *Toward North Brother Island*, 26; *Proceedings of the Board of Aldermen of the City of New York* 207 (1892): 315–24.

53. George M. Price "The Memoir of Doctor George M. Price," trans. Leo Shpall, *Pub. Amer. Jew. Hist. Soc.* 47 (1957): 105; *American Hebrew*, October 4, 1882, 95; October 20, 1882, 119.

54. D. Draper, "Meteorological Observations for the Health Department of the City of New York from the New York Meteorological Observatory at Central Park, for the week ending February 20, 1892," *Weekly Report of the Health Department of the City of New York* 2 (1892): 7; "Photographs of the *Massilia* Passengers en Route to North Brother Island," *Leslie's Illustrated Weekly*, March 24, 1892, 128.

55. *New York Tribune*, March 1, 1892, 4:4; *Ann. Rep. N.Y.C. Health Dept.* 30. The incubation period for typhus fever was well accepted as less than twelve days by most medical and public health officials. Cyrus Edson repeatedly asserted that no chances were to be taken and elected to adopt a quarantine period of twenty-one days. *New York Herald*, February 15, 1892, 3:3.

56. The board of health managed all of its activities on an annual budget of about $430,000, making the emergency appropriation—only 2.7 percent of the monies allotted to public health—rather paltry. See *Proceedings of the Board of Aldermen of the City of New York* (from January 4 to March 29, 1892) (New York: M. B. Brown,

1892), 205:213–16; *Proceedings, Board of Estimate and Apportionment, 1892 (New York City)*, 36–37.

57. Quote from p. 37, *Proceedings, Board of Estimate and Apportionment, 1892.*

Chapter 3. The Results of the Quarantine

1. *Ann. Rep. N.Y.C. Health Dept.*, 31. The mortality rates from typhus were higher among New York City residents (32%) than the *Massilia* passengers (9.4%). Overall, these mortality rates were comparable with those observed by other medical authorities. See William Osler, *The Principles and Practice of Medicine* (New York: Appleton, 1892), 39–43.

2. *New York Times*, August 7, 1892, 1:1; *New York Commercial Advertiser*, March 1, 1892, 4:2; *New York Sun*, February 17, 1892, 1:3; "Typhus Fever in New York," *Boston Med. & Surg. J.* 126 (1892): 173–74; J. W. Brannan and T. M. Cheesman, "A Study of Typhus Fever," *Medical Record* 41 (1892): 713–16; R. M. Wyckoff, "The Recent Incursion of Typhus Fever at New York," *Maryland Med. J.* 26 (1892): 463–65; *New York Tribune*, March 1, 1892, 2:1.

3. *Arbeiter Zeitung* (N.Y.), February 26, 1892, 2:1; *New York Tribune*, February 21, 1892, 4:2.

4. Howard Markel, "The Stigma of Disease: Implications of Genetic Screening," *Amer. J. Med.* 93 (1992): 209–15.

5. *Yiddish Tageblatt* (N.Y.), February 22, 1892, 1:2.

6. *New York Press*, February 16, 1892, 1:3; *Ann. Rep. N.Y.C. Health Dept.*, 130–31.

7. Etta died on March 7, 1892; her mother died two weeks earlier on February 21, 1892. *New York Sun*, February 13, 1892, 1:7; *Ann. Rep. N.Y.C. Health Dept.*, 128–29.

8. The Gouverneur Hospital was an emergency hospital, operated by the New York City Department of Public Charities and Correction. It was established in 1885 to handle accidents and emergencies frequently occurring among the workers along the docks and rivers. Moses King, ed., *King's Handbook of New York City* (Boston: Moses King, 1892), 461.

9. *New York Times*, February 15, 1892, 1:7; *New York Herald*, February 15, 1892, 3:3.

10. *New York Herald*, March 8, 1892, 5:6; March 9, 1892, 3:5.

11. *New York Herald*, March 4, 1892, 3:6.

12. *New York Tribune*, March 6, 1892, 5:4. Both father and son recovered.

13. *New York City Sanitary Code for 1892*, secs. 151–59, 54–62.

14. *New York Commercial Advertiser*, February 25, 1892, 8:1; *Annual Report of the Hebrew Benevolent Society of the City of New York, 1892* (New York: Cowen, 1893), 1–12; see also Hayim H. Donin, *To Be a Jew: A Guide to Jewish Observance in Contemporary Life* (New York: Basic Books, 1972), 297–99; Moses Rischin, *The Promised City: New York's Jews, 1870–1914* (Cambridge, Mass.: Harvard University Press, 1962), 230.

15. The "squirt gun" is described in the *New York Tribune*, March 1, 1892, 4:4; the weakness from hunger quote is in *Arbeiter Zeitung* (N.Y.), February 26, 1892, 2:1.

16. *New York Herald*, February 15, 1892, 3:3.

17. *New York Times*, March 1, 1892, 4:4. Henry Rice, president of the New York Hebrew Charities, appropriated $10,000 in food and supplies for the *Massilia* passengers. "Report of the President," *Annual Report of the United Hebrew Charities of New York City, 1892*, 10, 16–19.

18. Editorial, "Emigration Problem," *The Menorah* 12 (1892): 204; see also *New York Tribune*, March 1, 1892, for a sneering report on providing kosher food for the quarantined.

19. The Devlin family's bout with typhus and the differential treatment they received is described in *New York Herald*, March 9, 1892, 3:5; *New York Commercial Advertiser*, March 8, 1892, 1:3.

20. *New York Commercial Advertiser*, March 8, 1892, 1:3.

21. See, for example, *New York Times*, March 8, 1892, 4; *New York Herald*, March 8, 1892, 6; *New York Tribune*, March 8, 1892, 8; *New York World*, March 9, 1892, 4.

22. *New York Times*, February 13, 1892, 4:3; see *New York Times*, February 14, 1892, 2:1; *New York Tribune*, February 27, 1892, 4:2; *New York Commercial Advertiser*, February 16, 1892, 1:7 for similar articles.

23. Interview with Dr. Cyrus Edson, *New York Times*, February 14, 1892, 2:1; *New York Tribune*, February 27, 1892, 4:2.

24. Data extracted from the first two hundred cases of typhus fever in New York City during 1892, *Ann. Rep. N.Y.C. Health Dept.*, 122–42; Roy Lubove, *The Progressives and the Slums: Tenement House Reform in New York City, 1890–1917* (Pittsburgh: University of Pittsburgh Press, 1962), 262; Jacob A. Riis, *How the Other Half Lives: Studies among the Tenements of New York* (New York: Charles Scribner's Sons, 1890), 82–93; *New York Herald*, February 24, 1892, 3:6. Typhus data were recorded by the Health Department in terms of mortality and morbidity only. The numbers for the healthy contacts placed under quarantine are based on full occupancy rates for the eight tenement homes on the Lower East Side where the *Massilia* Jews were housed (approximately five hundred people) and the three cheap lodging houses on the Bowery (approximately five hundred people) that were placed under quarantine by the Health Department. The remaining two hundred inmates were former *Massilia* passengers.

25. *New York Commercial Advertiser*, February 16, 1892, 1:7. The reporter, Frederick J. Hamilton, developed typhus fever on March 2, 1892, most likely after a similar "scoophunting" visit to North Brother Island shortly after the February 15 lodging house visit. *New York Commercial Advertiser*, February 17, 1892, 3:3; *Ann. Rep. N.Y.C. Health Dept.*, 134–35. He died on March 14, 1892.

26. Irving Howe, *World of Our Fathers: The Journey of the East European Jews to America and the Life They Found and Made* (New York: Harcourt, Brace, Jovanovich, 1976), 519.

27. Mordechai Soltes, *The Yiddish Press: An Americanizing Agency* (New York: Teacher's College of Columbia University, 1925), 15–30. The anarchist newspaper *Freie Arbeiter Shtime* was sporadically published during the time of the typhus epidemic. Only two issues of this paper came out during this period (February to April 1892) and the epidemic was not mentioned.

28. Ronald Sanders, *The Downtown Jews: Portraits of an Immigrant Generation* (New York: Harper and Row, 1969), 108.

29. *Arbeiter Zeitung* (N.Y.), February 26, 1892, 2:1. *Lefl-leit,* or spoon-people, is a disparaging term for doctors that originates from the late-nineteenth-century physician's habit of using the reverse side of a table spoon for a tongue depressor. For an analysis of Cahan's life and journalism, see A. Cahan, *Bletter fun mein leben (Pages from My Life),* 3 vols. (New York: Forward, 1926), reprinted in English, *The Education of Abraham Cahan* (Philadelphia: Jewish Publication Society, 1969); Theodore Pollock, "The Solitary Clarinetist: A Critical Biography of Abraham Cahan 1860–1917" (Ph.D. diss., Columbia University, 1959), 132–92; Sanders, *Downtown Jews,* 148–276; Moses Richin, ed., *Grandma Never Lived in America: The New Journalism of Abraham Cahan* (Bloomington: University of Indiana Press, 1985); Tamara K. Hareven, "Un-American America and the *Jewish Daily Forward,*" *YIVO Annual of Jewish Social Science* 14 (1969): 234–50; Jules Chametsky, *From the Ghetto: The Fiction of Abraham Cahan* (Amherst: University of Massachusetts Press, 1977).

30. For an excellent analysis of the state of Yiddish journalism in the late nineteenth and early twentieth centuries, see Soltes, *The Yiddish Press,* 15–30, 51–75; Robert E. Park, *The Immigrant Press and Its Control* (New York: Harper and Brothers, 1922), 89–110, 166–92; Victor R. Greene, *American Immigrant Leaders, 1800–1910: Marginality and Identity* (Baltimore: Johns Hopkins University Press, 1987), 89–95.

31. *Leksikon fun de Nayer Yiddisher Literature (Biographical Dictionary of Modern Yiddish Literature)* (New York: Congress for Jewish Culture, 1960), 667–69; Sol Liptzin, *A History of Yiddish Literature* (New York: Jonathan David, 1972), 157–58.

32. *Yiddishe Tageblatt* (N.Y.), March 4, 1892, 1:4; *Yiddishe Gazetten,* March 4, 1892, 1:1.

33. For a cultural history of William Shakespeare in America, see Lawrence W. Levine, *Highbrow / Low Brow: The Emergence of Cultural Hierarchy in America* (Cambridge, Mass.: Harvard University Press, 1988), 13–81.

34. Gerald Sorin, *A Time for Building: The Third Migration, 1880–1920* (Baltimore: Johns Hopkins University Press, 1992), 55–60.

35. Anonymous, *The Talmud Jew: A True Exposure of the Doctrines and Aims of Judaism* (ten-cent pamphlet); John Higham, "Ideological Anti-Semitism in the Gilded Age," in *Send These to Me: Immigrants in Urban America,* rev. ed. (Baltimore: Johns Hopkins University Press, 1984), 95–116. I am grateful to Professor John Higham of the Johns Hopkins University for generously sharing his notes with me concerning this rare pamphlet.

36. *New York Tribune,* February 20, 1892, 1:4; *New York Sun,* February 25, 1892, 5:3.

37. *New York Evening Post,* February 16, 1892, 12:2; February 18, 1892, 1:3.

38. *New York Press,* February 18, 1892, 1; February 21, 1892, 1. For complaints by the Yiddish press of the *New York Press*'s coverage of Russian Jews, see *Arbeiter Zeitung* (N.Y.), February 19, 1892, 2:2; February 26, 1892, 2:1.

39. *New York Press,* February 18, 1892, 1; February 21, 1892, 1; *New York Sun,* February 12, 1892, 1:1.

40. *New York World,* February 15, 1892, 8:1; W. A. Swanberg, *Pulitzer* (New York:

Scribner's, 1967), 9. Anti-Semitic cartoons, like other forms of stereotypical dialect and racist humor, were staples of the American humor magazine and newspaper of the 1890s. The most casual perusal through an issue of *Puck, Life,* or *Judge,* the leading political humor magazines of the day, can easily confirm this statement. See, for example, *Judge,* November 12, 1892, 312–13; *Puck,* February 24, 1892, 6; *Life,* August 25, 1892, 104, for cartoons portraying Jews as avaricious, penurious, and the butt of humor. Such cheap satire was continually the source of injury and outrage among the Jewish American community. See, for example, an editorial entitled "Comic Journalism," *The Jewish Messenger,* February 26, 1892, 4:2, which attacks *Judge* magazine and similar periodicals for their "grotesque exaggeration" and "coarse lampoon" of Jews.

41. Letter to the editor from "A Reader," *New York Times,* February 21, 1892, 20:4; similar diatribes conflating typhus with the mass immigration of Russian Jews and the need to restrict their entry can be found in *New York World,* February 21, 1892, 4:2; *New York Sun,* February 22, 1892, 6:5; *Leslie's Illustrated Weekly* 4 (1892): 27.

42. *Boston Med. & Surg. J.* 126 (1892): 173–74.

43. *New York Times,* February 14, 1892, 2:1.

44. Ibid. The headline for this particular article reads: "The *Nevada*'s Hebrew Passengers Detained at Hoffman Island." For sanitary conditions of the Port of Liverpool during this time, see *Weekly Abst. San. Rep.* 7:83–87, 94–97.

45. *New York Times,* February 15, 1892, 1:7.

46. *New York Press,* February 16, 1892, 1:3; *New York Commercial Advertiser,* February 17, 1892, 3:3; *New York Herald,* February 16, 1892, 3:1. Quarantine stations in Boston, Philadelphia, Baltimore, and Port Charles, Maryland, are among those that adopted Jenkins' "Russian Jewish" policy.

47. *Immigration Investigation* (March 1892), 368.

48. Wyman later contradicted this action when summarizing the world's public health for the year; he announced by official circular in August 1892 that "no official information has been received from Odessa, or any other Russian port, announcing the prevalence in epidemic form, or to an alarming degree, of typhus fever." *Weekly Abst. San. Rep.,* 7:117. J. H. Volkmann, the acting U.S. consul at Odessa, did, however, report an epidemic of "typhus recurrens" (most likely recurrent fever, a spirochete infection) that winter among the poor but it was being well controlled by the chief surgeon and his staff. Other consulate reports, available in May 1892, from Warsaw, Riga, Helsingfors, Wilborg, and Ato confirmed that relatively few cases of typhus fever were noted in the Russian Pale of Settlement that year (ibid., 201–3).

49. "Collected Typhus Death Statistics for Jan. 1, 1891–March 11, 1892 as reported by the U.S. Consuls of Major Ports," *Weekly Abst. San. Rep.* 7: 118. This information was readily available to all health officers in the United States and was routinely provided for the health officers of the Ports of New York, Baltimore, and Boston, the major ports of entry for immigrants, via telegram to avoid delays; examples of the telegraphic communication between the surgeon general and local health officers in regard to the typhus epidemic can be found in the office letter books of the Marine

Hospital Service, Office of Supervising Surgeon General, 85:146, 170, 206–7, 220, 221, 300, 305–6, 344, 356, 375, 381, R.G. 90, National Archives, Washington, D.C.

50. *New York Times*, February 16, 1892, 1:5.

51. Frederic L. Paxson, "William Eaton Chandler," in A. Johnson, ed., *Dictionary of American Biography* (New York: Charles Scribner's Sons, 1929), 3:616–18; Leon B. Richardson, *William E. Chandler, Republican* (New York: Dodd, Mead, 1940), 408–58.

52. William E. Chandler, "Methods of Restricting Immigration," *The Forum* 13 (1892): 128–42; see also "Restricting Immigration," an editorial that appeared in the *New York Times*, March 6, 1892, 4:2, supporting Chandler's views.

53. Thomas J. Archdeacon, *Becoming American: An Ethnic History* (New York: Free Press, 1984), 145.

54. Richardson, *William E. Chandler, Republican*, 417; E. P. Hutchinson, *Legislative History of American Immigration Policy, 1798–1965* (Philadelphia: University of Pennsylvania Press, 1981), 100–103; J. Higham, *Strangers in the Land: Patterns of American Nativism, 1860–1925* (New York: Atheneum, 1963), 99–100.

55. Literacy of Russian Jews is also discussed in Peter Wiernik, "The Jew in Russia," in Charles Bernheimer, ed., *The Russian Jew in the United States* (Philadelphia: J. C. Winston, 1905), 27–28; and A. Cahan, "The Russian Jew in America," *Atlantic* 82 (1898): 128–39. For a general discussion of literacy tests as a means of immigration restriction, see Barbara Solomon, *Ancestors and Immigrants, A Changing New England Tradition* (Cambridge, Mass.: Harvard University Press, 1956), 79, 115–17, 124, 174, 180, 196–98, 202.

56. Philippa Strum, *Louis D. Brandeis: Justice for the People* (New York: Schocken, 1984), 10.

57. Letter from Lewis N. Dembitz, attorney at law, to Sen. W. E. Chandler, March 4, 1892, William E. Chandler Papers, vol. 85 (1892), items 5945–47, Library of Congress, Washington, D.C.

58. Higham, *Strangers in the Land*, 100.

59. *Congressional Record* (Senate), February 15, 1892, vol. 23, pt. 2 [52nd Cong., 1st sess.], 1132; *New York Times*, February 16, 1892, 1:5; *New York Tribune*, February 16, 1892, 1:4; *New York Herald*, February 16, 1892, 3:1; *New York Sun*, February 16, 1892, 2:1; William E. Chandler Papers, vol. 85, (January 13–March 31, 1892), vol. 86 (April 1–August 8, 1892), Library of Congress, Washington, D.C.

60. *New York Tribune*, March 5, 1892, 1:2; see also William Chandler Papers, vol. 85, items 5914–33.

61. *Immigration Investigation* (March 1892), 421.

62. Ibid., 422.

63. *New York Times*, March 7, 1892, 5:6; *New York Tribune*, March 7, 1892, 5:1.

64. *Immigration Investigation* (March 1892); Edson's testimony can be found on pp. 372–82; Biggs', pp. 382–89; Smith's, pp. 425–33; Jenkins', pp. 367–72.

65. Chandler, "Methods of Restricting Immigration," 128–42.

66. *New York Commercial Advertiser*, February 15, 1892, 1:3.

Chapter 4. Awaiting the Cholera

The title to Part 2 is quoted from a headline in the *New York Herald,* August 26, 1892, 1. The Godkin quote is from William Armstrong, ed., *The Gilded Age Letters of E. L. Godkin* (Albany: State University of New York Press, 1974), 439. The Yiddish curse (*"Choleria!"* — "A plague upon you!") cited in the subtitle to Chapter 4 can be found, for example, in Sholom Aleichem, "Cholera," in *The Great Fair: Scenes from My Childhood,* trans. Tamara Kahana (New York: Noonday, 1965), 165–71.

1. E. P. Hutchinson, *Legislative History of American Immigration Policy, 1798–1965* (Philadelphia: University of Pennsylvania Press, 1981), 106.

2. Ibid., 103–5.

3. Ronald Takaki, *Strangers from a Different Shore: A History of Asian-Americans* (New York: Penguin Books, 1989). A similar ease in legislating laws of separation was experienced by African Americans during this period. See, for example, C. Vann Woodward, *The Strange Career of Jim Crow,* 3rd ed. (New York: Oxford University Press, 1974); and Joel Williamson, *A Rage for Order: Black–White Relations in the American South since Emancipation* (New York: Oxford University Press, 1986).

4. Paul Krause, *The Battle for Homestead, 1880–1892: Politics, Steel and Culture* (Pittsburgh: University of Pittsburgh Press, 1992), 3, 5, 354–55.

5. Matthew Josephson, *The Robber Barons: The Great American Capitalists, 1861–1901* (New York: Harcourt, Brace, 1934), 371. Berkman is, perhaps, better known as Emma Goldman's erstwhile consort. Emma Goldman, *Living My Life,* 2 vols. (New York: Dover, 1970); Alice Wexler, *Emma Goldman in Exile: From the Russian Revolution to the Spanish Civil War* (Boston: Beacon, 1989).

6. Wim de Wit, "Building an Illusion: The Design of the World's Columbian Exposition," in Neil Harris, Wim de Wit, James Gilbert, and Robert W. Rydell, eds., *Grand Illusions: Chicago's World's Fair of 1893* (Chicago: Chicago Historical Society, 1993), 43–98; R. Reid Badger, *The Great American Fair: The World's Columbian Exposition and American Culture* (Chicago: Nelson Hall, 1979), 108.

7. The Adams quote is from *The Education of Henry Adams,* in Henry Adams, *Novels, Mont Saint Michel, The Education* (New York: Library of America, 1983), 1034. See also, The World's Congress Auxiliary of the World's Columbian Exposition of 1893, Department of Medicine and Public Health, "Preliminary Address of the Committee of the World's Congress Auxiliary on a Public Health Congress," 1893, Chicago World's Fair Collection, Harold Washington Archives and Historical Collections, Chicago Public Library, Chicago, Ill.; Isaac D. Rawlings, *The Rise and Fall of Disease in Illinois* (Springfield: Illinois State Department of Health, 1927), 325–27; testimony of John Rauch, M.D., to the U.S. Senate Committee on Immigration, January 6, 1893, *Congressional Record* (Senate) (52nd Cong., 2nd sess.), 363.

8. For summaries of the presidential platforms during the 1892 election, see Myron Berman, "The Attitude of American Jewry towards East European Immigration, 1881–1914" (Ph.D. diss., Columbia University, 1963), 162–93; Sheldon M. Neu-

ringer, "American Jewry and United States Immigration Policy, 1881–1953" (Ph.D. diss., University of Wisconsin, 1969), 1–37.

9. Over two million people died, worldwide, of cholera in 1892. Frank Clemow, *The Cholera Epidemic of 1892 in the Russian Empire* (London: Longmans, Green, 1893); J. G. Speed, "Cholera in Russia," *Harper's Weekly,* 36 (1892): 718; R. G. Robbins, *Famine in Russia, 1891–1892: The Imperial Government Responds to a Crisis* (New York: Columbia University Press, 1975), 170–71; John F. Hutchinson, *Politics and Public Health in Revolutionary Russia, 1890–1918* (Baltimore: Johns Hopkins University Press, 1990); Nancy Frieden, *Russian Physicians in an Era of Reform and Revolution, 1856–1905* (Princeton: Princeton University Press, 1981), 136–37; T. Donnelly and V. Gribabayedoff, "Famine Stricken Russia, Contemporary Scenes in the Volga Provinces," *Frank Leslie's Popular Monthly* 34 (1892): 37–48; W. C. Edgar, "Russia's Land System: The Cause of the Famine," *The Forum* 13 (1892): 578–82; E. B. Lanin, "Famine in Russia," *Fortnightly Review* 56 (1891): 636–52; editorial, "Famine and Disease in Russia," *Brit. Med. J.* 1 (1892): 974.

10. Charles Rosenberg, *The Cholera Years: The United States in 1832, 1849 and 1866* (Chicago: University of Chicago Press, 1987), 1; Richard Evans, *Death in Hamburg: Society and Politics in the Cholera Years, 1830–1910* (New York: Oxford University Press, 1987); Ilana Löwy, "From Guinea Pigs to Man: The Development of Haffkine's Anticholera Vaccine," *J. Hist. Med. Allied Sci.* 47 (1992): 270–309; Anne Hardy, "Cholera, Quarantine, and the English Preventive System, 1850–1895," *Med. Hist.* 37 (1993): 250–69. See also R. J. Morris, *Cholera, 1832: The Social Response to an Epidemic* (New York: Holmes and Meier, 1976); M. Durey, *The Return of the Plague: British Society and the Cholera, 1831–1832* (Dublin: Gill and Macmillan, 1979); F. Delaporte, *Disease and Civilization: The Cholera in Paris, 1832,* trans. A. Goldhammer (Cambridge, Mass.: MIT Press, 1986); C. J. Kudlick, *Cholera in Post-revolutionary Paris: A Cultural History* (Berkeley: University of California Press, 1996); M. Pelling, *Cholera, Fever, and English Medicine, 1825–1865* (Oxford: Oxford University Press, 1978); R. E. McGrew, *Russia and the Cholera, 1823–1832* (Madison: University of Wisconsin Press, 1965); Norman Longmate, *King Cholera: The Biography of a Disease* (London: H. Hamilton, 1966); F. Snowden, *Naples in the Time of Cholera, 1884–1911* (New York: Cambridge University Press, 1996).

11. For contemporary clinical descriptions of cholera, see William Osler, *The Principles and Practice of Medicine* (New York: Appleton, 1892), 118–24; Edmund C. Wendt, ed., *A Treatise on Cholera* (New York: William Wood, 1885).

12. Nancy Tomes, "The Private Side of Public Health: Sanitary Science, Domestic Hygiene, and the Germ Theory, 1870–1900," *Bull. Hist. Med.* 64 (1990): 509–39.

13. Evans, *Death in Hamburg,* 230.

14. *New York Times,* August 29, 1892, 1:1.

15. Evans documents the collusion in *Death in Hamburg,* 316–17. My examination of the cholera ships' manifests supports his conclusion. In order for a ship to set sail, the U.S. consul had to approve its "bill of health"; the federal representative, Charles H. Burke, was convinced by German health officials that cholera was

not a problem based upon their examination. The steamships *Moravia, Normannia,* and *Rugia* — all Hamburg-American steamers — were given a clean bill of health by Burke. These three ships brought the majority of cholera cases to America. *Passenger Lists of Vessels Arriving at New York, 1820–1897,* microcopy no. 237, reel no. 596, August 23–September 7, 1892; and reel no. 597, September 8–23, 1892, National Archives, Washington, D.C.

16. The scope and magnitude of the Hamburg cholera epidemic have been well described by Evans in *Death in Hamburg,* and need not be repeated here; *New York Tribune,* August 24, 1892, 1:1; see also *The 1893 Record of American and Foreign Shipping* (New York: American Shipmasters' Association, 1893); L. Cecil, *Albert Ballin: Business and Politics in Imperial Germany, 1888–1918* (Princeton: Princeton University Press, 1967), 24–25; "Hamburg-American Line, Pre-1914 File," Steamship Historical Society of America Collections, University of Baltimore, Baltimore, Md.

17. *Harper's Weekly* 36 (1892): 919.

18. *New York Times,* August 27, 1892, 4:4; August 28, 1892, 5:4; *New York Sun,* August 27, 1892, 6:2; *New York Evening Post,* August 25, 1892, 1:2; *New York Commercial Advertiser,* August 25, 1892, 1:2; *New York Daily Press,* August 24, 1892, 4:3; August 25, 1892, 1:1; August 28, 1892, 1:4; *New York World,* August 25, 1892, 4:2.

19. *New York Tribune,* August 31, 1892, 6:4. See also *The American Hebrew,* September 23, 1892, 659; *The Jewish Messenger,* September 9, 1892, 4:3.

20. *New York Herald,* August 21, 1892, 193. Specifically, the *Herald* stated that Russian and Polish Jews were "directly responsible for the appearance of cholera in Germany"; similar conclusions appear on the editorial pages of the *New York Times,* August 21, 1892, 5:4.

21. *New York Times,* August 29, 1892, 5:5.

22. *Judge,* September 17, 1892, 196.

23. *Baltimore Sun,* September 1, 1892, 8:6; "Quarantine and Congressional Legislation," December 20, 1892, Records of the House of Rep., 52nd Cong., R.G. 233, box 158, file HR52A-H9.3, National Archives, Washington, D.C.; E. O. Shakespeare, "The National Government Should Have Supreme Control of Quarantine at All Frontiers," *Medical News* 61 (1892): 281–87; Howard Markel, "Cholera, Quarantines, and Immigration Restriction: The View from Johns Hopkins," *Bull. Hist. Med.* 67 (1993): 691–95.

24. "An Ill-timed Exhibition of Selfishness and Malignity," *New York Sun,* September 12, 1892, 6:1; *New York Tribune,* August 25, 1892, 1:2.

25. *New York Times,* January 21, 1892, 5:1; January 30, 1892, 5:4; *Who's Who in New York City and State* (New York: L. R. Hamersly, 1904), 331.

26. Lothrop Stoddard, *Master of Manhattan: The Life of Richard Croker* (New York: Longmans, Green, 1931), 99–129; Hugh Grant Papers, (1891–92 File), New-York Historical Society. For a full-length study of patronage in the Coroner's Office, see Julie Johnson, "Speaking for the Dead: Forensic Scientists and American Justice in the 20th Century" (Ph.D. diss., University of Pennsylvania, 1992).

27. During his tenure as deputy coroner, Jenkins performed over three thousand autopsies and pronounced the cause of death on over ten thousand New Yorkers.

While Jenkins did not contribute greatly to the intellectual development of autopsy pathology in the form of experimental work, this workload represents a significant accomplishment in its practice. *New York Herald,* February 12, 1892, 20:4; *New York Tribune,* February 12, 1892, 4:5.

28. *New York Times,* January 21, 1892, 5:1.

29. *The Nation* 55 (1892): 214–15; *N.Y. Med. J.* 56 (1892): 470; *New York Evening Post,* September 26, 1892, 2:1. John Duffy describes the history of the health officer of the Port of New York in his *History of Public Health in New York City* (New York: Russell Sage Foundation, 1974), 1:330–35; 2:200–207.

30. The typhus epidemic of New York City in 1892 comprises chaps. 1, 2, and 3 of this book. For examples of newspaper editorials blaming Jenkins for the epidemic, see *New York Commercial Advertiser,* February 12, 1892, 4:1; *New York Evening Post,* February 12, 1892, 1:5; Jenkins' order regarding the disinfection of all entering Russian Jews can be found in "Report of the Health Officer," *Ann. Rep. Comm. Quar.,* 38.

31. "Report of the Health Officer," *Ann. Rep. Comm. Quar.* 47; *New York Herald,* August 28, 1892, 19:3; *New York Times,* August 29, 1892, 5:5; *New York Tribune,* August 29, 1892, 1:2.

32. *New York Times,* August 30, 1892, 5:4.

33. *New York Herald,* August 30, 1892, 7:4. It should be noted that most of Jenkins' quarantine policies were markedly similar to his predecessors' at the quarantine station in terms of cursory examination, rapid steam and chemical disinfection, and preferential treatment for the cabin class. What was decidedly different was the focus on Russian Jewish immigrants.

34. *New York Times,* August 28, 1892, 4:1; August 26, 1892, 5:4; *New York Herald,* August 26, 1892, 3:5; August 30, 1892, 7:4.

35. *New York Tribune,* September 1, 1892, 1:3; D. Haws, *Merchant Fleets in Profile* (Cambridge: P. Stephens, 1980), 4:41.

36. *New York Tribune,* September 1, 1892, 1:4; *New York Times,* September 1, 1892, 1:7; *New York Herald,* September 1, 1892, 3:1.

37. *Yiddishe Tageblatt,* September 4, 1892, 1:6; *svartzer immigrantka* literally means "the black immigrant." Jewish burial rituals are among the most strict for Orthodox Jews, and many believe that refusal to comply with them affects the dead's afterlife. They include great care in handling the dead body and specific instructions for the rapid interment of the dead in the ground using a simple pine box for the casket. Most likely, all of these burial laws were violated in the understandable rush to throw a dead cholera victim overboard; for a brief summary of such rituals, see Hayim H. Donin, *To Be a Jew: A Guide to Jewish Observance in Contemporary Life* (New York: Basic Books, 1972), 296–310.

38. *New York Times,* September 1, 1892, 1:7.

39. *New York Herald,* September 1, 1892, 3:1; "Report of the Health Officer," *Ann. Rep. Comm. Quar.,* 41–65.

40. *Cholerine* was a nebulous term used by nineteenth-century physicians. At times, it was a euphemism for Asiatic cholera used "to conceal the truth from people so as not to alarm them as cholerine did not sound so terrible as Asiatic cholera."

Most physicians, however, classified cholerine as a mild form of diarrhea; a benign and noncontagious variant of cholera (e.g., *cholera morbus* or *cholera nostras*); a prodrome to Asiatic cholera; or a variant of influenza accompanied by intestinal symptoms. "Cholera and Cholerine," *New York Times*, September 1, 1892, 2:3; Osler, *Principles and Practice of Medicine*, 122–23. See also *New York Tribune*, September 1, 1892, 1:1; John S. Billings, *The National Medical Dictionary* (Philadelphia: Lea Brothers, 1890), 1:272.

41. Evans, *Death in Hamburg*, 289, 298, 492. At least three Hamburg-American ships, the *Moravia, Bohemia,* and *Scandia,* carried contaminated water from the Elbe River for the steerage passengers' consumption.

42. *Arbeiter Zeitung* (N.Y.), September 2, 1892, 1:2.

43. Quotes are from Edmund Morris, *The Rise of Theodore Roosevelt* (New York: Coward, McCann and Geoghegan, 1979), 399. See also Thomas C. Platt, *The Autobiography of Thomas Collier Platt* (New York: B. W. Dodge, 1910), 215; Joseph B. Foraker, *Notes of a Busy Life* (Cinncinati, Ohio: Stewart and Kidd, 1916); J. S. Wise, *Recollections of Thirteen Presidents* (New York: Doubleday, Page, 1906), 200.

44. Harrison's wife died on October 25, 1892, turning the rest of the president's reelection campaign into "almost a desire for defeat." *New York Tribune*, October 25, 1892, 1:5.

45. Harrison's views on Russian Jews can be found in his third annual address to the U.S. Congress (December 9, 1891) and his fourth and final annual message to Congress (December 6, 1892) in J. D. Richardson, ed., *A Compilation of the Messages and Papers of the Presidents, 1789–1897,* vol. 9, *1889–1897* (Benjamin Harrison and Grover Cleveland) (Washington, D.C.: U.S. Congress, 1899), 188, 330.

46. "An Act to Prevent the Introduction of Contagious or Infectious Diseases into the United States, April 29, 1878" (20 Stat.L, 37). For an excellent review on the complex division of power among federal, state, and municipal public health agencies, see Laurence F. Schmeckebier, *The Public Health Service: Its History, Activities and Organization* (Baltimore: Johns Hopkins University Press, 1923), 111–13; Howard Kramer, "Agitation for Public Health Administration in the 1870s, Part II, The National Board of Health of 1879," *J. Hist. Med. Allied Sci.* 4 (1949): 75–89; Margaret Humphreys, *Yellow Fever and the South* (New Brunswick, N.J.: Rutgers University Press, 1992). The problems of local versus national quarantine administration, the economic hardships incurred by one port with stricter quarantine regulations than another port, and other issues were also heatedly discussed before the Civil War. See *Minutes from the National Quarantine and Sanitary Conventions, 1857–1860* (New York: Arno, 1977).

47. This anecdote (and the quote) are from *New York Herald*, September 1, 1892, 5:2.

48. *New York Tribune*, August 31, 1892, 1:2. For an essay on the history of states' rights in the United States, see Arthur Meier Schlesinger Sr., "The State Rights Fetish," in *New Viewpoints in American History* (New York: Macmillan, 1948), 220–43. Schlesinger defined the doctrine as a "desire of the state government to enhance their power, or, at least, to resist encroachments of the federal authority" (p. 220).

49. *New York Herald,* September 1, 1892, 5:3; "Confidential Telegram" to Dr. W. A. Wheeler from Surgeon General W. Wyman, September 1, 1892 (item 1266, p. 116), letter books of the surgeon general, vol. 89, R.G. 90, National Archives, Washington, D.C. Upon receiving the president's circular, Wyman wired Wheeler, "Unnecessary to follow instructions wired today"; September 1, 1892 (item 1298, p. 131), letter books, vol. 89, R.G. 90; National Archives, Washington, D.C.; *New York Herald,* September 1, 1892, 1:2; Fitzhugh Mullan, *Plagues and Politics: The Story of the U.S. Public Health Service* (New York: Basic Books, 1989), 35; Wyman's political savvy is discussed in Victoria Harden, *Inventing the N.I.H.: Federal Biomedical Research Policy, 1887–1937* (Baltimore: Johns Hopkins University Press, 1986), 16.

50. *New York Times,* September 1, 1892, 1:1; *New York Herald,* September 1, 1892, 5:3; *New York Tribune,* September 1, 1892, 1:6; circular: "Quarantine Restrictions Upon Immigration to Aid in the Prevention of the Introduction of Cholera in the United States," *Weekly Abst. San. Rep.,* 7:445. Upon signing the circular, Harrison left Washington immediately for Loon Lake to be with his dying wife.

51. The application of these directives specifically to immigrants, especially Russian Jews, is made clear in a "Memorandum to President Harrison from the Secretary of the Treasury, Charles Foster, Sept. 1, 1892," Benjamin Harrison Papers, Library of Congress (reel 36, ser. 1), Washington, D.C. The ports mentioned in the circular were among the most frequently used exits by East European Jewish immigrants. See Howe, *World of Our Fathers,* 28. Incubation periods for Asiatic cholera are derived from Osler, *Principles and Practice of Medicine,* 121–22; and Nathan Brill, "Cholera and a Federal Quarantine," January 9, 1893, R.G. 233, box 197, file HR52A-H28.1, National Archives, Washington, D.C.

52. "Steerage Traffic Stops," *New York Times,* December 14, 1892, 12:1; Hutchinson, *Legislative History of American Immigration Policy, 1798–1965,* 95–103.

53. *New York Tribune,* September 2, 1892, 6:3.

54. *New York Herald,* September 2, 1892, 3:1; *New York Times,* September 2, 1892, 4:2. Local quarantine efforts, across the nation, ranged from blockading railway stations to Russian Jews to actual physical harassment. *New York Tribune,* September 2, 1892, 3:6; September 3, 1892, 3:3; *New York Herald,* September 3, 1892, 4:4; *13th Annual Report of the State Board of Health, New York (1892)* (Albany: J. B. Lyon, 1893), 16–17; *Annual Report of the State Board of Health for the Commonwealth of Pennsylvania for 1892,* 14–28; *New York Times,* September 2, 1892, 5:4; September 5, 1892, 5:1; *New York Tribune,* September 2, 1892, 3:5; Rawlings, *The Rise and Fall of Disease in Illinois,* 325–27.

55. *New York Times,* September 2, 1892, 5:4; *New York Tribune,* September 2, 1892, 3:5; *New York Times,* September 5, 1892, 5:1.

56. *New York Tribune,* September 5, 1892, 1:5.

57. *New York Herald,* September 2, 1892, 3:4.

58. "Report of the Health Officer," *Ann. Rep. Comm. Quar.,* 56–62.

59. *New York Tribune,* September 3, 1892, 1:3; E. O. Shakespeare, *Report on Cholera in Europe and India* (Washington, D.C.: U.S. Government Printing Office, 1890), 851; Alan I. Marcus, "Disease Prevention in America: From a Local to a National

Outlook," *Bull. Hist. Med.* 53 (1979): 184–203; M. Kagan, "Federal Public Health: A Reflection of a Changing Constitution," *J. Hist. Med. Allied Sci.* 16 (1961): 256–79; Howard Kramer, "Agitation for Public Health Reform" (in two parts), *J. Hist. Med.* 3 (1948): 473–78; 4 (1949): 75–89; idem, "Early Municipal and State Boards of Health," *Bull. Hist. Med.* 24 (1950): 503–29. Assumption of control of immigration by the federal government in 1890 only further confounded the blurred domains over public health.

60. *New York Herald,* February 12, 1893, 20:4; *New York Tribune,* February 12, 1893, 4:5; February 25, 1893, 4:1; February 26, 1893, 6:3.

61. S. W. Rosendale, "Report of the Attorney General of the State of New York on Quarantine Regulations," (September 2, 1892), *Assembly Documents of New York State,* 1893, 3:275–79; *New York Times,* September 3, 1892, 1:5; *New York Herald,* September 3, 1892, 3:1; *New York Tribune,* September 3, 1892, 1:3.

62. W. J. Hartman, "Politics and Patronage: The New York Custom House, 1852–1902" (Ph.D. diss., Columbia University, 1952), 315–18; DeAlva S. Alexander, *Four Famous New Yorkers: The Political Careers of Cleveland, Platt, Hill, and Roosevelt* (New York: Henry Holt, 1923), 85.

63. *New York Tribune,* September 7, 1892, 5:1.

64. Throughout the epidemic, Jenkins displayed a resentful attitude toward the federal public health effort. Telegrams between Secretary Charles Foster and President Harrison and between the surgeon general and his subordinate officers stationed in New York at this time document a careful handling of Jenkins and tacit agreement that he was "foolish." Benjamin Harrison Papers, Library of Congress (August 31–September 16, 1892; reel 36, ser. 1), Washington, D.C.; letter books of the surgeon general, August 31–September 31, 1892, vol. 89, R.G. 90, National Archives, Washington, D.C.

Chapter 5. "Knocking Out the Cholera!"

The headline in the chapter title is from *New York World,* September 10, 1892, 1. It was inspired by the John L. Sullivan–"Gentleman Jim" Corbett heavyweight boxing championship match on September 7, 1892. Corbett knocked out Sullivan after twenty-one rounds. An accompanying cartoon in the *World* depicted a pugilistic Dr. Jenkins, complete with boxing gloves and shorts, boxing an anthropomorphized cholera germ.

1. *Ann. Rep. Comm. Quar.,* 46.

2. Richard Evans, *Death in Hamburg: Society and Politics in the Cholera Years, 1830–1910* (New York: Oxford University Press, 1987), 317.

3. *New York Times,* September 4, 1892, 1:7.

4. David Haws, *Merchant Fleets in Profile* (Cambridge: P. Stephens, 1980), 4:46; "Hamburg-American Pre-1914 File," Steamship Historical Society of America, University of Baltimore, Baltimore, Md.; John M. Brinnin, *The Sway of the Grand Saloon: A Social History of the North Atlantic* (London: Arlington, 1986), 326–27.

5. Philip Taylor, *The Distant Magnet: European Emigration to the U.S.A.* (London: Eyre and Spottiswoode, 1971), 145; *New York Times,* September 4, 1892, 1:5.

6. "Interview with William T. Jenkins," *New York Herald,* September 4, 1892, 13:2.

7. *New York Herald,* September 4, 1892, 13:3; "Report of the Health Officer," *Ann. Rep. Comm. Quar.,* 48. There were no culture confirmations of any of the deaths aboard the *Normannia,* but the opinion of many physicians, including Jenkins, and my own retrospective diagnosis point to cholera.

8. Jenkins diagnosed Hegert's and Heynemann's deaths empirically as due to Asiatic cholera. He defended the decision of quarantining all the *Normannia's* passengers because of the "grave risk" and to "give the public the benefit of the doubt." "Report of the Health Officer," *Ann. Rep. Comm. Quar.,* 61; *New York Tribune,* September 4, 1892, 13:1; *New York Times,* September 4, 1892, 1:1.

9. *New York Times,* September 5, 1892, 1:7; the thirteen-day detention refers to the cabin-class passengers; steerage passengers were detained on Hoffman Island for six additional days.

10. Evans, *Death in Hamburg,* 282–83.

11. "Report of the Health Officer," *Ann. Rep. Comm. Quar.,* 30; William Osler, *The Principles and Practice of Medicine* (New York: Appleton, 1892), 118–24; "Report of the Health Officer," *Ann. Rep. Comm. Quar.,* 90–122.

12. *New York Tribune,* September 2, 1892, 6:2; Walter Vought, *A Chapter on Cholera for Lay Readers: History, Symptoms, Prevention, and Treatment of the Disease* (Philadelphia: F. A. Davis, 1893).

13. The concept that historians should not assume a "normative" model for public health was pointed out to me by Dr. Daniel M. Fox of the Milbank Memorial Fund. Instead, when interpreting the history of public health, one needs to pay close attention to the spectrum of responses, between the extremes of what science dictates and public desires that may contradict scientific theory. I am also grateful to the Albert Einstein-SUNY Stonybrook-CUNY-Columbia History of Medicine consortium for helping me sort out these ideas.

14. Letter from T. Mitchell Prudden to William H. Welch, September 8, 1892, general correspondence, box 1, file 1, T. Mitchell Prudden Papers, Yale University, New Haven, Conn.

15. Letter from W. H. Welch to T. Mitchell Prudden, September 13, 1892, general correspondence, box 1, file 1, T. M. Prudden Papers, Yale University. C.-E. A. Winslow, *The Life of Hermann Biggs* (Philadelphia: Lea and Febiger, 1929), 50–52, 78, 99–104; correspondence between Surgeon General Wyman and Joseph J. Kinyoun, September 15–October 30, 1892, *Letterbooks of the Supervising Surgeon General of the M.H.S.,* National Archives, Washington, D.C.

16. *New York Evening Post,* September 20, 1892, 1:2; September 26, 1892, 2:1.

17. George M. Sternberg, *A Manual of Bacteriology* (New York: William Wood, 1892). This prodigious volume has 900 pages and classifies approximately 500 species of bacteria, including 158 pathogens.

18. Arnold H. Eggerth, *A History of the Hoagland Laboratory* (Brooklyn, N.Y.,

privately printed, 1960), 19–43. I am indebted to the anonymous reviewer of this chapter for pointing out this reference.

19. Martha Sternberg, *George Miller Sternberg, A Biography by His Wife* (Chicago: American Medical Association, 1921); Eggerth, *History of the Hoagland Laboratory,* 27–32.

20. Sternberg performed a number of exacting experiments assessing the cultures, temperatures, nutrients, and many other conditions needed for cholera to propagate. See George M. Sternberg, "The Biological Character of the Cholera Spirillum," *Med. Rec.* 42 (1892): 387–91; idem, "Disinfection at Quarantine Stations— especially against Cholera," *N.Y. Med. J.* 57 (1893): 57–62; idem, "Bacteriological Report on Cholera," *Amer. J. Med. Sci.* 105 (1893): 388–93; idem, "The Destruction of Cholera Germs," in Edmund C. Wendt, ed., *A Treatise on Asiatic Cholera* (New York: William Wood, 1885), 325–35.

21. George Sternberg, "How Can We Prevent Cholera?" *Medico-Legal Journal* 11 (1893): 1–8 (quote from pp. 1–2).

22. For published interviews Jenkins and his assistant, Dr. John Byron, gave on how bacteriological methods, including cholera cultures, would be applied to prevention of a cholera epidemic, see *New York Herald,* September 1, 1892, 3:1; *New York Times,* September 2, 1892, 1:5. For similar claims that New York was protected by modern science and bacteriology, see *New York Tribune,* September 20, 1892, 3:1; Wade Oliver, *The Man Who Lived for Tomorrow: A Biography of William Hallock Park, M.D.* (New York: E. P. Dutton, 1941), 71–74; Winslow, *Life of Hermann Biggs,* 96– 99; Charles F. Boulduan, *Over a Century of Health Administration in New York City,* Monograph no. 13, New York City Health Department, March 1916; Lillian Prudden, ed., *Biographical Sketches and Letters of T. Mitchell Prudden* (New Haven: Yale University Press, 1927), 79–94.

23. "Report of the Health Officer," *Ann. Rep. Comm. Quar.,* 66; *New York Herald,* September 1, 1892, 3:1; Patricia P. Gossel, "The Emergence of American Bacteriology, 1875–1900" (Ph.D. diss., Johns Hopkins University, 1989), 44–55. Gossel has described the many technical problems in conducting a bacteriological laboratory and how easily cultures failed to produce reliable clinical data in the 1890s.

24. "Report of the Health Officer," *Ann. Rep. Comm. Quar.,* 52; "Chamber of Commerce of the State of New York. Report of the Special Committee on Quarantine at the Port of New York During the Cholera of 1892," 20–40, Special Collections of the New York Academy of Medicine; *35th Annual Report of the Corporation of the Chamber of Commerce of the State of New York for the year 1892–1893* (New York: Press of the Chamber of Commerce, 1893), 74–116. The committee consisted of Drs. Stephen Smith, Abraham Jacobi, Edward G. Janeway, Hermann Biggs, Allan M. Hamilton, T. Mitchell Prudden, and Richard H. Derby.

25. This propensity has been well described by a number of scholars. See, for example, Richard Shyrock, "The Early American Public Health Movement," *Amer. J. Pub. Health* 27 (1937): 965–71; see also idem, "The Origins and Significance of the Public Health Movement in the United States," *Ann. Med. Hist.* n.s. 1 (1929): 645–65;

Judith W. Leavitt, *The Healthiest City: Milwaukee and the Politics of Health Reform* (Princeton: Princeton University Press, 1982), 240–64.

26. "Health Officer's Report," *Ann. Rep. Comm. Quar.*, 46–63; Advisory Committee on Quarantine Reports to the New York Chamber of Commerce for 1888 and for 1892, Collections of the New York Academy of Medicine. The deficiencies of the stations' physical plant found in both these reports, four years apart, are all too similar. See also A. N. Bell, "The Need of National Legislation for the Protection of Life," *JAMA* 19 (1892): 424–29; *New York Herald*, September 1, 1892, 3:1; *New York Times*, September 2, 1892, 1:5. For strikingly familiar pleas for increased funding to the quarantine station, see *Ann. Rep. Comm. Quar.*, 1881–1901.

27. *Annual Report of the New York Chamber of Commerce, 1892*, 13–23; *New York Tribune*, September 6, 1892, 5:2; *New York Herald*, September 5, 1892, 3:1; Frank Abbott, "The Treatment of Asiatic Cholera Based on Observations Made at Swinburne Island during September and October, 1892," *Med. Rec.* 43 (1893): 363–64; John M. Byron, "Asiatic Cholera at Lower Quarantine in 1892," *Trans. N.Y. Acad. Med.* 9, 2nd ser. (1892): 289–99.

28. *New York Herald*, September 4, 1892, 13:1.

29. *New York Herald*, September 7, 1892, 6:6; September 22, 1892, 5:1; *New York Sun*, September 10, 1892, 6:5; *New York Times*, September 7, 1892, 5:5; *New York Tribune*, September 22, 1892, 3:3.

30. The Columbus statue story is reported in *New York Herald*, September 4, 1892, 13:1; September 5, 1892, 1:5; *New York Tribune*, September 4, 1892, 1:1. Kenneth T. Jackson, ed., The *Encyclopedia of New York City* (New Haven, Conn.: Yale University Press, 1995), 261, reports that only the Carrara marble pedestal was delivered in 1892 with the actual statue being erected in 1894. The most energetic reporters in the bay were, undoubtedly, from Joseph Pulitzer's *New York World;* the *World* correspondents were so successful in "scooping" the other dailies that its reporters were accused of smuggling themselves aboard the ships for a story and bringing the germ of cholera with them into New York City. *New York World*, September 1–20, 1892, 1; *Annual Report of the Police Department, N.Y.C., 1892* (New York: M. B. Brown, 1893), 55–59. For a firsthand account of the media-circus in New York Bay by the *New York Herald* correspondent covering the event, see Charles Edward Russell, *These Shifting Scenes* (New York: Hodder and Stoughton/George H. Doran, 1914), 245–57; *New York Times*, September 5, 1892, 1:4.

31. *New York Herald*, September 5, 1892, 3:1; *Harper's Weekly*, September 24, 1892 (cover); *Leslie's Illustrated Weekly*, September 22, 1892 (cover); excerpts of foreign newspaper accounts can be found in *New York Times*, September 14, 1892, 10:1.

32. Allan Nevins, *The Evening Post: A Century of Journalism* (New York: Russell and Russell, 1968), 476; E. L. Godkin letters, James Wright Brown and Silas Burt Collection, New-York Historical Society; William M. Armstrong, ed., *The Gilded Age Letters of E. L. Godkin* (Albany: State University of New York Press, 1974), 439–40; ironically, Godkin unleashed his vitriol against the New York City board of health during the cholera epidemic of 1865–66 for *not* quarantining the Port of New York.

33. *New York Evening Post,* September 12, 1892, 2:1; September 26, 1892, 2:1; *New York Tribune,* September 6, 1892, 5:4; Godkin continued his attacks on Jenkins well after the cholera crisis was over, choosing always to assail the health officer's character on the printed page. See E. L. Godkin, "A Month of Quarantine," *N. Amer. Rev.* 155 (1892): 737–43. The *Normannia* was quarantined from September 3 to September 16, 1892. For Jenkins' rebuttal, see W. Jenkins, "Quarantine at New York," *N. Amer. Rev.* 155 (1892): 585–91; "Report of the Health Officer," *Ann. Rep. Comm. Quar.,* 47–52. Many other observers, such as Charles A. Dana of the *New York Sun* and the editorial board of *Puck* and *Life* magazines, called Godkin's behavior petulant and childish. *New York Sun,* September 12, 1892, 6:1; September 13, 1892, 6:1; September 14, 1892, 6:6; *Life,* September 29, 1892, 172; *Puck,* September 28, 1892, 82.

34. "Ta-ra-ra Boom-de-ay" was the major hit song of 1891–92. First sung in the British music halls by Lottie Collins during the spring of 1891, the catchy tune soon became an international standard. Lottie Collins scrapbooks, Robinson Locke Collection of Theatrical Scrapbooks, New York Public Library for the Performing Arts, vol. 77, ser. 2.

35. *New York World,* September 4, 5, 6, 9, 1892, 1; Lottie Collins scrapbook, New York Public Library for the Performing Arts, Research Division. For other passengers' letters to the editor, see *New York Herald,* September 7, 1892, 6:6; *New York Sun,* September 10, 1892, 6:5; *New York Times,* September 7, 1892, 5:5; *New York Tribune,* September 22, 1892, 3:3; *New York Herald,* September 22, 1892, 5:1.

36. *New York Times,* September 10, 1892, 9:1.

37. *Arbeiter Zeitung* (N.Y.), September 9, 1892, 1:5.

38. *New York Herald,* September 7, 1892, 5:2; September 8, 1892, 11:2; September 9, 1892, 3:1; *New York Times,* September 8, 1892, 1:6, 4:2; *New York Tribune,* September 8, 1892, 1:3; September 9, 1892, 1:4. The yellow journalists, especially those on the *Herald,* had a field day reporting the supposed sale of counterfeit "entry passes" by a teenage clerk in the U.S. Customs Office of New York. The passes, which sold for twenty-five cents, gave "clearance" for ships to enter the harbor. The ruse was quickly aborted by the federal authorities.

39. John B. Hamilton, "The Establishment of a National Quarantine Station near New York Harbor," *JAMA* 19 (1892): 443–45; "Report of the Health Officer," *Ann. Rep. Comm. Quar.,* 56; *New York Tribune,* September 8, 1892, 1:6. One of the major private contributors to the development of the national quarantine station at Sandy Hook, New Jersey, was Long Island Railroad president Austin Corbin. Corbin, it may be recalled, established the first American summer resort at Manhattan Beach, New York, in 1888 that restricted the potential visits of Jews and other "undesirables." See Louise A. Mayo, *The Ambivalent Image: Nineteenth-Century America's Perception of the Jew* (Rutherford, N.J.: Fairleigh Dickinson University Press, 1988), 98–101.

40. *New York Tribune,* September 8, 1892, 1:3; September 9, 1892, 1:4; September 10, 1892, 1:2; *New York Times,* September 8, 1892, 1:6, 4:2, 2:4; September 9, 1892, 2:1, 4:5; *New York Herald,* September 8, 1892, 3:1, 11:2.

41. *New York Times,* September 9, 1892, 2:1; September 10, 1892, 4:2; September 11,

1892, 2:2; October 1, 1892, 4:2; *New York Herald,* September 10, 1892, 4:3; *New York Tribune,* February 16, 1893, 5:2.

42. *Arbeiter Zeitung* (N.Y.), September 16, 1892, 1:5.

43. Godkin, "Month of Quarantine," 740.

44. Russell, *These Shifting Scenes,* 254.

45. Robert A. Caro, *The Power Broker: Robert Moses and the Fall of New York* (New York: Vintage-Random House, 1975), 147–48.

46. *New York Times,* September 9, 1892, 2:2; September 11, 1892, 2:1; *New York Tribune,* September 9, 1892, 3:1; September 10, 1892, 1:2; September 11, 1892, 5:3; "Report of the Health Officer," *Ann. Rep. Comm. Quar.,* 50–56.

47. *New York Times,* September 12, 1892, 1:6; *New York Tribune,* September 12, 1892, 2:1; *New York Herald,* September 12, 1892, 3:1.

48. *New York Herald,* September 13, 1892, 5:1. The *London Standard* called the affair "a piece of savagery more worthy of Central Asia than America." For a summary of international coverage on the event, see *New York Times,* September 14, 1892, 2:2. Mob responses to quarantines in the New York area commonly occurred during the nineteenth and early twentieth centuries. See F. H. Garrison, "The Destruction of the Quarantine Station on Staten Island in 1858," *Contributions to the History of Medicine* (New York: Hafner, 1966), 467–79; Guenter Risse, "Revolt Against Quarantine: Community Responses to the 1916 Polio Epidemic, Oyster Bay, New York," *Trans. Stud. Coll. Physicians of Phila.* 14 (1992): 23–50.

49. *New York Tribune,* September 14, 1892, 1:5; *New York Times,* September 14, 1892, 1:5, 2:2; *New York Herald,* September 14, 1892, 5:1.

50. "Letters from Passengers of the *Scandia,*" *New York Herald,* September 14, 1892, 2:5.

51. *New York Herald,* September 14, 1892, 5:1.

52. Allan McLane Hamilton, *Recollections of an Alienist: Personal and Professional* (New York: George H. Doran, 1916), 105; *New York Herald,* September 14, 1892, 5:1. For a discussion of Hamilton's work as a late-nineteenth-century psychiatrist, see Charles E. Rosenberg, *The Trial of Assassin Guiteau: Psychiatry and Law in the Gilded Age* (Chicago: University of Chicago Press, 1968), 171.

53. *New York Tribune,* December 24, 1892, 2:2. The biblical quotation supposedly attributed to Jenkins is most appropriately from Job 3:17.

54. *New York Times,* August 24, 1892, 7:3; *New York Tribune,* August 25, 1892, 1:2; *New York Times,* August 25, 1892, 1:1.

55. Evans, *Death in Hamburg,* 285–327. Evans describes three major factors in the Hamburg cholera epidemic of 1892: (1) attempts at concealing cases and improper planning by Hamburg public health officials; (2) a lack of sanitary water and sewage treatment systems in Hamburg; and (3) malnourished, poor immigrants or urban dwellers who might be more likely to be exposed to cholera.

56. *Minutes of the New York City Board of Health,* entries for August 16–September 27, 1892, Municipal Archives of the City of New York.

57. Joseph B. Bishop, *A Chronicle of 150 Years: The Chamber of Commerce of the State of New York, 1768–1918* (New York: Charles Scribner's Sons, 1918), 95.

58. These precautions and their estimated budgets are detailed in a number of New York City documents. See *Ann. Rep. N.Y.C. Health Dept.*, 34–64; *New York City Board of Health Minutes* (August 16–October 4, 1892), 146–67; *New York City Board of Estimate and Apportionment, Annual Report, 1892*, 303–13, 351–53, 512–21; *New York City Department of Public Works, Annual Report, 1892*, 8–11; *New York City Aqueduct Commission: Report to the Aqueduct Commissioners, 1892*, 1; *New York City Police Department Annual Report, 1892*, 40–49, 55–59; "Annual Report of the New York City Street Cleaning Dept., 1892," *The City Record*, May 9, 1893, 1570–75; *Journal of the Board of Education of the City of New York, 1892* (Meeting for September 14, 1892), 945–47; *Proceedings of the Board of Aldermen of the City of New York, 1892*, 207:112, 159, 314–24.

59. *New York Times*, September 15, 1892, 1:7; *New York World*, September 15, 1892, 5:1; *New York Tribune*, September 15, 1892, 1:5.

60. *Ann. Rep. N.Y.C. Health Depart.*, 34–35; *Yiddishe Tageblatt* (N.Y.), March 18, 1892, 1:3. Edson's lack of popularity among the Jewish Quarter is discussed in chap. 2.

61. *New York Times*, September 5, 1892, 5:1; September 7, 1892, 2:2; September 16, 1892, 2:2; *New York Tribune*, September 5, 1892, 1:5.

62. *Arbeiter Zeitung* (N.Y.), September 2, 1892, 4:1. Despite the socialist "spin," this reporter's observation of public health initiatives has been echoed by a number of public health historians. See Judith W. Leavitt, *The Healthiest City: Milwaukee and the Politics of Health Reform* (Princeton: Princeton University Press, 1982).

63. *Ann. Rep. N.Y.C. Health Dept.*, 118–20; Oliver, *The Man Who Lived for Tomorrow*, 65–74; Winslow, *Life of Hermann Biggs*, 91–99; Hermann Biggs, "History of the Recent Outbreak of Epidemic Cholera in New York," *Amer. J. Med. Sci.* 105, n.s. (1893): 63–72.

64. McAvoy's clinical case has been presented in a variety of places, including *Ann. Rep. N.Y.C. Health Dept.*, 107, 111. See also Hermann Biggs' account of the epidemic ("History of the Cholera Epidemic in New York"); and Robert Deshon, "Clinical History of the First Case of Cholera in New York," *Med. Rec.* 42 (1892): 420.

65. Winslow, *Life of Hermann Biggs*, 70–106; "Hermann Biggs," *Dictionary of National Biography* (New York: Charles Scribner's Sons, 1929), 2:262–63. For an example of applying germ theory technology to maritime quarantine, see Hermann Biggs, "The Diagnostic Value of the Cholera Spirillum as Illustrated by the Investigation of a Case at the New York Quarantine Station," *N.Y. Med. J.* 66 (1887): 548.

66. Oliver, *Man Who Lived for Tomorrow*, 73; Winslow, *Life of Hermann Biggs*, 98–99; *New York Times*, September 15, 1892, 2:3; James J. Walsh, *History of Medicine in New York: Three Centuries of Medical Progress* (New York: National Americana Society, 1919), 4:78–80; letter from Hermann Biggs to Hugh Grant, September 9, 1892, Mayor's Papers, (1892) Municipal Archives of New York City; letter from Cyrus Edson to Clarence Johnson, clerk of the Senate Immigration Committee, (Vol. 87, 6453–54), December 3, 1892, William E. Chandler Papers, Library of Congress, Washington, D.C.

67. *New York Times*, September 9, 1892, 2:4; September 15, 1892, 1:7; *New York Herald*, September 9, 1892, 3:6; September 15, 1892, 5:1; *New York Tribune*, Septem-

ber 9, 1892, 5:1; September 15, 1892, 1:5; *Minutes of the New York City Board of Health,* September 8, 1892.

68. E. K. Dunham, "The Bacteriological Examination of Recent Cases of Epidemic Cholera in the City of New York," *Amer. J. Med. Sci.* 103, n.s. (1892): 72–80.

69. *New York Herald,* September 15, 1892, 5:1. See also *New York Tribune,* September 15, 1892, 1:5; and *New York Times,* September 15, 1892, 2:3. Matters become even more unclear in Wade Oliver's account of the diagnostic process. Oliver insisted that Biggs' original diagnosis of cholera nostras in McAvoy was "a provisional one," yet the language of Biggs' September 8, 1892 announcement stating that the findings were "not at all suggestive of cholera asiatica" seems to refute such a claim. Oliver, *Man Who Lived for Tomorrow,* 71–72.

70. *New York Herald,* September 18, 1892, 17:4.

71. *New York Herald,* September 15, 1892, 5:1.

72. *Ann. Rep. N.Y.C. Health Dept.,* 106–21; *Sanitary Code of the City of New York, 1892,* 54–57 (secs. 151–58).

73. Charles F. Roberts, "Report of the Cholera Epidemic in New York in 1892," *Ann. Rep. N.Y.C. Health Dept.,* 106–21; Biggs, "History of the Recent Outbreak of Epidemic Cholera in New York," 69–70.

74. *New York Herald,* September 15, 1892, 1:1; *New York Times,* September 15, 1892, 1:7; *New York Tribune,* September 15, 1892, 1:6; *New York Herald,* September 16, 1892, 3:1.

75. Biggs, "History of the Recent Outbreak of Epidemic Cholera in New York," 63–72.

76. *New York Times,* September 15, 1892, 2:1.

77. *New York Herald,* September 17, 1892, 2:3, 4:2, 8:2; *New York Sun,* September 14, 1892, 6:6; *New York Press,* September 15, 1892, 1.

78. *New York Herald,* September 18, 1892, 17:1; *Ann. Rep. N.Y.C. Health Dept.,* 121. Telegrams from Emmons C. Clark to the Supervising Surgeon General Walter Wyman, September 29, 1892, U.S. Marine Hospital Service, incoming correspondence, R.G. 90, National Archives, Washington, D.C.

79. The heading of this section was the title of an editorial in the *New York Times,* September 27, 1892, 4:4.

80. The *Heligoland* was allowed to deliver its cargo and then went back to sea. *New York Times,* September 17, 1892, 1:7; *New York Herald,* September 16, 1892, 4:5.

81. *Report of the Advisory Committee on Quarantine, 1892,* 39.

82. Ibid., 23. Horrid conditions and treatment of steerage passengers were not limited to those aboard the *Bohemia.* Literally every detained steerage passenger was probably subjected to increased exposure to the germ of cholera. For eyewitness accounts, see "The Women of the *Normannia,*" *New York Times,* September 18, 1892, 2:5; and "Trials of *Wyoming* Passengers," *New York Times,* September 22, 1892, 2:5.

83. *Report of the Chamber of Commerce Quarantine Committee,* 30–31.

84. Letter books of the surgeon general of the Marine Health Service, vol. 89 (August 31–September 30, 1892), 409, 471, 478, 479; vol. 90 (October 1892), 14, 36, 37, 41, 53, 55, 125–26, R.G. 90, National Archives, Washington, D.C.; Joseph J. Kinyoun,

"Ship Sanitation and Modern Treatment of Infected Vessels," *Trans N. Y. Acad. Med.* 9, 2nd ser. (1893): 351–91. Kinyoun was the Marine Health Service bacteriologist and founder of the Hygienic Laboratory in Washington, D.C., which ultimately became the National Institutes of Health. He was eventually transferred to San Francisco, where he became involved in a bitter battle over his handling of a bubonic plague epidemic and the subsequent quarantining of Chinese in 1901. Victoria Harden, *Inventing the NIH: Federal Biomedical Research Policy, 1887–1937* (Baltimore: Johns Hopkins University Press, 1986), 10–15. For documentation on the rivalry between Surgeon General Wyman and Dr. John Hamilton, see *Boston Globe,* April 3, 1893, 29.

85. Appendix E, *Ann. Rep. Comm. Quar.,* 88–122; *Ann. Rep. N.Y.C. Health Dept.,* 121, 179–80. There was one other cholera death, a boat captain in New Brunswick, New Jersey.

86. Jon C. Teaford, *The Unheralded Triumph: City Government in America, 1870–1900* (Baltimore: Johns Hopkins University Press, 1984), 248; Winslow, *Life of Hermann Biggs,* 98; *Ann. Rep. N.Y.C. Health Dept.,* 38; "Report of the Health Officer," *Ann. Rep. Comm. Quar.,* 73; *Annual Report of the Superising Surgeon General of the Marine Hospital Service, 1892,* 35–38.

87. The average temperature of the city of New York during September 1892 was 66°F. Cholera grows best in more temperate climates, with temperatures in the 80s to 90s. For meteorological data on the city of New York during the 1892 epidemic, see *Weekly Reports of the Health Department of New York City* for September 3, 1892, to October 1, 1892 (New York: M. B. Brown, 1892).

88. The Croton aqueduct water system was truly one of the great civil engineering projects of the nineteenth century. For details on this important topic in public health and urban history, see *New York City Aqueduct Commission: Report to the Aqueduct Commissioners for the Year 1892–1893* (New York: M. B. Brown, 1893); Timothy M. Cheesman, "Report of a Recent Sanitary Inspection of One of the Sources of the Croton Water Supply," *Trans. N.Y. Acad. Med.* 10, 2nd ser. (1893): 181–95; "Report of the Committee on the Croton Water Supply of N. Y. Acad. Med.," *Trans. N.Y. Acad. Med.* 10, 2nd ser. (1893): 196–209; Neil Fitzsimons, ed., *The Reminiscences of John B. Jervis, Engineer of the Old Croton* (Syracuse, N.Y.: Syracuse University Press, 1971); *Report of the Department of Public Works of the City of New York, for 1893* (New York: M. B. Brown, 1893), 69–72.

89. Charles Rosenberg, *The Cholera Years: The United States in 1832, 1849 and 1866* (Chicago: University of Chicago Press, 1987), 65–98, 133–50, 192–212.

90. *Medical News* 61 (1892): 523–24; *American Hebrew,* September 23, 1892, 659; *Deutsche Medicin. Wochenschr.* 36 (1892); Frank Clemow, *The Cholera Epidemic of 1892 in the Russian Empire* (London: Longmans, Green, 1893), 51–67; W. C. Burns, "President's Address of the Michigan State Sanitary Convention," *Proceedings and Addresses at a Sanitary Convention under the Direction of the Michigan State Board of Health* (Lansing, Mich.: Robert Smith, 1893), 10; Fred Rosner, "Communicable Diseases and the Physician's Obligation to Heal," in Fred Rosner, ed., *Medicine and Jewish Law* (Northvale, N.J.: Jason Aronson, 1990), 79–87; idem, *Modern Medicine and Jewish Ethics* (New York: Ktav, 1986).

Chapter 6. Maintaining the Quarantine

The epigraph for Part III comes from William E. Chandler, "Shall Immigration Be Suspended?" *N. Amer. Rev.* 156 (1893): 1.

1. Charles Rosenberg, "What Is an Epidemic? AIDS in Historical Perspective," in Charles Rosenberg, *Explaining Epidemics and Other Studies in the History of Medicine* (New York: Cambridge University Press, 1992), 286–87.

2. Robert Sullivan, *Goodbye Lizzie Borden* (Brattleboro, Vt.: Stephen Greene, 1974).

3. *Weekly Abst. San. Rep.*, 7:696–720.

4. See, for example, *Official Catalogue of the United States Government Building (Part XVI) at the 1893 World's Columbian Exposition* (Chicago: W. B. Conkey, 1893), 31–32; Isaac D. Rawlings, *The Rise and Fall of Disease in Illinois* (Springfield: Illinois Board of Health, 1927), 325–27; "No Fear of Cholera," *JAMA* 20 (1893): 164.

5. Walt Whitman, "By Blue Ontario's Shore," *Leaves of Grass and Selected Prose* (New York: Modern Library, 1950), 270.

6. *Speeches Made on the Occasion of the Annual Banquet of the Chamber of Commerce of the State of New York, November 15, 1892* (New York: Chamber of Commerce Press, 1892), 24–27.

7. Samuel Joseph, *Jewish Immigration to the United States from 1881 to 1910* (New York: Columbia University Press, 1914), 163–65; Simon Kuznets, "Immigration of Russian Jews to the United States: Background and Structure," *Perspectives in American History* 9 (1975): 35–124. Total immigration to the United States during 1892–93 was less directly affected by the short-lived Harrison quarantine order. Total immigration in 1892 was 579,660 and fell to 440,000 in 1893. Immigration rates continued to dip to the 200,000 to 300,000 mark for the remainder of the nineteenth century.

8. *New York Sun*, March 3, 1893, 6:4.

9. Harold Frederic, *The New Exodus: A Study of Israel in Russia* (New York: G. P. Putnam's Sons, 1892), 3.

10. *New York Times*, November 5, 1892, 2:7; November 6, 1892, 3:1; November 7, 1892, 3:4, 3:6; November 11, 1892, 8:6.

11. Philip Taylor, *The Distant Magnet: European Migration to the U.S.A.* (London: Eyre and Spottiswoode, 1971), 145. Overall, during 1891, there were 448,000 steerage arrivals in New York, 41,000 in Baltimore, 31,000 in Boston, and 26,000 in Philadelphia; see also House Executive Document 235, pt. 1, 52nd Cong., 1st sess. (Washington, D.C.: U.S. Government Printing Office, 1891), 323.

12. *New York Times*, November 15, 1892, 3:4. Foster stated that given the upcoming World's Fair in the spring of 1893 and the threat of cholera returning to the United States at that time, there would be no "modification" in the policy, or at least none during the waning months of the Harrison administration; *New York Herald*, November 17, 1892, 7:1.

13. *New York Herald,* November 23, 1892, 12:1; *New York Times,* November 23, 1892, 8:2; *New York Post,* November 23, 1892, 3:1; "Testimony of Steamship Owners and Agents," *Immigration Report,* February 22, 1893, Accompanying S. 3786, 52nd Cong., 2nd sess.; Establishing additional regulations concerning immigration to the United States, with history of immigration, investigation, legislation, etc., 52nd Cong., 2nd sess., Senate Report 1333 (ser. #3073), [Y4.IM6:IM6] (Washington, D.C.: U.S. Government Printing Office, 1893), 14–15, 41–55. For specific details of the abridgment of steamship line traffic between Europe and America in the aftermath of the epidemic and the twenty-day rule, see *New York Times,* November 6, 1892, 3:1; November 8, 1892, 3:6; November 23, 1892, 8:2; *New York Herald,* November 23, 1892, 12:1; *New York Evening Post,* November 30, 1892, 1:5.

14. *New York Evening Post,* November 17, 1892, 3:3.

15. Schwab discusses this plan in a variety of places, including his testimony before the Senate Immigration Committee (Senate Report 1333, pp. 15–38); *New York Times,* December 4, 1892, 20:1; December 18, 1892, 15:4; "A Practical Remedy for Evils of Immigration," *The Forum,* February 1893, 803–14. This was not the first time a German shipping concern promised to provide more sanitary service. Dr. Hermann Biggs received similar assurances from the Hamburg American Packet Company only one month before the 1892 cholera epidemic. C.-E. A. Winslow, *The Life of Hermann M. Biggs* (Philadelphia: Lea and Febiger, 1929), 93–94.

16. Schwab, "A Practical Remedy for Evils of Immigration," 807.

17. *New York Sun,* November 16, 1892, 6:3; *New York Evening Post,* November 16, 1892, 6:4.

18. *New York Evening Post,* November 16, 1892, 6:4. Godkin's plea for such a lawsuit seems especially futile given that those most affected by the Harrison order were, for the most part, newly arrived immigrants with little knowledge of English, let alone the American judicial system, and those on the other side of the Atlantic Ocean eagerly awaiting passage.

19. *New York Times,* November 7, 1892, 3:4.

20. The Chinese Restriction Act of 1882 was signed into law by President Chester Arthur. Some immigration historians trace its origins to the Naturalization Act of 1870, which limited naturalization to "white persons and persons of African descent" and placed Chinese immigrants in a different class. Roger Daniels, *Coming to America: A History of Immigration and Ethnicity in American Life* (New York: Harper Perennial, 1990), 245.

21. Benjamin Harrison, "Third Annual Address to the Congress, December 9, 1891," in J. D. Richardson, ed., *A Compilation of the Messages and Papers of the Presidents, 1789–1897* (Washington, D.C.: U.S. Congress, 1899), 9:188; E. P. Hutchinson, *Legislative History of American Immigration Policy, 1798–1965* (Philadelphia: University of Pennsylvania Press, 1981), 97–114.

22. In actuality, all three major party platforms during the 1892 presidential campaign, Republican, Democratic, and Populist, called for some form of immigration restriction. Not surprisingly, the Democrats, who held a great many immigrants in their fold, made the mildest plea. Meyer Berman, "The Attitude of American Jewry

toward East European Jewish Immigration, 1881–1941" (Ph.D. diss., Columbia University, 1963), 171–72.

23. Benjamin Harrison, "Fourth Annual Address to the Congress, December 6, 1892," in Richardson, ed., *A Compilation of the Messages and Papers of the Presidents,* 9:330.

24. James Blaine to Charles E. Smith, U.S. Minister to Russia, February 18, 1891, *Papers Relating to the Foreign Relations of the United States* (Washington, D.C.: U.S. Government Printing Office, 1891), 737–39; Berman, "Attitude of American Jewry towards East European Jewish Immigration," 171–72; Simon Wolf, *Selected Addresses and Papers of Simon Wolf* (Cincinnati: Union of American Hebrew Congregations, 1926), 203–14; Oscar Straus, *Under Four Administrations: From Cleveland to Taft* (Boston: Houghton Mifflin, 1922), 104–9; Cyrus Adler, *Jacob H. Schiff: His Life and Letters* (Garden City, N.Y.: Doubleday, Doran, 1928), 2:95, 114–16.

25. L. B. Richardson, *William E. Chandler, Republican* (New York: Dodd, Mead, 1940), 437.

26. Charles Dickens, *Little Dorrit* (New York: Penguin Books, 1976 edition, originally published in 1857), 627.

27. Ismar Elbogen discusses American immigration law and East European Jews in the early 1890s in *A Century of Jewish Life* (Philadelphia: Jewish Publication Society, 1946), 326–52 (quote from p. 335).

28. *Arbeiter Zeitung* (N.Y.), September 2, 1892, 2:1.

29. Oscar Handlin, "American Views of the Jew at the Opening of the Twentieth Century" *Pub. Amer. Jew. Hist. Soc.* 40 (1951): 323–44. John Higham has refuted Handlin's previously widely accepted view of anti-Semitism in the United States during the Gilded Age; see John Higham, "Ideological Anti-Semitism in the Gilded Age," and "Social Discrimination against Jews, 1830–1930," in Higham, *Send These to Me: Immigrants in Urban America* (rev. ed. Baltimore: Johns Hopkins University Press, 1984), 116–29, 130–73. As Higham notes, even if there existed no overt programs designed to promote racist policies against American Jews, as there were in Nazi Germany, the popular Jewish stereotypes and various degrees of social discrimination nevertheless had a distinct effect on these people's lives.

30. Leonard Dinnerstein, *Anti-Semitism in America* (New York: Oxford University Press, 1994), 48; Dinnerstein discusses anti-Semitism in America during the Gilded Age on pp. 35–57; see also Frederic Cople Jaher, *A Scapegoat in the New Wilderness: The Origins and Rise of Anti-Semitism in America* (Cambridge, Mass.: Harvard University Press, 1994); Louise A. Mayo, *The Ambivalent Image: Nineteenth Century America's Perceptions of the Jew* (Rutherford, N.J.: Fairleigh Dickinson University Press, 1988); David A. Gerber, ed., *Anti-Semitism in American History* (Urbana: University of Illinois Press, 1986); Naomi Cohen, "Anti-Semitism in the Gilded Age," in Naomi Cohen, ed., *Essential Papers on Jewish–Christian Relations in the United States: Imagery and Reality* (New York: New York University Press, 1990); Michael Selzer, ed., *"Kike!" A Documentary History of Anti-Semitism in America* (New York: World, 1972), 40–114.

31. William Harvey, *Coin's Financial School,* ed. Richard Hofstadter (Cambridge:

Belknap Press of Harvard University Press, 1963), 1–70. Hofstadter's introduction to this 1892 best-selling book on finance discusses the resentment Populists and others had toward Jews with regard to the world's money and gold supply. The original version sold well over a million copies. International financiers such as the Rothschilds and immigration philanthropist Maurice de Hirsch were frequent targets of these diatribes. The role anti-Semitism and conspiracy theories played in the Populist movement and among other social groups during the Gilded Age is discussed in Michael Dobkowski, *The Tarnished Dream: The Basis of American Anti-Semitism* (Westport, Conn.: Greenwood, 1979); and Irwin Unger, *The Greenback Era: A Social and Political History of American Finance, 1865–1879* (Princeton: Princeton University Press, 1964). Perhaps the most infamous casting of the "Jewish money conspiracy" was its twentieth-century reincarnation as *The Protocols of the Elders of Zion,* a book created by members of the Russian secret police at the turn of the century, documenting a conspiracy among the Jewish bankers and the devil to control the world's money supply and to undermine Christian civilization. Industrialist Henry Ford was especially fond of this anti-Semitic treatise and reproduced its tenets in his newspaper, *The Dearborn Independent,* between 1920 and 1927. See Dinnerstein, *Anti-Semitism in America,* 80–83, 111–15; Norman Cohn, *Warrant for Genocide: The Myth of the Jewish World-Conspiracy and the Protocols of the Elders of Zion* (London: Eyre and Spottiswoode, 1967).

32. Henry Adams, *Democracy, A Novel* (New York: Henry Holt, 1880). For a summary of Adams' anti-Semitism, see Dobkowski, *Tarnished Dream.*

33. Ignatius Donnelly, *Caesar's Column: A Story of the Twentieth Century* (Chicago: F. J. Schulte, 1890).

34. Camille Flammarion, "Omega: The Last Days of the World," *Cosmopolitan Magazine* 15 (1892): 200–213.

35. For discussions of the politics and ideology of William Jennings Bryan, see Richard J. Hofstadter, *The American Political Tradition and the Men Who Made It* (New York: Vintage Books, 1961), 186–206; see also idem, *The Age of Reform, from Bryan to FDR* (New York: Alfred Knopf, 1955), 80; and idem, "Introduction," *Coin's Financial School,* 1–70; Roy Ginger, ed., *William Jennings Bryan: Selections* (Indianapolis: Bobbs-Merrill, 1967), 37–46. Bryan's views on immigrants are more clearly expressed in William J. Bryan, "Foreign Influences in American Politics," *The Arena* 19 (1898): 433–38; Stephen Bloore, "The Jew in American Literature, 1794–1930," *Pub. Amer. Jew. Hist. Soc.* 40 (1951): 345–60.

36. The derogatory epithet *kike* supposedly has its roots during this period in U.S. history. Although many scholars of anti-Semitism, such as Leonard Dinnerstein, have traced the word's etymology to the anti-Semitic slur "Christ Killer," other historians, such as Edward Robb Ellis, claim that the word was actually coined by German Jewish Americans who were making fun of the propensity of Russian Jewish names to end in the suffix *ki.* Originally "kikis" in the early 1880s, the name was soon shortened to the even more harsh "kike." See Dinnerstein, *Anti-Semitism in America,* 35–57; Edward Robb Ellis, *The Epic of New York City: A Narrative History from 1524 to Present* (New York: Coward-McCann, 1966), 417.

37. Handlin, "American Views of the Jew at the Opening of the Twentieth Century," 340. It seems likely that Handlin was reflecting upon the most dangerous forms of anti-Semitism, the Nazi extermination of 6 million Jews, as he wrote this essay in the 1950s. Yet the process of dehumanization through prejudice and cultural perceptions probably served their negative function in representing American or foreign Jews as dangerous and expendable far earlier, but with markedly different results, than during World War II. See also Hannah Arendt, *Eichmann in Jerusalem: A Report on the Banality of Evil* (New York: Viking, 1963).

38. Higham, "Ideological Anti-Semitism in the Gilded Age," 116–37.

39. Abram S. Isaacs, "The Danger Signal," *The Jewish Messenger,* September 16, 1892, 4:2. Isaacs was a well-connected writer and editor, a Reform rabbi, and a professor of Hebrew and Germanic literature at New York University; for similar editorials by Isaacs, see the September 2, 9, 24, 31 issues of the *Messenger.*

40. *The American Israelite,* March 3, 1892, 4:6. Isaac Wise originally wrote this editorial in response to the typhus epidemic of 1892, but its sentiments were reprised that fall during and after the cholera epidemic. See, for example, *American Israelite,* September 21, 1892, 4:5.

41. "News from Detroit," *The American Israelite,* September 29, 1892, 2:6.

42. *The American Hebrew,* December 30, 1892, 292–93. Philip Cowen, American publisher and editor, had a distinguished career as a journalist and was an astute advocate for immigration. See Philip Cowen, *Memories of an American Jew* (New York: International Press, 1932).

43. See Wolf, *Selected Addresses and Papers of Simon Wolf,* 203–14; idem, *The Presidents I Have Known from 1860–1918* (Washington, D.C.: Byron S. Adams, 1919), 152–66; Adler, ed., *Jacob H. Schiff,* 2:81–95, 114–17; Straus, *Under Four Administrations from Cleveland to Taft,* 105–9; Lewis L. Straus, "Oscar S. Straus: An Appreciation," *Pub. Amer. Jew. Hist. Soc.* 60 (1950): 1–16; *American Israelite,* December 8, 1892, 4:5.

44. See *Annual Reports of the United Hebrew Charities for 1892–1893,* 7–22; *Annual Report of the International Order of the B'nai B'rith for 1892–1893,* 67–71; *Minutes of the New York City Board of Health for 1892–1893,* entries for meetings dated September 1–October 5, 1892. These Jewish charities served a similarly helpful and financial role in the typhus epidemic of 1892 in New York City.

45. President's report for the Baron de Hirsch Fund, New York, January 1893 (manuscript); Baron de Hirsch Fund Papers, box 1, American Jewish Historical Society, Waltham, Mass.

46. William Sparger, "Editorial," *The Menorah* 12 (1892): 112. *Hassidism* is a particularly Orthodox sect of East European Judaism. Founded in the eighteenth century by a mystic named Israel ben Eliezer (later renamed the *Baal Shem Tov*), *Hassidism* emphasizes joyous prayer, devout adherence to Jewish law, and life apart from Gentiles. For similar worries by the German Jewish American community about the effects of unrestricted immigration of the Russian Jews, see *Annual Report of the United Hebrew Charities of the City of New York, 1893,* 16, 22; *Proceedings, Report of the Board of Delegates, Union of American Hebrew Congregations for 1891,* 2820; ibid., for 1892, 3007.

47. Letter from Oscar Straus to Baron Maurice de Hirsch, January 20, 1893, Oscar Straus Papers, Library of Congress, Washington, D.C.

48. Abraham Cahan, *The Education of Abraham Cahan* (originally published in Yiddish in 1926 under the title *Bletter Fun Mein Leben*) (Philadelphia: Jewish Publication Society, 1969), 396.

49. "Men of Three Races. How They Would Solve the Puzzling Problem of Immigration," *New York World*, December 15, 1892, 1:1. The other "races" consulted were representatives of the Italian, Swedish, and Polish communities in New York. Not surprisingly, they were reluctant to support Jewish immigration in the face of the epidemic but, nevertheless, made strong pleas for the admission of their own ethnic groups. Rabbi Joseph's career continued to progress in relative obscurity until, ironically, his death. During the funeral procession, Irish American laborers began pelting the Orthodox Jewish mourners with refuse from their lunches. The mourners became indignant and violent. The group of long-bearded, Yiddish-speaking Jewish men stormed the door of the factory that employed the Irish laborers and proceeded to fight with them, using stones, bricks, and other projectiles to make their point. The riot, which was the most serious one involving New York's Jews until, perhaps, the 1991 riots at Crown Heights, Brooklyn, was especially controversial for the lack of help rendered to the Jewish mourners by the New York City Police Department. See obituaries and description of the funeral of Rabbi Jacob Joseph, *New York Times*, July 31, 1902, 1:7, 2:1; August 1, 1902, 8:2, 14:1; August 2, 1902, 3:1; August 4, 1902, 8:1; August 5, 1902, 14:1; and August 7, 1902, 14:1. See also Abraham J. Karp, "New York Chooses a Chief Rabbi," in A. J. Karp, ed., *The Jewish Experience in America*, vol. 4, *The Era of Immigration* (New York: Ktav, 1969), 126–84; Moses Rischin, *The Promised City: New York's Jews, 1870–1914* (Cambridge, Mass.: Harvard University Press, 1962), 148; Howard Sachar, *A History of the Jews in America* (New York: Alfred Knopf, 1992), 192, 274–75.

50. *Arbeiter Zeitung* (N.Y.), December 7, 1892, 1:1; December 16, 1892, 2:3; December 23, 1892, 1:4; January 13, 1893, 1:1, 4:1.

51. *Yiddishe Tageblatt* (N.Y.), January 13, 1893, 4:5; February 17, 1893, 4:1.

52. See, for example, editorials in *The American Hebrew*, December 30, 1892, 292, and *The Jewish Messenger*, December 9, 1892, 1; See also Adler, ed., *Jacob Schiff*, 2: 68–120; Sheldon Neuringer, "American Jewry and United States Immigration Policy, 1881–1953" (Ph.D. diss., University of Wisconsin, 1969), 29–30.

Chapter 7. The Doctors' Prescription for Quarantine

1. See, for example, Gerald L. Gieson, *Michael Foster and the Cambridge School of Physiology: The Scientific Enterprise in Late Victorian Society* (Princeton: Princeton University Press, 1978); François Delaporte, *Disease and Civilization: The Cholera in Paris, 1832*, trans. A. Goldhammer (Cambridge, Mass.: MIT Press, 1986); William Rothstein, *American Physicians in the 19th Century, from Sects to Science* (Baltimore: Johns Hopkins University Press, 1972), 261–81; Alexandra Oleson and John Voss,

eds., *The Organization of Knowledge in Modern America, 1860–1920* (Baltimore: Johns Hopkins University Press, 1979), to name but a few studies exploring how medical knowledge passes through a filter of social and historical context.

2. For example, see letter from Dr. Edward Snader on behalf of the Homeopathic Society of Pennsylvania to the president of the United States, February 3, 1893, petitioning for improved sanitary regulations at American seaports, R.G. 233, papers of the U.S. House of Representatives, 52nd Cong., box 158, National Archives, Washington, D.C.. The famed hydropathist Simon Baruch, M.D., wrote reassuring editorials in his journal, the *Hygienic and Dietary Gazette* (8 [1892]: 170–71, 189–90) on the value of good sanitation and effective public health regulations in the control of the cholera epidemic; see also Patricia Spain Ward, *Simon Baruch: Rebel in the Ranks of Medicine, 1840–1921* (Tuscaloosa: University of Alabama Press, 1994), 176–83.

3. This definition, and those for miasmatic contagion, chemical (or zymotic) contagion, and contingent contagionism, are taken from Alfred L. Loomis's *A Textbook of Practical Medicine Designed for the Use of Students and Practitioners of Medicine* (New York: William Wood, 1890) (quote from p. 610). For more positive discussions of the germ theory of disease causation, see William Osler, *The Principles and Practice of Medicine* (New York: Appleton, 1892), 1–263.

4. See, for example, some of the older, more positivistic histories of the early years of American bacteriology, such as C.-E. A. Winslow, *The Life of Hermann Biggs* (Philadelphia: Lea and Febiger, 1929); Wade Oliver, *The Man Who Lived for Tomorrow: A Biography of William Hallock Park, M.D.* (New York: E. P. Dutton, 1941).

5. Abraham Jacobi, "Inaugural Address, Feb. 5, 1885," *Miscellaneous Addresses and Writings* (New York: Critic and Guide, 1909), 7:170. Jacobi became a strong and vociferous supporter of germ theory not long after making this speech.

6. Minutes of the Section on Public Health, Legal Medicine, Medical and Vital Statistics, New York Academy of Medicine (manuscript in folio), vol. 1, 1891–1911, 51–56.

7. For excellent examples of a contingent contagionist explanation of various contagious diseases, such as yellow fever, cholera, and diphtheria, see Loomis, *Textbook of Practical Medicine* (1890 ed.), 609–710. For excellent discussions of the zymotic theory of disease, the role fermentation was thought to play in contagious diseases by Victorian era physicians, and other nineteenth-century etiologic theories, see John M. Eyler, *Victorian Social Medicine: The Ideas and Methods of William Farr* (Baltimore: Johns Hopkins University Press, 1979), 97–122; Margaret Pelling, *Cholera, Fever, and English Medicine, 1825–1865* (Oxford: Oxford University Press, 1978); Richard Evans, *Death in Hamburg: Society and Politics in the Cholera Years, 1830–1910* (New York: Oxford University Press, 1987).

8. William James, *Essays in Pragmatism* (New York: Hafner, 1968), ix. James originally wrote these essays between 1879 and 1907.

9. See the testimonies of Cyrus Edson, George F. Shrady, Alfred Loomis, and Joseph E. Winters in *Immigration Report Accompanying S. 3786*, 52nd Cong., 2nd sess., no. 1333, ser. 3073, Y4.Im6:Im6 (Washington, D.C.: U.S. Government Printing

Office, 1893), 9–14. Shrady repeats his nativist comments in an editorial in *The Medical Record*, January 14, 1893, 48–49.

10. George E. Waring Jr., "Cholera and Quarantine" (letter to the editor) *New York Evening Post*, January 11, 1893, 2:3. For biographical information on the sanitarian's life, see James H. Cassedy, "The Flamboyant Colonel Waring: An Anticontagionist Holds the American Stage in the Age of Pasteur and Koch," *Bull. Hist. Med.* 36 (1962): 163–76; Richard Skolnik, "George Edwin Waring, Jr., A Model for Reformers," *New-York Historical Society Quarterly* 52 (1968): 354–78; Martin V. Melosi, *Pragmatic Environmentalist: Sanitary Engineer George E. Waring, Jr.* (Washington, D.C.: Public Works Historical Society, Essays in Public Works History, no. 4, 1977).

11. See, for example, A. C. Abbott, "Prophylactic Measures against Asiatic Cholera," *Medical News* 61 (1892): 287–90; A. L. Carroll, "How Long Shall a Cholera-Infected Vessel Be Detained at Quarantine?" *N.Y. Med. J.* 56 (1892): 350–54; George M. Sternberg, "Bacteriology of Cholera and Methods of Disinfection," *Brooklyn Med. J.* 6 (1892): 10–16; E. C. Wendt, ed., *A Treatise on Asiatic Cholera* (New York: William Wood, 1885).

12. Prudden was a consistent advocate for the separate consideration of immigration and quarantine policy and a national system of quarantine, maintaining that scientific knowledge of cholera's transmission and disinfection along with careful medical scrutiny were more than ample to prevent a cholera epidemic. See T. Mitchell Prudden, "Some Hygienic Aspects of Asiatic Cholera," *The Christian Union* 46 (1892): 487–88; idem, *The Story of the Bacteria and Their Relations to Health and Disease* (New York: G. P. Putnam's Sons, 1889), 90–95; unsigned piece, "Cholera and Our Quarantine," *Harper's Weekly* 36 (1892): 890. In "Bound Pamphlets and Reprints of T. Mitchell Prudden, presented to the New York Academy of Medicine by the Author," New York Academy of Medicine Historical Collection, New York. William Welch was also a strident opponent of quarantine as an immigration restriction. See W. H. Welch, "Asiatic Cholera in Its Relation to Sanitary Reform," *Popular Health Magazine* 1 (1893–94): 6–12.

13. Henry P. Walcott, *The Physician, the College and the Commonwealth* (New Haven: Yale University Press, 1893), 8. For a summation of Walcott's career as a sanitarian, see Barbara G. Rosenkrantz, *Public Health and the State: Changing Views in Massachusetts, 1842–1936* (Cambridge, Mass.: Harvard University Press, 1972), 91–96.

14. Henry P. Walcott, "National Health Legislation and Quarantine," *Boston Med. & Surg. J.* 127 (1892): 307–8.

15. "Politics and the Public Health," *Medical News* 61 (1892): 687–88. The editorial is unsigned but has been attributed to John Shaw Billings by William H. Welch in Welch's personal copy of the journal, which is in the collections of the William Henry Welch Library of the Johns Hopkins University School of Medicine, Baltimore, Md. This is confirmed by a telegram to Billings from the editor of the *Medical News*, George Gould, thanking Billings for composing an editorial on the subjects of cholera and the "restriction of immigration," dated December 27, 1892. John Shaw Billings Papers, New York Public Library, microfilm reel 14 (December 1892–April 1, 1893).

16. Letter to Oscar S. Straus, chairman of the quarantine committee, New York Board of Trade and Transportation, December 7, 1892, John Shaw Billings Papers, New York Public Library, microfilm reel 25, general correspondence, 1884–95.

17. Edward O. Shakespeare, *Report on Cholera in Europe and India*, U.S. Senate, 49th Cong., misc. doc. 92 (Washington, D.C.: U.S. Government Printing Office, 1890). This copious text synthesizes the world's literature about the bacteriology, disinfection, transmission, epidemiology, and prevention of cholera as it was understood in 1890.

18. Edward O. Shakespeare, "International Sanitation," *Dietetic and Hygienic Gazette* 9 (1893): 244–46 (quote from p. 246); see also idem, "Cholera and Quarantine," *Dietetic and Hygienic Gazette* 9 (1893): 189–92; idem, "The Total Mortality Materially Reducible by Thorough Disinfection of Baggage of Immigrants," *Dietetic and Hygienic Gazette* 9 (1893): 293–94; idem, "The National Government Should Have Supreme Control of Quarantine at All Frontiers," *Medical News* 61 (1892): 281–87.

19. For a description of the marvels of bacteriology by Bryant, see, for example, *New York Times*, September 15, 1892, 2:1; for Bryant's comments advocating immigration restriction as one means of preventing another cholera epidemic, see *Immigration Report, Feb. 22, 1893, Accompanying S. 3786, 52nd Congress, 2nd Session: Establishing Additional Regulations Concerning Immigration to the United States*, Senate Report no. 1333, series 3073, Y4.Im6:Im6 (Washington, D.C.: U.S. Government Printing Office, 1893), 9–10.

20. A. L. Gihon, "The Hygiene of Cholera," *Brooklyn Med. J.* 6 (1892): 16–21.

21. I cover this episode in a brief article: Howard Markel, "Cholera, Quarantines, and Immigration Restriction: The View from Johns Hopkins, 1892," *Bull. Hist. Med.* 67 (1993): 691–95.

22. *Congressional Record*, January 10, 1893, 472.

23. Allan McLane Hamilton, *Recollections of an Alienist: Personal and Professional* (New York: George H. Doran, 1916), 15, 105–6. Hamilton, the grandson of Alexander Hamilton, enjoyed a fabulously successful career bridging newspaper writing, medicine, psychiatry, and politics. Hamilton's appointment to this committee, aside from his social prominence and professional reputation as an alienist, was probably a function of his friendship with Abraham Jacobi, who was once Hamilton's pediatrician.

24. Philip Van Ingen, *The New York Academy of Medicine, Its First Hundred Years* (New York: Columbia University Press, 1949), 211, 237, 262–74. Dr. Janeway, among other accomplishments, was one of Hermann Biggs' medical role models. Winslow, *Life of Hermann Biggs*, 44.

25. The correspondence of T. Mitchell Prudden for 1892 confirms his leadership role in both the Chamber of Commerce and, subsequently, the New York Academy of Medicine Quarantine Committees. See general correspondence files, 1892–93, T. Mitchell Prudden Papers, Sterling Library Rare Book and Manuscript Collections, Yale University, New Haven, Conn.

26. T. Mitchell Prudden and Francis Delafield, *Handbook of Pathological Anatomy,*

4th ed. (New York: William Wood, 1892); and Prudden, *Manual of Practical Normal Histology,* 4th ed. (New York: G. P. Putnam's Sons, 1892).

27. Quote from *Harper's Weekly* 36 (1892): 890. Prudden's three popular books, all published by G. P. Putnam's Sons in New York, are: *The Story of the Bacteria and Their Relations to Health and Disease* (1889), *Dust and Its Dangers* (1890), *Drinking Water and Ice Supplies and Their Relations to Health and Disease* (1891).

28. Letter from Seth Low to Alexander Orr, October 27, 1892, Seth Low Papers, box 13, file June–December 1892, Columbia University Rare Book and Manuscript Library. See *Report of the Special Advisory Committee on Quarantine to the New York State Chamber of Commerce, 1892.*

29. *New York Times,* February 1, 1893, 2:1; *Med. Rec.* 43 (1893): 175. The committee consisted of Drs. T. G. Thomas (chair), R. H. Derby (secretary), A. Jacobi, E. B. Bronson, C. L. Dana, J. H. Girdner, E. G. Janeway, L. Johnson, C. C. Lee, D. Lewis, T. M. Prudden, A. H. Smith, S. Smith, D. D. Webster, C. McBurney, M. A. Starr, C. C. Rice, L. A. Sayre, W. T. Lusk, S. B. Ward, and T. M. Markoe.

30. Loomis first reported his typhus fever experience as "The History of Typhus Fever, as It Occurred in Bellevue Hospital, Together with Some Results of the Non-Stimulating Plan of Treatment in that Disease," *Bull. N.Y. Acad. Med.* 2 (1865): 348–67. The quote is from A. L. Loomis, *Lectures on Fevers* (New York: William Wood, 1877), 212–13. See also, Loomis, *Textbook of Practical Medicine,* 714.

31. Loomis, *Lectures on Fevers,* 212–13.

32. See *Immigration Hearings,* U.S. Senate doc. 1333, 10–11.

33. These anecdotes appear in Simon Flexner and James T. Flexner, *William Henry Welch and the Heroic Age of American Medicine* (New York: Viking, 1941), 67, 119, 142, 159 (quote from p. 119); Robert J. Carlisle, ed., *An Account of Bellevue Hospital with a Catalogue of the Medical and Surgical Staff from 1736 to 1894* (New York: Society of the Alumni of Bellevue Hospital, 1893), 118.

34. Letter from Stephen Smith and T. M. Prudden on behalf of the quarantine committee to Alexander Orr, of the N.Y. Chamber of Commerce, October 19, 1892, T. Mitchell Prudden Papers, Yale University.

35. This memorandum documenting the relationship of Prudden and Loomis is in box 5, file 78, T. Mitchell Prudden Papers, Yale University; for published accounts of the meetings of the New York Academy of Medicine where the debate took place, see *Med. Rec.* 43 (March 4, 1893): 272, 277, 285; 43 (March 18, 1893): 35, 247; see also *Medical News* 62 (1893): 247; *N.Y. Med. J.* 57 (1893): 141, 202–3. The president of the New York Academy of Medicine, D. B. St. John De Roosa, suggested still another reason for Loomis's political machinations: "It is all a scheme of Tammany Hall, and you [Loomis] are working in its interest"; *New York Tribune,* February 25, 1893, 5:3. Loomis heatedly denied such allegations.

36. For the opinions and subsequent strategies of the National Quarantine Committee in regard to the passage of the National Quarantine Act of 1893, see "The Harris Quarantine Bill: Opinions of the Advisory Medical Board," *New York Evening Post,* January 14, 1893, 2:1. The committee objected to the bill's clauses giving the president, rather than an impartial health board, authority to suspend immigration

and the role the Marine Hospital Service was to play in administering a national quarantine system.

37. *New York Times*, February 25, 1893, 1:1.

Chapter 8. The Congress Responds

1. Letter to Simon Wolf from William E. Chandler, April 25, 1893, in Simon Wolf, *Selected Addresses and Papers of Simon Wolf* (Cincinnati: Union of American Hebrew Congregations, 1926), 204–7.

2. Ibid., 205–7; letter from Schiff to President Benjamin Harrison, in Cyrus Adler, ed., *Jacob Schiff: His Life and Letters* (Garden City, N.Y.: Doubleday, Doran, 1928), 2:76.

3. See "Speech of Senator Chandler of New Hampshire in the United States Senate on the 6th Day of January, 1893 on the Subject of the danger from cholera in 1893 and the state and national quarantine systems and in favor of all immigration for one year," 27–29, Collections of the New-York Historical Society.

4. Philip Taft, *The A.F. of L. in the Time of Gompers* (New York: Harper and Brothers, 1957), 302–7; Samuel Gompers, *Seventy Years of Life and Labor: An Autobiography* (New York: E. P. Dutton, 1925), 2:151–73; Elias Tcherikower, ed., *Geshikhte Fun Der Yidisher Arbeter-Bavegung In Di Fareyniket Shtatn* (*The History of the Jewish Labor Movement in the United States*), 2 vols. (New York: Forward, 1943, 1945); David Montgomery, *The Fall of the House of Labor: The Workplace, the State, and American Labor Activism, 1865–1925* (New York: Cambridge University Press, 1987).

5. "Labor's View of Immigration," *New York World*, December 17, 1892, 2:2.

6. Ibid.

7. Ibid., 2:3; *Report of the Proceedings of the 12th Annual Convention of the A.F.L.*, *1892*, 14, 28.

8. *The Jewish Messenger*, December 23, 1892, 1.

9. Quote from letter to Chandler from "An American," dated February 16, 1892, William Eaton Chandler Papers, vol. 85, Library of Congress, Washington, D.C. Chandler's letter books contain literally hundreds of such letters advocating immigration restriction of Russian Jews and other undesirable new immigrants. What makes the letters between February 1892 and January 1893 so interesting is that reasons of public health and the threat of imported disease are used most frequently as the pressing need for such legislation. Prior to this period and right after, the concerns routinely given are those of immigrants taking much-needed jobs from native-born Americans, the economic cost of supporting people who arrived impoverished, and vague concern about the future of the "American stock." Other letters asserting Jewish conspiracies to overtake the nation also appear frequently before, during, and after the epidemics. Similarly, in a review of petitions sent to the House of Representatives during the Fifty-first through Fifty-third Congresses (1889–95), those originating from private citizens, local Chambers of Commerce, and various interest groups urging restriction take a distinctly different tack after the typhus epidemic and especially after the cholera epidemic. For example, the San Francisco Chamber

of Commerce petitioned the Congress to halt immigration: "With the probable advent of the World's greatest scourge, Asiatic cholera, from European ports whence this undesirable immigration departs for this country, it has become a question of self preservation to prohibit immigration while such risk exists." See Memorial from the San Francisco Chamber of Commerce to the House of Representatives, January 17, 1893, House of Representatives Records, 52nd Cong., R.G. 233, box 201, file 52A-H28.3, National Archives, Washington, D.C. The petitions citing the older reasons (jobs, etc.) for restricting immigrants begin to reappear in late 1893, after the passage of the National Quarantine Act of 1893 and the failure of cholera to return to the United States that year. See House of Representatives Records, 53rd Cong., Immigration Committee Papers, R.G. 233, National Archives, Washington, D.C.

10. Letter from J. W. Van Buskirk to Chandler, June 15, 1892, vol. 86, items 6167–72, William Chandler Papers, Library of Congress, Washington, D.C.

11. Letter to Chandler from C. M. Ready, November 30, 1892, Chandler Papers, vol. 87, items 6432–33.

12. Letter to Chandler from Phillip Mulligan, December 18, 1892, Chandler Papers, vol. 87, item 6498.

13. Letter to Chandler from Sarah Gaylord, January 8, 1893, Chandler Papers, vol. 87, items 6582–83.

14. John Higham, *Strangers in the Land: Patterns of American Nativism, 1860–1925* (New York: Atheneum, 1963), 100.

15. See, for example, *New York Herald*, November 14, 1892, 6:3. See also *New York Times*, November 27, 1892, 4:2; *New York Sun*, December 1, 1892, 6:1.

16. Speech of Senator Chandler, 3; See also *Congressional Record*, vol. 24, pt. 1 [52nd Cong., 2nd sess.], January 6, 1893, 357–77; "Suspension of Immigration" File, HR52A.F50.1, Administrative Papers, House of Representatives, 52nd Cong., box 137, National Archives, Washington, D.C.; *New York Times*, January 1, 1893, 9:7; January 5, 1893, 3:3; January 7, 1893, 4:6; *New York Sun*, January 2, 1893, 1:3; January 5, 1893, 5:1; January 7, 1893, 5:1; *New York Herald*, January 4, 1893, 4:1; January 5, 1893, 5:1; January 7, 1893, 5:3.

17. Speech of Senator Chandler, 3.

18. Speech of Senator Chandler, 23–25; *Congressional Record*, January 6, 1893, 363–66.

19. Naomi W. Cohen, *A Dual Heritage: The Public Career of Oscar S. Straus* (Philadelphia: Jewish Publication Society, 1969), 39–54; Charles A. Madison, *Eminent Jewish Americans, 1776 to the Present* (New York: Frederick Ungar, 1970), 86–98; Oscar S. Straus, *Under Four Administrations: From Cleveland to Taft* (Boston: Houghton Mifflin, 1922), 105–8; *New York Times*, November 29, 1892, 9:3; *New York Tribune*, November 29, 1892, 5:2.

20. Erwin H. Ackerknecht, "Anticontagionism between 1821 and 1867: The Fielding H. Garrison Lecture," *Bull. Hist. Med.* 22 (1948): 562–93.

21. Robert Greenhalgh Albion (with the collaboration of Jennie Barnes Pope), *The Rise of New York Port, 1815–1860* (New York: Charles Scribner's Sons, 1939), 349–51.

22. "Report of the Special Committee of the New York Board of Trade and Trans-

portation on Quarantine, Adopted January 6, 1893, with the Correspondence," 6, Collection of the A. Alfred Taubman Medical Library (Rare Book Division), The University of Michigan at Ann Arbor; Memorial to the president of the United States of America from the New York Board of Trade and Transportation, January 7, 1893, "Incoming Correspondence, New York, 1893," Marine Hospital Service Records, box 96, R.G. 90, National Archives, Washington, D.C. The other members of this special committee were Ambrose Snow, E. H. Cole, E. S. A. de Lima, and Jeremiah Fitzpatrick, all prominent New York merchants and importers.

23. Transcript of "Speech by John B. Weber, Commissioner of Immigration, Port of New York, at Cooper Union, New York City, January 4, 1893," file I-80, box 37A (general correspondence regarding immigration), Collection of the American Jewish Historical Society, Waltham, Mass.

24. *Congressional Record,* 366.

25. Ibid., 370–71.

26. *New York Times,* January 1, 1893, 9:7.

27. A "very much softened" version of Chandler's 1893 immigration bill made its way into law. Instead of expanding the excludable classes of immigrants to include the illiterate, the impoverished or those "likely to become a public charge," the blind, the crippled, the "otherwise physically imperfect," and the anarchist or politically untoward, the act confined itself to regulations pertaining to the recording of ships' manifests, their transmission to U.S. inspection officials, and similar requirements. As immigration law historian E. P. Hutchinson noted: "It brought no new developments of immigration policy but rather a reinforcement of existing laws." E. P. Hutchinson, *Legislative History of American Immigration Policy, 1798–1965* (Philadelphia: University of Pennsylvania Press, 1981), 108.

28. *New York World,* December 12, 1892, 1; December 13, 1892, 3; December 14, 1892, 1; December 15, 1892, 1.

29. Wyndham Miles, *History of the National Board of Health,* unpublished manuscript, History of Medicine Division, National Library of Medicine (MS C237), 230–35.

30. The short-lived National Board of Health and attempts to nationalize quarantine policy in the United States during the late 1870s and 1880s is discussed in Margaret Humphreys, *Yellow Fever and the South* (New Brunswick, N.J.: Rutgers University Press, 1992); John H. Ellis, *Yellow Fever and Public Health in the New South* (Lexington: University Press of Kentucky, 1992); Khaled J. Bloom, *The Mississippi Valley's Great Yellow Fever Epidemic of 1878* (Baton Rouge: Louisiana State University Press, 1993); John Duffy, *The Sanitarians: A History of American Public Health* (Urbana: University of Illinois Press, 1990). The expanding role of the U.S. Marine Hospital Service and, after 1902, its successor agency, the U.S. Public Health Service, is described in Ralph C. Williams, *The United States Public Health Service, 1798–1950* (Washington, D.C.: Commissioned Officers Association of the U.S.P.H.S., 1951); Laurence F. Schmeckebier, *The Public Health Service: Its History, Activities, and Organization* (Baltimore: Johns Hopkins University Press, 1923); Robert D. Leigh, *Federal Health Administration in the United States* (New York: Harper and Brothers,

1917); Alan Marcus, "Disease Prevention in America: From a Local to a National Outlook, 1880–1910," *Bull. Hist. Med.* 53 (1979): 203.

31. Clipping from *Washington Republic,* December 28, 1892, 18–19. From the U.S. Marine Health Service clipping scrapbook, vol. 4, 1892–93, National Library of Medicine, Bethesda, Md.

32. *Annual Report of the Supervising Surgeon General of the Marine Hospital Service of the United States, for the fiscal year of 1892* (Washington, D.C.: U.S. Government Printing Office, 1893), 35–52.

33. *Congressional Record* (Senate), January 10, 1893, 464–65.

34. "An Act Granting Additional Quarantine Powers and Imposing Additional Duties upon the Marine Hospital Service, February 15, 1893" (27 Stat.L. 449); Schmeckebier, *The Public Health Service,* 19–20, 214–18; Leigh, *Federal Health Administration in the United States,* 295–300.

35. Higham, *Strangers in the Land,* 100. It should also be noted that during the years 1880 to 1924, rarely were more than 2 percent of *all* immigrants seeking entry to the United States denied based upon physical abnormality or disease. The annual average of immigrants turned away for reasons of health was about 1 percent of all those seeking entry. See "Aliens debarred at all United States ports during the fiscal years 1892 to 1910, inclusive by cause," in U.S. Senate Immigration Commission, *Statistical Review of Immigration, 1820–1910,* 61st Cong., 3rd sess., doc. 756, vol. 20 (Washington, D.C.: U.S. Government Printing Office, 1911), 366–67; Alan M. Kraut, *Silent Travelers: Germs, Genes, and the "Immigrant Menace"* (New York: Basic Books, 1994; Baltimore: Johns Hopkins University Press, 1995), 66.

36. "Act of February 15, 1893 (27 Stat. L. 449) — An Act Granting Additional Quarantine Powers and Imposing Additional Duties Upon the Marine Hospital Service" (sec. 7), reprinted in Schemeckebier, *Public Health Service,* 216; Higham, *Strangers in the Land,* 100.

37. *Congressional Record* (Senate), January 10, 1893, vol. 24, pt. I, 52nd Cong., 2nd sess., 473.

38. John Duffy has described federal quarantine policy and state rights issues as being "inextricably intertwined" during the nineteenth century. *Sanitarians,* 162.

39. Arthur M. Schlesinger Sr., "The State Rights Fetish," in *New Viewpoints in American History* (New York: Macmillan, 1922), 222–23.

40. *New York Herald,* January 22, 1893, 19:5; January 24, 1893, 5:3, 6:3; *New York Tribune,* January 24, 1893, 2:1, 6:2.

41. *Dictionary of American Biography* (New York: Charles Scribner's Sons, 1929), 2:256–57.

42. For examples of the frequent string-pulling Croker ordered Cockran to do, see the Hugh Grant Papers (1890–92 files), of the New-York Historical Society, New York City; Cockran lost reelection in 1888, but returned to Congress for two terms in 1890–94 and three more from 1904 to 1909.

43. "Dr. Jenkins Heard From: All Tammany Men Ordered to Oppose the Quarantine Bill," *New York Tribune,* January 20, 1893, 4:4; "A Legislative Botch," *New York Tribune,* January 24, 1893, 2:1.

44. *Congressional Record* (House), January 21, 1893, 758.

45. *Congressional Record* (House), 761. Specifically, the Cockran amendment, which the anti-Tammany press derided as "the Jenkins amendment," provided that nothing in the act could "relax, modify, or suspend any rule, precaution, or regulation" that either was in effect or was put into effect by state or municipal quarantine officials in regard to the exclusion of contagious diseases from a U.S. port.

46. "Tammany and Quarantine," *New York Tribune,* January 24, 1893, 6:2. For similar diatribes against the politics of Tammany Hall and their attempts to protect their control of the New York quarantine station, see *Baltimore Sun,* January 20, 1893, 2:1; January 21, 1892, 4:1; *New York Herald,* January 22, 1892, 19:5; January 24, 1893, 5:3, 6:3, 6:4; *New York Tribune,* January 24, 1893, 2:1, 6:2; January 26, 1893, 6:2, 11:5; *New York Evening Post,* January 24, 1893, 6:1; January 25, 1893, 6:4.

47. *New York Herald,* January 31, 1893, 6:1; "Congress and Quarantine," *New York Evening Post,* January 31, 1893, 6:4.

48. *New York Tribune,* February 10, 1893, 6:4; *New York Herald,* February 16, 1893, 7:6.

49. Leigh, *Federal Health Administration in the United States,* 318–19; see also James A. Tobey, *The National Government and Public Health* (Baltimore: Johns Hopkins University Press, 1926), 31, 88. The efforts of the federal government to coordinate and harmonize its public health efforts on a national basis has been discussed by a number of historians. See, for example, Victoria Harden, *Inventing the N.I.H.: Federal Biomedical Research Policy, 1887–1937* (Baltimore: Johns Hopkins University Press, 1986), 9–70; Williams, *United States Public Health Service, 1798–1950,* 113–75. Another critical issue that often impeded this centralization process was inadequate financial appropriations to carry out the public health regulations enacted into federal law during this period.

50. Hugh Cumming, "The United States Quarantine System during the Last Fifty Years," in Mazÿck P. Ravenel, ed., *A Half Century of Public Health* (New York: American Public Health Association, 1921), 118–32.

51. Marcus, "Disease Prevention in America," 203.

52. Robert H. Wiebe, *The Search for Order, 1877–1920* (New York: Hill and Wang, 1967), 111–32.

53. See, for example, Oleg P. Schepin and Waldemar V. Yermakov, eds., *International Quarantine* (Madison, Conn.: International Universities Press, 1991); N. Howard-Jones, "The Scientific Background of the International Sanitary Conferences, 1851–1938," *WHO Chronicle* 28 (1974): 119–47, 269–84, 455–70, 495–508.

54. The role eugenic theory played in supporting the immigration restriction movement during the first decades of the twentieth century and the resulting Immigration Restriction Act of 1924 are described in Kenneth M. Ludmerer, *Genetics and American Society: A Historical Appraisal* (Baltimore: Johns Hopkins University Press, 1972); Daniel J. Kevles, *In the Name of Eugenics: Genetics and the Uses of Human Heredity* (New York: Alfred Knopf, 1985); Garland Allen, "The Eugenics Record Office at Cold Spring Harbor, 1910–1940: An Essay in Institutional History," *OSIRIS,* 2, 2nd ser. (1986): 225–64.

Epilogue: "The Microbe as Social Leveller"

The epilogue title comes from Cyrus Edson, "The Microbe as Social Leveller," *N. Amer. Rev.* 161 (1895). The opening epigraph is cited from Sholom Aleichem, *The Adventures of Mottel the Cantor's Son,* trans. I. Schor (New York: Henry Schuman, 1953), 242–44.

1. François Delaporte, *Disease and Civilization: The Cholera in Paris, 1832,* trans. A. Goldhammer (Cambridge, Mass.: MIT Press, 1978), 6.

2. Myron E. Wegman, "Using Vital Statistics in Pediatric Practice, Education, and Research," Grand Rounds, Department of Pediatrics, The University of Michigan Medical Center, June 6, 1995; see also Myron E. Wegman, "Annual Summary of Vital Statistics—1993," *Pediatrics* 94 (1994): 792–803.

3. *New York Times,* February 12, 1893, 3:1.

4. Alan M. Kraut, *Silent Travelers: Germs, Genes, and the "Immigrant Menace"* (New York: Basic Books, 1994; Baltimore: Johns Hopkins University Press, 1995), 254–72.

5. Michael Seltzer, *Kike! A Documentary History of Anti-Semitism in America* (New York: World, 1972), 40–62.

6. Frederic Cople Jaher, *Doubters and Dissenters: Cataclysmic Thought in America, 1885–1918* (New York: Free Press, 1964).

7. For specific descriptions of the medical and supportive treatments attempted at the quarantine station during the cholera epidemic, see *Annual Report of the Health Officer of the Port of New York, 1892, 1893;* for similar documentation of the treatment plans at Riverside Hospital-North Brother Island, see minutes of the medical board, Riverside Hospital, New York Academy of Medicine Collections.

8. See, for example, reports on quarantine by the Special Advisory Committee of the New York Academy of Medicine and the New York State Chamber of Commerce for 1888 and 1892; *Arbeiter Zeitung* (N.Y.), September 16, 1892, 1:5.

9. "Averting a Pestilence" (interview with Dr. Cyrus Edson), *New York Times,* August 7, 1892, 1:1. The heated contention between immigrants and public health officials (and police officers) is well documented in Lincoln Steffens, *The Autobiography of Lincoln Steffens* (New York: Harcourt, Brace, 1931), 206–7, 208–14; Jacob Riis, *How the Other Half Lives: Studies among the Tenements of New York* (New York: Charles Scribner's Sons, 1890), 118–19; Edward King, *Joseph Zalmonah, A Novel* (New York: Lee and Shepard, 1893).

10. Charles McClain, "Of Medicine, Race, and American Law: The Bubonic Plague Outbreak of 1900," *Law and Social Inquiry* 13 (1988): 447–513; L. G. Lipson, "Plague in San Francisco in 1900: The United States Marine Hospital Service Commission to Study the Existence of Plague in San Francisco," *Ann. Intern. Med.* 77 (1972): 303–10; Kraut, *Silent Travelers,* 78–97; Guenter B. Risse, "'A Long Pull, A Strong Pull, and All Together': San Francisco and Bubonic Plague, 1907–1908," *Bull. Hist. Med.* 66 (1992): 260–86.

11. Arthur J. Viseltear, "The Pneumonic Plague Epidemic of 1924 in Los Angeles," *Yale J. Bio. Med.* 47 (1974): 40–54; George J. Sanchez, *Becoming Mexican American: Ethnicity, Culture and Identity in Chicano Los Angeles, 1900–1945* (New York: Oxford University Press, 1993).

12. Mirko Grmek, *History of AIDS: Emergence and Origin of a Modern Pandemic,* trans. Russell C. Maulitz and Jacalyn Duffin (Princeton: Princeton University Press, 1990), 158–59.

13. John Higham, *Strangers in the Land: Patterns of American Nativism, 1860–1925* (New York: Atheneum, 1963), 330.

14. Edson, "Microbe as Social Leveller," 422–23.

15. Ibid., 425.

16. For examples of the current wave of nativism, circa 1993–95, see *New York Times,* October 25, 1993, A1; January 14, 1995, A15; April 2, 1995, A1; April 23, 1995, B3; June 15, 1995, A1.

17. Peter Brimelow, *Alien Nation: Common Sense about America's Immigration Disaster* (New York: Random House, 1995), 187.

18. Matthew T. McKenna, Eugene McCray, and Ida Onorato, "The Epidemiology of Tuberculosis among Foreign-Born Persons in the United States, 1986–1993," *New Engl. J. Med.* 332 (1995): 1071–76; Michael D. Iseman and Jeffery Starke, "Immigrants and Tuberculosis Control," *New Engl. J. Med.* 332 (1995): 1094–95; Michael D. Lemonick, "Return to the Hot Zone," *Time,* May 22, 1995, 62–63; editorial, "Who Will Be the World's Doctor?" *New York Times,* May 12, 1995, A18; Steven Aasch, Barbara Leake, and Lillian Gelberg, "Does Fear of Immigration Authorities Deter Tuberculosis Patients from Seeking Care?" *Western J. Med.* 161 (1994): 373–76; Tal Ann Ziv and Bernard Lo, "Denial of Care to Illegal Immigrants: Proposition 187 in California," *New Engl. J. Med.* 332 (1995): 1095–98.

19. *New York Times,* November 21, 1993, A1.

20. Tim Golden, "Patients Pay a High Price in Cuba's War on AIDS," *New York Times,* October 16, 1995, A1.

21. For journalistic accounts of the 1995 Ebola virus epidemic in Zaire, see *New York Newsday,* May 30, 1995, A4–5, A16–17; *New York Times,* May 12, 1995, A6, A18; May 13, 1995, A1; May 31, 1995, A6; *Time,* May 22, 1995, 62–63; May 29, 1995, 44–47; Richard Preston, "Back in the Hot Zone," *The New Yorker,* May 22, 1995, 43–45; Howard W. Frech, "Sure, Ebola Is Bad: Africa Has Worse," *New York Times,* June 11, 1995, E2. Ebola virus is a particularly intriguing epidemic disease for comparison in that it has a rapid rise and fall not unlike the nineteenth-century scourges of typhus and cholera; AIDS and tuberculosis, on the other hand, are contagious but chronic illnesses.

22. Historians are, by nature, hesitant to predict the future. The complex mix of nativism, public health, and scapegoating is impossible to predict in its specific manifestations. There have been, however, some reports suggesting that public health authorities are developing isolation policies that take into account their responsibilities to consider individual rights as much as possible in epidemic con-

tainment. See, for example, United Hospital Fund of New York, *The Tuberculosis Revival: Individual Rights and Societal Obligations in the Time of AIDS* (New York: United Hospital Fund, 1992), which describes humane considerations in the isolation of tuberculosis patients as well as issues of screening, reporting, and treatment.

23. For examples of this literary device, see Sholom Aleichem, *The Old Country*, trans. Julius and Frances Butwin (New York: Crown, 1946); idem, *Tevye's Daughters*, trans. Frances Butwin (New York: Crown, 1949). The doctrine of *an der anter hant* was most widely popularized in the successful Broadway musical by Joseph Stein, Jerry Bock, and Sheldon Harnick, *Fiddler on the Roof* (New York: Crown, 1964).

Index

Page numbers in italics refer to illustrations; those in boldface refer to tables.

Library of Congress Cataloging-in-Publication Data
Markel, Howard.
  Quarantine : East European Jewish immigrants and the New York City epidemics of
1892 / Howard Markel.
     p.   cm.
  Includes bibliographical references and index.
  ISBN 0-8018-5512-8 (alk. paper)
     1. Quarantine—New York (State)—New York.   2. Jews, East European—Health and
hygiene—New York (State)—New York.   3. Immigrants—Health and hygiene—New
York (State)—New York.   4. Typhus—New York (State)—New York.   5. Cholera—
New York (State)—New York.   6. Epidemics—New York (State)—New York.
I. Title.
RA667.N7M37   1997   96-43095
                                                                     CIP